THE
BONUS
YEARS
DIET

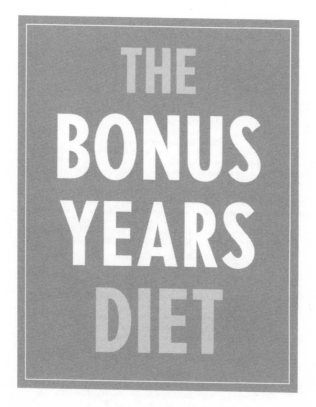

THE BONUS YEARS DIET

7 miracle foods including Chocolate,
Red Wine, and Nuts that can add
6.4 years on average to your life

Ralph Felder, M.D., Ph.D., and Carol Colman

OSCAR H. FRANCO, M.D., PH.D., SCIENTIFIC ADVISER

G. P. PUTNAM'S SONS
NEW YORK

ı||P

G. P. PUTNAM'S SONS
Publishers Since 1838
Published by the Penguin Group
Penguin Group (USA) Inc., 375 Hudson Street, New York, New York 10014, USA •
Penguin Group (Canada), 90 Eglinton Avenue East, Suite 700, Toronto, Ontario M4P 2Y3, Canada
(a division of Pearson Penguin Canada Inc.) • Penguin Books Ltd, 80 Strand,
London WC2R 0RL, England • Penguin Ireland, 25 St Stephen's Green, Dublin 2, Ireland
(a division of Penguin Books Ltd) • Penguin Group (Australia), 250 Camberwell Road,
Camberwell, Victoria 3124, Australia (a division of Pearson Australia Group Pty Ltd) •
Penguin Books India Pvt Ltd, 11 Community Centre, Panchsheel Park, New Delhi—110 017, India • Penguin Group (NZ),
67 Apollo Drive, Mairangi Bay, Auckland 1311,
New Zealand (a division of Pearson New Zealand Ltd) • Penguin Books (South Africa)
(Pty) Ltd, 24 Sturdee Avenue, Rosebank, Johannesburg 2196, South Africa

Penguin Books Ltd, Registered Offices:
80 Strand, London WC2R 0RL, England

Library of Congress Cataloging-in-Publication Data

Felder, Ralph.
The bonus years diet : 7 miracle foods including chocolate, red wine, and nuts that can
add 6.4 years on average to your life / Ralph Felder and Carol Colman.
p.   cm.
Includes bibliographical references and index.
ISBN 978-0-399-15432-4
1. Materia medica, Vegetable—Therapeutic use.   2. Chocolate—Therapeutic use.
3. Nuts—Therapeutic use.   I. Colman, Carol.   II. Title.
RM236.B6675   2007   2007000545
615'.321—dc22

Printed in the United States of America
1   3   5   7   9   10   8   6   4   2

Book design by Stephanie Huntwork

ACKNOWLEDGMENTS

A toast to my close friends and colleagues, whose care and encouragement shine through every page of this book.

First to Ellen, Stan, and Elizabeth Ferris, whose friendship over the past twenty years has sustained and nourished me like no others'.

To my coauthor, Carol Colman, and agent, Laurie Bernstein, who have shown unwavering confidence in my vision, and without whom this book would still be only a dream.

To Dr. Oscar Franco, my brilliant colleague, whose unmatched insight into diet and nutrition is the beacon that lights the road to the Bonus Years.

To my colleague and close friend Dr. Kenneth Desser, chief of cardiac training at Good Samaritan Hospital in Phoenix, whose advice and good humor have guided me over the past two years.

To the chef instructors at the Art Institute of Phoenix, without whose patience and help I could never have attempted writing this book. To chefs Bill Sy and Walter Leible, the codirectors of the culinary program, who gave me every opportunity to learn at their side. To Chef Joe Lavilla, who suggested many of the wine pairings outlined in the book. And to Chef Eric Watson, my first instructor at the Institute, whose teaching continues to guide me every time I pick up a knife in the kitchen.

To Shauna Halawith, owner of Kitchen Classics in Phoenix, who has been one of our greatest cheerleaders and who through her classes has allowed us to validate the Bonus Years approach to diet and nutrition.

To Jeanette Egan, whose recipe testing and guidance on menu development made her an integral part of the Bonus Years team, and who has now, along with her husband, John, become a much appreciated friend.

To my grade school colleague and now attorney Charles Taylor, who continues to provide good advice and cheer as he has always done over the past forty years.

To John Duff, my editor and publisher at Putnam, who has given us unparalleled freedom to pursue our vision on the Bonus Years.

CONTENTS

PART 2
IS THERE A DOCTOR IN THE KITCHEN?

THE
BONUS
YEARS
DIET

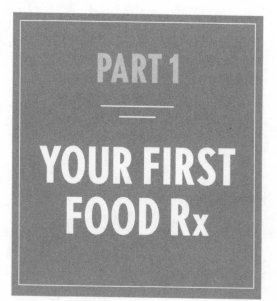

PART 1

YOUR FIRST
FOOD Rx

CHAPTER 1

The Bonus Years
Your First Food Rx

Would you like to extend your life by six years?

Of course you answered yes. Who wouldn't want to live longer, especially if you could do it in a healthy body? We all want to enjoy some "bonus" years traveling, playing with grandchildren, pursuing a second or even third career, or just doing all those things that we never had time to do before.

But, you think, this is a trick question, there's a catch. "What," you're wondering, "do I have to give up to get those bonus years?"

"Do I have to follow a starvation diet?"

"Do I have to eat awful 'health food' for the rest of my life?"

"Do I have to kiss bread and pasta good-bye?"

"Do I have to forgo dessert forever?"

Put your fears to rest, the answer to all these questions is an emphatic "No!"

True, I'm a physician, but I don't expect people to follow a strict and boring diet to gain a few years of life. If that were what I had in mind, I would not be writing this book, and you would not be reading it.

Frankly, I like eating as much as the next guy, probably more. You see, medicine is my profession, but food is my passion. I'm not just a physician, I'm a trained chef. In fact, in Phoenix, Arizona, where I practice medicine and run Bonus Years cooking classes, I'm known locally as Dr. Chef.

And trust me, if eating bland, tasteless food was the only way to earn those bonus years, I might well be the first to say, "It's just not worth it."

But that's not the way it is.

The really great news is that living longer has never tasted better.

The Bonus Years Diet features a revolutionary eating plan that I designed in collaboration with Dr. Oscar Franco, M.D., Ph.D., a prominent London-based, Colombian-born epidemiologist, who is renowned for his research on the prevention of cardiovascular disease. His work on the role of nutrition in preventing heart disease, which provided the inspiration for *The Bonus Years,* has been published in the *British Medical Journal,* a highly respected, peer-reviewed scientific journal.

And because of the solid science behind the Bonus Years Diet, we are able to make a claim that other diet plans cannot: other diet plans have promised to make you thinner or healthier, but none can also make the claim that you will *live longer.* We can. If you follow the Bonus Years Diet, odds are you will live a longer and healthier life.

I'm not kidding. To be scientifically precise, men who follow the Bonus Years Diet can add on average an extra 6.4 years of life. Women can add an extra 4.6 years.

And there's yet another bonus to the Bonus Years Diet: by following this eating plan, you can decrease your risk of developing heart disease—the number-one killer of both men and women in the Western world—by a remarkable 76 percent.

Let's be clear, these are *extra* years you would not otherwise get to enjoy. And *enjoy* truly is the operative word, because we are talking about adding healthy years, extending the prime of your life!

And you can put your fears to rest. You get to eat great stuff every day, including your favorite treats such as a glass of wine, nuts by the handful, and even a bar of chocolate *every day* for dessert. This not just an eating plan you can *live with.* It's an eating plan that you can *live it up with.*

How is it possible that simply by eating some favorite foods you can actually prolong life and extend your healthy years? The Bonus Years Diet represents a true paradigm shift in how we think about food, and, equally important, how we *use* food.

Taking Food to a New Level

For years there's been speculation and anecdotal evidence suggesting that longevity may be linked to diet. Of course, everyone's grandmother has advised that an apple a day keeps the doctor away. And from time to time the popular press has, for example, touted the health benefits of red wine, or reported that blueberries can make your brain sharper, or most recently, suggested that chocolate might be good for your heart.

These news reports did not just catch *your* eye. They also made some serious scientists wonder whether what we eat might actually explain why some of us are more robust and live longer than others. Thanks to years of painstaking research, scientists now have a real understanding of how foods work and have precisely identified the life-enhancing properties that give certain foods the power to restore our health and extend our lives.

One of the things scientists have proven is that our grandmothers were right about apples. But unlike Granny, who had a vague sense that some foods were better for you than others, scientists have pinpointed exactly which nutrients, in which foods, and in what "doses" can deliver these health benefits. Indeed, some of these benefits are the same as those that you might derive from some cutting-edge pharmaceutical treatments.

The idea of dosing food, just like we dose drugs, is an important new concept that is unique to the Bonus Years Diet, and I will explain more about it later, but let me give you a brief overview of what I mean here. In recent years, we've made great strides in treating heart disease with the use of new pharmaceutical therapies. We now have sophisticated statin drugs that can lower cholesterol levels. We have antihypertension drugs that can reduce high blood pressure. We have anticoagulant drugs to prevent blood clots, which can trigger a heart attack. These are great drugs, but they are not without side effects and can be quite costly. The fact is, we now know that by eating certain amounts of certain foods, you can significantly reduce your risk of ever having to take any of these drugs in the first place. *The same kind of rigorous, peer-reviewed, cutting-edge research that is employed in pharmaceutical studies has identified seven foods that alone, or in combination, can do the same job as these drugs just as well, or even better.*

These seven foods—the Bonus Years foods—are the foundation for the Bonus Years Diet.

In Chapter 2, I will explain more about the science behind the Bonus Years foods, but I understand that you are curious to know what the prescription is right away.

YOUR BONUS YEARS FOODS Rx

1 5-ounce glass of red wine daily
2 ounces of dark chocolate daily
4 cups of fruits and vegetables daily
3 5-ounce servings of your favorite fish or seafood weekly
1 clove of garlic daily
2 ounces of nuts (about 2 handfuls) daily

As good as these foods are, don't think that this is all you can eat. If you are like me, you want a bit more variety in your diet, and the good news is that on the Bonus Years eating plan, you can have your proverbial cake and eat it too. As long as you get your full daily dose of Bonus Years foods, you can incorporate other foods into your meals, and I show you how to do that in Part 2, Is There a Doctor in the Kitchen?

Given the choice, wouldn't you really rather have a real cocktail or a shrimp cocktail than a drug cocktail? Wouldn't you prefer a fresh strawberry dipped in chocolate, or a handful of almonds, to a handful of pills, which make you groggy or upset your stomach or have even worse side effects? Who wouldn't? But, you may wonder, how can this be true? How can food work as well as a drug?

So How Does It Work?

Bonus Years foods work individually and synergistically to protect your entire cardiovascular system, the very lifeline of your body, by keeping your blood vessels healthy and well functioning. By protecting your cardiovascular system, this dietary plan not only helps prevent and postpone heart disease and stroke, but also helps prevent a myriad of other diseases that you probably don't even associate with cardiovascular function. In fact, our cardiovascular system not only affects the health of our heart and lungs, but is also critical to the health of our brain, kidneys, and practically every organ and tissue in the body that relies on a steady flow of blood and oxygen. Cardiovascular health is so fundamental to overall health that simply by targeting each branch of the cardiovascular tree this dietary plan is able to guarantee Bonus Years to everyone who follows the program. (In Chapters 2 and 3, I explain more about how Bonus Years foods save your heart and extend your life.)

Many of you may be thinking, "What about cancer? Can the Bonus Years Diet protect me against the number-two killer in the Western world?" Medical science still has not discovered how to prevent many cancers, but it is common wisdom that a fruit-and-vegetable-rich diet will help. Even here the Bonus Years Diet is your friend, because we do know that many of the same mechanisms that trigger heart disease also trigger cancer. So by reducing your risk of heart disease, you may also be reducing your risk of cancer.

Medicine Is Important, Too!

The Bonus Years foods will go a long way in helping to prevent heart disease, but what if you already suffer from it? Don't get the wrong idea: I'm not telling you to stop taking the heart medications that your doctor has prescribed for you. These medicines, including statin drugs that lower cholesterol, or other drugs that lower blood pressure, are proven lifesavers. Once you have established heart disease, you may need drugs regardless of how well you eat or how much you exercise. Yet, medicine alone is not enough to protect your heart. You may be surprised to learn that diet and lifestyle can have *twice* the impact of preventing heart disease than simply taking drugs. The effect of both can be synergistic. And if you are at very high risk of having a heart attack or stroke, you will need to do both. In other words, simply popping a pill is not going to make you immune to poor lifestyle choices.

Food: The Neglected Medicine

I know that many of you are thinking, "If food is such a powerful tool in preventing disease and extending life, why doesn't my doctor spend more time talking about what I should be eating and less time prescribing drugs, or at least do both with equal zeal?"

I know that I'm unusual in that I'm a doctor who truly believes that food is the best medicine. Despite lip service paid to the role of nutrition in health, many of my colleagues are, in truth, shockingly ignorant and untrained in matters of nutrition. If they refer to nutrition at all, many doctors will typically advise their patients in only the most general terms: "You need to eat better" or "You should be getting more good carbs" or "You need to go on a low-fat diet." But most doctors don't know enough about nutrition to actually explain what they mean or how patients can implement this vague advice.

So, already patients are getting a mixed message, because they intuitively understand that if their doctors were serious about diet, if their doctors really thought diet was imperative to their patients' health, they would be more informed, more specific, and more involved. Can you imagine a doctor recommending that you pursue a course of chemotherapy but then not personally overseeing your progress on that treatment? Of course not. But when it comes to nutrition, doctors are essentially leaving their patients to fend for themselves, abandoning them to navigate a sea of books, media stories, and experts offering starkly contradictory messages.

Doctors do agree in principle that nutrition is important, even vital, to health. Nevertheless, although medical schools train our doctors to be exceedingly knowledgeable in the science of pharmaceuticals, they don't do as well when it comes to educating them about nutrition. Until very recently, the vast majority of medical schools did not require their medical students to take even a single course in nutrition in order to graduate. As a result, doctors are much more confident when it comes to prescribing drugs than they are at offering practical advice on nutrition.

Not surprisingly, doctors in the Western world, and especially in the United States, are doing what they do best. According to the U.S. Centers for Disease Control, Americans are the most medicated people in the world, with more than half the adult population on prescription medication.

Despite our constant pill popping, obesity is the leading public health problem in the United States and the Western world. More than 60 million Americans—nearly one-third of the adult population—are considered obese. We westerners are more overweight than ever, and, as a result, we are suffering from more diabetes, heart disease, cancer, and other life-shortening conditions than ever before.

The answer is not new and better drugs. Rather, it is a new and better approach that gets to the underlying problem that is causing these epidemics in the first place: our poor diet. The typical Western diet is high in calories and rich in heart-clogging fat. About two-thirds of all Americans do not eat the five daily servings of fruits and vegetables recommended by virtually every health organization, including the U.S. Department of Agriculture in its new official Food Pyramid. Instead, many of us are eating highly processed foods that have been stripped of much of their nutritive value. Here's a really shocking statistic: of the calories consumed daily in the United States, 20 percent of them come from sweetened beverages, such as soda or fruit drinks—"liquid junk food," one public health group calls it. As a physician, I believe that we doctors cannot practice good medicine until we give nutrition its due and take it as seriously as we do drugs. That is why I feel my work in the kitchen is every bit as important as my work in the hospital. If more doctors felt as I do, we would be writing far fewer prescriptions for drugs to undo the damage caused by poor diet. (Lifestyle is also an important factor that I address in Chapter 11, "The Bonus Years Lifestyle.")

How the Doctor Ended Up in the Kitchen

People often ask me what motivated me to trade my white coat for a white apron. How did I go from Dr. Felder to Dr. Chef? Well, first of all, I still practice medicine. But my interest in food goes back more than thirty years to the time when I was completing work on my M.D. and Ph.D. in the medical scientist training program at Stanford University. Stanford had one of the world's leading cardiac research centers, and I was thrilled to be part of it. The first heart transplants were being performed at the hospital where I was training. When we employed costly space-age technology to replace a broken heart, our efforts made front-page news. With much less fanfare, but with equal enthusiasm, other researchers at Stanford were pursuing another approach, trying to figure out how to prevent hearts from breaking in the first place. At that time, Dr. John Farquahr was in the process of establishing the Stanford Heart Disease Prevention Program, based on the "revolutionary" concept that changes in diet, exercise, and weight control might be able to reverse the epidemic in heart disease. I attended lectures by Dr. Gerald Reaven, the first medical researcher to discern a disturbing trend: Americans were developing a new disorder that he called Syndrome X, or metabolic syndrome, which he linked to poor diet and a sedentary lifestyle. Metabolic syndrome is a constellation of problems, including high blood pressure, obesity (especially around the waist), abnormal blood lipids, and insulin resistance. Insulin resistance occurs when your pancreas produces plenty of insulin, but your body doesn't utilize it correctly. Dr. Reaven first identified metabolic syndrome in the early 1980s, and since that time it has become a virtual epidemic in the United States. Today, as many as 40 percent of the adult population is destined to suffer some form of this problem, which dramatically increases the risk of having a heart attack or stroke and shortens life.

In retrospect, though, it wasn't the time that I spent in the laboratory, but the time that I spent in the kitchen that was to have the greatest impact. Before coming to Stanford, I was enthusiastic about eating, but I had always left the cooking to others. That all changed when I met Chef Tong, who came to the United States from mainland China and opened a Chinese restaurant in Palo Alto, California, that soon became my favorite. To break the grind of laboratory research, I began working in his restaurant on the weekends, first as a busboy clearing tables, and later as an apprentice chef. Chef Tong became my culinary mentor. He taught me the basics of cooking. I learned how to quickly chop and prepare meats and vegetables (lots and lots of vegetables) with the ubiquitous Chinese cleaver. The Chinese, who are typically slim and healthy, have a clear preference for vegetables, seafood, and soy dishes. Compared to American cuisine, Chinese cuisine is much lower in fat. Many dishes are simply steamed. Even stir-fry recipes require only a tablespoon or so of oil. And yet, everything tastes great, proof that you don't have to drown food in fat to get flavor. Whenever I had a chance, I would go with Chef Tong to Chinatown in San Francisco and watch how he carefully selected the produce and seafood for the day. At Tong's side, I learned how to use these ingredients to create the simple but elegant dishes that distinguish the Chinese kitchen. As a doctor, I was intrigued by the obvious health benefits of Chinese cuisine, but as a food aficionado, I was absolutely delighted by the delicious meals I was learning how to cook.

After I left the Bay Area, I continued to cook at home. When I came to Phoenix, I enrolled in the Culinary Arts Program at the Art Institute, where

I learned the basics of classic French cooking, adding to my background in Asian cooking. I loved the technique of French cooking, but not the high saturated fat content. And so I often reinvented recipes, using healthier fats and figuring out ways to streamline the calories without losing the flavor.

I began my career as an internist in a medical practice where, unfortunately, time was money. And I was spending too much time with my patients, which was a good thing for my patients, but a bad thing for a busy group practice. I knew that in order to restore the health of my patients I needed to talk with them in depth about their lifestyle habits, especially their diets, but I quickly learned that this was impossible within the narrow confines of managed-care office visits. I was expected to see several patients an hour, but in reality, it could take an hour to teach a patient what cooking oils are best for the heart, and how to cook vegetables so that they stayed so firm and succulent that no one would feel the need to drown them in butter. I would try to convince my patients to eat more fish, only to be met with blank stares and comments like, "I don't know how to cook fish. Cooking fish is scary." And I would offer some suggestions. As a result, my patient visits were taking far longer than the allotted time.

It became clear to me that it was futile—and inefficient—to try to educate patients about healthy eating one at a time. Instead, I began teaching cooking classes to small groups of people who needed to learn how to prepare healthy, wholesome, and delicious food at home. At the same time, I devoted much of my professional time to research on nutrition, trying to devise an eating plan that would not only be heart healthy, but satisfy the most demanding of palates—mine!

The result—the Bonus Years Foods Rx—is the culmination of my thirty years of nutritional research and recipe development merged with today's cutting-edge science. In the chapters to come, I will show you how easy it is to build a delicious, life-enhancing and life-extending eating plan around the Bonus Years foods. You will learn about the scientific studies supporting the Bonus Years Foods Rx, and how each of these foods can have a profound impact on your health and longevity.

I will also teach you simple techniques that I have developed to help home cooks prepare easy and delicious dinners that rival the best restaurant fare. And speaking of restaurants, I know that many of you probably eat one or more meals out every day, but don't worry. Once you learn the basics, you will be able to fill your Bonus Years Foods Rx whether you eat most of your meals out, on the run, or in a restaurant.

THE BONUS YEARS DIET Q&A

Will the Bonus Years Diet help me shed excess pounds?

Here's the skinny on weight loss with the Bonus Years Diet. If you are already at your desired weight, the Bonus Years prescription will help you *stay* trim for life and make it possible for you to fend off the dreaded weight-creep associated with middle-age spread in men and women alike. For those of you who are interested in trimming your waistline substantially while extending your lifeline simultaneously, the Bonus Years Diet is just what the doctor ordered.

If you are looking to shed excess pounds, see page 99 for tips on how to modify the eating plan to accelerate weight loss until you have successfully reached your target weight goal. Once you have achieved your desired weight, you can switch to the standard Bonus Years eating plan, which will help enable you to maintain that ideal weight for life.

Why do women gain fewer Bonus Years than men do?

Although women and men are at equal risk for developing heart disease, it tends to strike women about ten years later than it strikes men. Scientists believe that the female hormone estrogen may somehow protect younger women from heart disease. However, as a woman's estrogen levels drop as she enters menopause, that protection dissipates. Since women typically are free from heart disease for a decade longer than men, and tend to live longer than men, they gain fewer Bonus Years. Nevertheless, 4.8 extra years of life is still a significant amount of time, especially if it can be lived in a healthy body.

Is it ever too late to reap the benefits of the Bonus Years promise? Might I have missed the boat?

The best news of all is that even a late start won't hamper your ability to reap the full rewards of the Bonus Years. That's right, it isn't necessary for you to have been following the Bonus Years plan from childhood to reap these stunning results. You will still be able to earn your full Bonus Years allotment even if you are starting the program in your fifties (or later).

CHAPTER 2

How the Bonus Years
Keep You Young

You're savoring an elegant dinner of pan-roasted salmon over rice pilaf served with oven-roasted asparagus and shiitake mushrooms. You're sipping a glass of California Pinot Noir, a full-bodied red wine that holds up well against the bold flavors of the fish. You're feasting on a dessert of fresh pears poached in red wine, topped with chocolate sauce and slivered almonds.

With every delicious morsel, you're lowering your blood pressure, keeping your cholesterol levels in check, preventing blood clots that can cause a heart attack, and reducing inflammation throughout your body.

HAS MEDICINE EVER TASTED BETTER?

How is it possible that a great-tasting meal can do so many good things for your body? What's the secret behind the seven Bonus Years foods?

To answer those questions, you need to know a bit about the history and the science behind the Bonus Years. You may be surprised to learn that the Bonus Years did not come about because the medical community suddenly recognized the power of food, but because of the medical community's fixation on drugs, and specifically a drug cocktail called the Polypill.

If you were told that by taking a combination of six drugs every day you could prevent heart disease, would you do it? That's exactly what some scientific researchers want you to do. The authors of an article published in 2003 in the *British Medical Journal* created quite a stir when they proposed the development of a Polypill that would consist of a cocktail of six cardiac drugs. The authors suggested that such a Polypill be taken daily, not just by people with existing heart conditions, but by everyone in the general population over age fifty-five, because virtually everyone in that age group is considered high risk for cardiovascular disease.

What would such a Polypill contain? It would be composed of six already existing drugs, each targeted to lower the four major risk factors for heart disease: elevated cholesterol, high blood pressure, high homocysteine blood levels, and sticky blood platelets (which lead to blood clots). The six drugs are: aspirin, folic acid (a B vitamin), a statin drug to lower cholesterol, and three different blood pressure medications. Each drug tackles atherosclerosis (hardening of the arteries) from a different angle; the six drugs combined would pack a powerful punch against cardiovascular heart disease. Aspirin helps prevent blood clots that can block an artery delivering blood to the heart or brain. Folic acid reduces levels of homocysteine, an amino acid (a building block of protein) in the body that, if elevated, promotes the buildup of plaque in the arteries. Statin drugs help lower bad cholesterol, raise good cholesterol, and reduce inflammation. Reducing inflammation is important because it is a very destructive process that injures blood vessels. The three blood pressure medicines lower blood pressure and help prevent heart arrhythmias, abnormal heart rhythms that can lead to sudden death.

The multidrug approach is already being used to treat people who have had heart attacks or are at high risk of having one. Proponents of the Polypill hypothesize that if this drug combination is taken daily by *everyone* over age fifty-five, it will reduce their risk of heart disease by 80 percent and extend their life expectancy by up to six years.

The downside to all this is that with the Polypill, as with any medication, there is risk of side effects. Statin drugs can cause liver problems and muscle pain; medications that lower blood pressure can make you feel poorly and can even cause heart failure; and even medications we consider to be benign, such as aspirin, can cause abdominal bleeding and ulcers. Not to mention the fact that some of these drugs (notably statins and blood pressure–lowering drugs) are very expensive.

I agree that these medications are truly lifesaving for those sick enough to need them, but the question is, should they be our first line of defense? Does *everybody* really need to take them?

A Dietary Equivalent to the Polypill

The article on the Polypill caught the attention of Dr. Oscar Franco, who was then completing his Ph.D. at the Department of Public Health at Erasmus Medical Center in the Netherlands. Dr. Franco questioned the premise that the entire population over age fifty-five needed to be medicated, regardless of health status or risk factors. He wondered whether there was a better alternative. He asked whether it was possible to get similar results by eating certain foods instead of taking drugs.

Dr. Franco took on the challenge of identifying the precise nutritional equivalent to the Polypill, and proving that the right combination of foods would produce precisely the same health benefits of the six-drug cocktail. Dr. Franco recognized that to compete with the Polypill, his "Polymeal" would have to exert the same powerful effect as the drug cocktail in terms of lowering cholesterol and other bad blood lipids, normalizing high blood pressure and homocysteine levels, and preventing blood clots.

Dr. Franco assembled an impressive team of European scientists and relied on the same research techniques used to develop the Polypill. Dr. Franco pored over hundreds of scientific studies to determine which foods would produce the desired results. A stickler for evidence-based medicine, Dr. Franco established strict criteria for what he would accept as a valid study. All the scientific studies that were used to develop the Polymeal had to have been performed by reputable scientists at established research centers using generally accepted scientific techniques. In lay terms, Dr. Franco was only interested in the real deal. Furthermore, these studies had to have been published in peer-reviewed, well-respected scientific journals. Finally, the data collected from these studies had to come from experiments in which human subjects had been placed on diets requiring specified quantities of a particular food and in which results were then measured against a control group of subjects who did not eat the particular food being tested. For example, if the researchers were looking at the effect of chocolate on blood pressure, they would compare the change in blood pressure of the subjects who ate chocolate to the blood pressure of the subjects who did not. In this way, the researchers could determine whether chocolate was the factor that was influencing blood pressure.

Using this approach, Dr. Franco identified the seven foods his Polymeal comprises: red wine, chocolate, fruits and vegetables, fish, garlic, and nuts, especially almonds. Next, he devised a mathematical model to determine the correct dose for each food, that is, how much of each ingredient would be necessary to reduce the risk of heart disease and extend life for people age fifty and over.

In December 2005, the results of Dr. Franco's work were published in the *British Medical Journal* in "The Polymeal: A More Natural, Safe and Probably Tastier (Than the Polypill) Strategy to Reduce Cardiovascular Disease by More Than 75%." In the article, which received a lot of press attention, Dr. Franco reported that his Polymeal, like the hypothetical Polypill, would reduce the risk of heart disease by an average of 75 percent and significantly increase life span. The study was groundbreaking, because it provided scientific evidence that food, if dosed like medicine, could be just as effective in improving health and extending life.

Six thousand miles away, in Phoenix, I read about the Polymeal with intense interest. Dr. Franco's tongue-in-cheek suggestion that if the plan put too many cardiologists out of work they "could be retrained as Polymeal chefs and wine advisers" made me think, "Wait a minute! That's me!"

As a doctor, I appreciated the measurable health benefits offered by the Polymeal. As a chef (and a person who really enjoys food), I recognized that the Polymeal wasn't a practical eating plan that the average person could follow every day. Food choices were limited, and some foods were overrepresented while others were ignored. Intrigued by his research, I immediately contacted Dr. Franco and suggested that we team up to create an eating plan that offered the same longevity benefits as the Polymeal, but was much more user friendly. Dr. Franco knew immediately that my love of food and cooking as well as my medical background made me the right person for the job.

Over the next few months, Dr. Franco and I developed a full-spectrum eating plan with the original Polymeal foods—chocolate, nuts, red wine, garlic, fish, and unlimited fruits and vegetables—at its core. We understood from the outset that just giving people a list of seven Bonus Years foods is not sufficient, that people must also see how to incorporate these foods into their daily menu plans. We also understood that these menu plans had to provide the same benefits that were reported in the Polypill and Polymeal studies.

The result is a menu of seven Bonus Years foods dosed in precisely the right amount to offer maximum cardiovascular benefits. They are:

RED WINE

One 5-ounce glass of red wine daily reduces the overall risk of cardiovascular disease by 32 percent. Red wine contains potent chemicals called polyphenols that reduce cholesterol, prevent blood clots, and lower blood pressure. The effect is similar to the combined action of statin drugs, blood pressure-lowering medicines, and aspirin in the Polypill.

DARK CHOCOLATE

A 2-ounce serving of dark chocolate daily reduces systolic blood pressure (the top number) by 5.1 and diastolic blood pressure (the bottom number) by 1.8, resulting in a 21 percent reduction in cardiovascular risk. Dark chocolate is a rich source of flavonoids, chemicals that help prevent the collapse and rupture of blood vessels. This, for reasons that I will explain later, is key to preserving cardiovascular health. By the way, milk chocolate won't do; it doesn't contain enough flavonoids to lower blood pressure.

FRUITS AND VEGETABLES

Eating four cups (measured raw) of any kind of fruit or vegetable daily reduces systolic blood pressure by 5 and diastolic blood pressure by 1.8, resulting in a 21 percent risk reduction in heart disease. Combined with red wine and dark chocolate, fruits and vegetables can control high blood pressure as well as the need for medical intervention.

FISH

Eating three 5-ounce servings of fish each week reduces the risk of cardio-vascular disease by 14 percent. The omega-3 fatty acids in fish are natural blood thinners that work like aspirin to prevent blood clots and like statin drugs to normalize cholesterol.

GARLIC

Eating 2.7 grams of garlic, about one clove of fresh or frozen garlic daily, re-duces cholesterol levels by seventeen points, resulting in a heart disease risk reduction of 25 percent. Garlic contains sulfur compounds that inhibit the production of cholesterol by the liver. (Statin drugs also affect cholesterol production, but do it through a different chemical pathway.) Cooked garlic is preferable because heat releases its most potent health-enhancing chemicals.

NUTS

Eating two ounces of nuts daily (particularly almonds) reduces cholesterol and results in a 10 percent reduction in heart disease. Almonds combined with red wine, garlic, and fish have the same impact on lowering cholesterol as statin drugs do. Walnuts and pistachios have also been shown to lower cholesterol, although they are not quite as effective as almonds.

How Bonus Years Foods Protect the Heart

The job of the heart is to pump blood to the rest of the body, but it can't do its job well if blood flow to the heart is impaired. The way to keep the heart working well is to make sure that the coronary arteries that are feeding it blood stay in good working order.

This sounds easy, but a lot can go wrong and often does. Your arteries are particularly vulnerable to atherosclerosis, a disease characterized by the for-mation of deposits of plaque, a thick yellowish, waxy substance consisting of cholesterol and other types of cells. Plaque deposits can narrow an artery, compromising the flow of blood.

The real danger, though, is that some plaques have a tendency to rupture and create a blood clot that can completely block the flow of blood to the heart. This is what causes a heart attack. Elevated levels of cholesterol, especially a bad type of cholesterol, called low-density lipoprotein, or LDL, can promote the formation of plaque. LDL cholesterol is vulnerable to oxidation. In other words, it gets rancid much the way a piece of fat left in the open air will get rancid over time. Oxidized LDL interacts with white blood cells to form foamy deposits that in turn form the basis of plaque in the artery walls. These foamy deposits then attract blood-clotting cells (platelets) to further grow the plaque. They also release chemicals that are toxic to the delicate lining of the blood vessel wall, the endothelium.

You may never have heard about the endothelium before, but scientists have just recently discovered that it is critical to our health. The endothelium is the thin protective barrier that surrounds the lumen, the opening in your coronary arteries through which blood flows to the heart. When I was in medical school, the endothelium was considered to be just part of the background scenery in the body. Back then we didn't know its critical role in regulating blood flow. Although the endothelium is just 1/1,000 the width of a human hair, it plays a crucial role in keeping your heart healthy. A healthy endothelium is vital to maintain the function of the artery.

The endothelial cells protect your arteries from unwanted guests that may be floating through the bloodstream, such as excess cholesterol and those foamy cells that cause so much trouble. For example, if LDL cholesterol (bad cholesterol) gets past the endothelium into the artery wall, it can cause the formation of plaque, and it is the plaque that starts out in the endothelium that can rupture and cause a heart attack. Therefore, you need to keep the endothelium barrier strong so that LDL can't do its dirty work. The best strategy is to protect the endothelium from potential troublemakers, and that's precisely how the Bonus Years foods work. Too much LDL can eventually wear the endothelium down, which is why you want to keep your LDL cholesterol low. Two Bonus Years foods, nuts and wine, keep LDL in check. Two Bonus Years foods—garlic and wine—also control LDL by encouraging the production of HDL, also known as good cholesterol. HDL is important because it shuttles excess LDL cholesterol to the liver so it can be excreted in the bile from the body. This is nature's way of naturally creating the right cholesterol balance in our bodies. I should also mention that regular exercise also boosts HDL levels.

The Antioxidant Connection

I'm sure many of you have heard of antioxidants, and probably some of you are taking them in supplement form. Antioxidants are compounds that are produced by the body and occur naturally in many foods, particularly Bonus Years foods. Antioxidants prevent oxidation of LDL, but they also protect our bodies from the free radicals that are a by-product of oxidation. Free radicals are not all bad, in fact, many are required for the normal function of the body. In excess, however, free radicals can be dangerous. The body manufactures free radicals in the normal course of energy production, but there are also substances in our environment that can trigger the production of free radicals. These include toxic chemicals, cigarette smoke, solar radiation, and pollutants. Free radicals can also damage the endothelium, so you want to eat enough antioxidant-rich foods to keep them under control. The Bonus Years foods derived from plants are rich in phytochemicals, many of which are antioxidants. Flavonoids, a type of phytochemical found in chocolate, wine, and many fruits and vegetables, are particularly potent antioxidants.

High blood pressure also harms the endothelium. If you have high blood pressure, it means that your heart is working harder than it should to pump blood, and that puts a strain on your arteries. Over time, the strain can injure the endothelium, making it more vulnerable to infiltration by LDL. The flavonoids contained in fruits and vegetables, chocolate, and wine substantially lower blood pressure by promoting the production of nitric oxide, a colorless, odorless gas produced by the cells that relaxes the lining of the arteries, promoting easy blood flow. Naturally, that causes blood pressure to drop.

Fish plays a unique Bonus Years foods role because many types of fish—particularly cold water, fatty fish—are rich in omega-3 fatty acids. These are good fats that prevent the formation of blood clots and have natural anti-inflammatory properties. Eating fish helps protect the endothelium by reducing inflammation, and helps prevent heart attacks by reducing the likelihood that plaque will form a blood clot. And fish does something else: it appears to prevent fatal arrhythmias that can be caused by irregular heartbeats.

More on Your Plate

Although they were not incorporated in the original Polymeal, Dr. Franco noted in his study that if other scientifically proven foods, such as soy, legumes (all beans), tea, oat bran, flaxseed, and whole grains were added to the Polymeal, they would only enhance the health benefits and increase variety. We did just that and created a separate category of Booster foods that may not meet Dr. Franco's demanding standard for Bonus Years foods, but come close.

What about neutral foods? These are the ones that don't do any harm but haven't been shown to do any good either. To round out this full-service eating plan, Dr. Franco and I devised a list of Bonus Compatible foods to incorporate into the meal plans. The Bonus Compatible foods complement the Bonus Years foods, but do not themselves share their proven medicinal properties. We have included Bonus Compatible foods not because they themselves will add Bonus Years, but because they will help you round out meals without undercutting the beneficial effects of Bonus Years foods.

And what about foods that can be harmful, particularly if eaten often? The Bonus Years eating plan features a Penalty Box, designed to help you steer clear of foods that might rob you of your bonus years by undermining the positive health impact of the Bonus Years foods. This feature will help you identify bonus-robbing foods and will also help you calibrate how much is being stolen from your bonus years tally. The foods you'll find in the Penalty Box are typically those loaded with bad fats such as saturated and trans fats, highly processed foods, and those containing carcinogenic preservatives like nitrates. The Bonus Years eating plan will help you learn to spot these Bonus Years stealers and will offer guidelines about how often these foods can be introduced into your meal plans before they eat away at your bonus years.

In the next chapter, you will learn more about each of the Bonus Years foods and how they work.

THE BONUS YEARS FOODS Q&A

What if I'm allergic to nuts or if I just don't like one of the Bonus Years foods? Can I still follow the Bonus Years foods prescription and reap those extra years?

If you have sensitivity to a particular Bonus Years food, or if you just don't like it, don't panic. If you eat all the right foods together in the right dosages, you will experience a 76 percent reduction in your risk of heart disease. But even if you have to eliminate an entire food group, such as nuts or wine, you're still way ahead of the game in terms of heart disease risk reduction, and your loss of Bonus Years is negligible. For example, if you don't drink wine, your risk reduction for heart disease goes down to 65 percent, but that is still a significant benefit. To put it in perspective, even without drinking wine, you are still 65 percent less likely to have a heart attack following the diet than if you were not. If you omit nuts from the eating plan, your reduction in risk for cardiovascular disease dips to 72.5 percent—not exactly a huge difference. If you omit fish, your risk reduction goes down to 73 percent. If you can't eat chocolate, your risk reduction drops to 70 percent. And it goes down to 68 percent if you can't eat garlic. The bottom line is, even if you have to eliminate one of the food groups from the Bonus Years Diet, you can still reap most of its benefits.

CHAPTER 3

The Bonus Years Foods

W hen Hippocrates said, "Let food be your medicine and medicine be your food," he could only speculate about the healing power of food. Today, we are light-years ahead in our knowledge of the chemistry of food and its impact on our bodies.

As you read about each of the Bonus Years foods, you will get a better understanding of this exciting new science and why food is indeed powerful medicine.

The Bonus Years Foods

Wine

Dark chocolate

Fruits and Vegetables

Fish

Garlic

Nuts

WINE

BONUS YEARS RX: *One 5-ounce glass of wine, preferably red*
BONUS YEARS BENEFIT: *Reduces the overall risk of cardiovascular disease by 32 percent*
Note: *Wine is the "broad spectrum" Bonus Years Food—it offers a wide range of cardiovascular benefits.*

- Decreases LDL (bad cholesterol) and boosts HDL (good cholesterol)
- Prevents the oxidation of LDL cholesterol, which injures the delicate lining of the blood vessels (the endothelium) and promotes the formation of artery-clogging plaque, and lowers blood pressure
- Makes blood cells less sticky, which prevents dangerous blood clots

The French Paradox

To your health, and *Salud* (Spanish for "health"), *L'chaim* (Hebrew for "To life"), and *À votre santé* (French for "To your health") are common toasts that suggest that people worldwide have long known about the health benefits of wine. For more than six thousand years, wine has been used as both a common beverage and a medicine. The planting of vineyards is mentioned in Genesis, the first book of the Old Testament, making it the first known crop in recorded history. Yet, despite centuries of folklore, it wasn't until fairly recently that we've been able to pinpoint the specific ingredients that make wine such potent medicine.

About a decade ago, researchers from the University of Alabama set out to study a phenomenon that is called the French Paradox. They wondered why relatively few people in the south of France died from heart disease, despite the fact that they ate a diet high in saturated fat, got little exercise, and were moderate to heavy smokers. Not only were deaths from heart disease about a third lower in southern France than they were in England at the time, but also deaths from heart disease were lower in the south of France than in any other country, except for China and Japan, where diets are known for being low in saturated fats.

The researchers were stumped. They looked at comparative levels of stress; they wondered whether deaths from heart disease were simply under-reported in the south of France. Then they hypothesized that maybe there was a lag between heart disease–related deaths and this lifestyle, similar to the lag between smoking and the onset of lung cancer. But none of their theories could explain the lower incidence of heart disease in people with such apparently unhealthy habits.

When they started looking at the population's consumption of red wine, the lightbulb went on. As it turned out, France has the highest per capita consumption of wine of any developed country. The French routinely drink a glass of wine—usually red—with their meals. This had to be the key to the low incidence of heart disease. But how?

We now know far more about why wine is protective and the mechanism that offers us that protection. Simply stated, flavonoids, the antioxidants found in the skin and seeds of grapes, can protect our cardiovascular system from disease. Flavonoids are part of a family of plant chemicals (phyto-chemicals) called polyphenols. The polyphenol family contains some of the most powerful antioxidants found in nature.

Researchers have determined that the flavanoids found in wine work in three ways to reduce heart disease: by reducing LDL cholesterol, by enhanc-ing the production of HDL cholesterol, and by improving circulation. There are about four thousand phytochemicals that are part of the flavonoids group. Flavonoids give foods deep rich color: the skins of grapes, the bright orange of a cantaloupe, the deep purples, reds, and blues of berries, the fire-engine red of red peppers.

Wine's Powerful Disease Fighters: Flavonoids

Flavonoids are abundant in both the skin and the seeds of grapes. The an-tioxidants in grape skin and seeds act like a fighting front-line force, pre-venting the oxidation process whereby free radicals cause damage to healthy cells. And here's good news for red-wine drinkers: red wine packs even more antixoxidant power than white wine due to the way the wine is made. The skins are retained in the process of making red wine, whereas they are typically not used in making white wine. As a result, although white wine still has some flavonoids, red wine contains about ten to twenty times more flavonoids.

Does this mean that you can never drink white wine? Absolutely not. But try to drink red wine whenever possible.

Flavonoids protect the heart in other ways beyond their antioxidant properties. It appears that flavonoids also promote the production of nitric oxide in the body. Nitric oxide is a gas produced by the lining of the arteries (and other cells of the body) that plays an important role in promoting good circulation. Nitric oxide helps your blood vessels relax, which keeps the flow of blood through the vessels and arteries smooth. It also keeps blood from sticking to the vessel and artery walls, which can cause clots. The overall effect of nitric oxide is to promote the smooth and regular flow of blood with reduced pressure on the artery walls (what we refer to as blood pressure).

How Much Wine Gives Us the Optimal Benefits?

The healthy compounds in red wine function much in the same way as would a medication that a physician might prescribe for you. Just as is the case with medication, the right amount gives us benefits, but too much either negates the benefits or can even be harmful. This is especially true for wine, which of all the Bonus Years foods is the most potent. Dr. Franco wrote the following caution in his original Polymeal study regarding wine. He notes it "should not be combined with additional consumption of alcohol, in order to avoid intoxication and conflicts with friends, relatives, and authorities." Although it is written tongue in cheek, his admonition should not be taken lightly. In addition to causing impaired judgment, excess alcohol consumption can raise blood pressure, which can increase your risk of having a heart attack. So when it comes to wine, it is particularly important not to exceed the recommended dose of one 5-ounce glass daily.

Which Wines Are the Most Heart-Healthy?

The drier and darker the red wine, the higher the concentration of flavonoids. Conversely, the sweeter the wine, the lower the flavonoid level.

The composition of flavonoids varies among wines, depending on factors such as fermentation conditions and grape selection.

To get the highest flavonoid level out of your red wine, choose a Cabernet Sauvignon, which ranks at the top, followed by Petit Syrah and Pinot Noir reds, then the Merlots and red Zinfandels.

What Is Resveratrol—and Why Does It Matter?

Resveratrol is a remarkable type of polyphenol called a phytoalexin, a substance produced by plants as part of their defense system against disease. Red wine contains high levels of resveratrol, as do grapes, raspberries, peanuts, allium vegetables (these vegetables include garlic), broccoli, spinach, blueberries, strawberries, tea, and chocolate, all of which are Bonus Years foods.

Resveratrol appears to be the specific antioxidant in wine to which many health benefits are attributed, including the ability to keep blood from being sticky, thus reducing the likelihood of blood clots; preventing plaque from building up on blood vessel walls by limiting the oxidation of LDL cholesterol, helping to enhance production of nitric oxide which keeps muscles relaxed and blood flowing smoothly, and even functioning as an anti-inflammatory agent in the body.

According to published studies, resveratrol has the ability to thin out the blood because it makes the individual blood cells (platelets) less sticky, thus preventing dangerous blood clots. When blood clots form and become lodged in the smaller vessels of the heart or brain, they prevent oxygen from reaching these vital organs. This lack of oxygen is called *ischemia*. In fact, a heart attack (also called myocardial infarction, or MI) is a result of severe ischemia, just as severe ischemia in the brain is called a stroke.

Resveratrol has also been shown to limit the oxidation of low-density lipoproteins (LDL). When LDL cholesterol is oxidized, it sets into motion the first step of creating plaque on the inside of blood vessels. Any reduction in the levels of LDL, or in its oxidation, can potentially decrease the buildup of plaque.

Resveratrol has also demonstrated abilities in regulating nitric oxide, a gas that enables smooth muscles to relax and allow blood to flow smoothly. One French study of men who had already suffered heart attacks indicates that the effects of resveratrol, via moderate red wine consumption, may help prevent future heart attacks.

Evidence also exists that resveratrol can function as an anti-inflammatory. The resveratrol in red wine is the same substance as is found in the yucca (*Yucca schidigera*), a medicinal plant native to the deserts of the southwestern United States and northern Mexico whose extract has been treasured for its anti-inflammatory properties. Native Americans used the yucca plant to treat a variety of ailments, including arthritis. Recently it has been recognized that yucca contains other physiologically active constituents, particularly polyphenols, such as resveratrol, which has been identified in yucca bark.

DARK CHOCOLATE

BONUS YEARS Rx: *Two ounces of dark chocolate with a minimum 60 percent cocoa content, but preferably 70 percent, daily*

BONUS YEARS BENEFIT: *Reduces risk of cardiovascular disease by an average of 11 percent*

- Can reduce high blood pressure as effectively as some prescription blood pressure–lowering medications when eaten with your daily dose of wine, and fruits and vegetables
- Reduces systolic blood pressure (the top number) by 5.1 and diastolic pressure (the bottom number) by 1.8

- Increases nitric oxide production, which relaxes the artery wall and lowers blood pressure

BOOSTER BENEFITS
- May improve insulin sensitivity, thus helping to prevent metabolic syndrome (prediabetes) and diabetes
- Prevents the oxidation of LDL cholesterol, which promotes the formation of artery-clogging plaque
- Reduces inflammation
- A powerful antioxdiant

You've heard the saying, or maybe seen it on a T-shirt, "Life is uncertain. Eat dessert first." Well, it turns out that may be some pretty good health advice, that is, if what you eat first is dark chocolate.

Here's why: the cacao bean, which is what chocolate is made from, is an excellent source of flavonoids. In terms of overall heart health, the particular type of flavonoids in chocolate that have caught the attention of scientists and researchers are the flavon-3-ols, known as flavonols. Flavonols are derived from plants as are all flavonoids.

Interestingly, of all the plant-derived foods and beverages, cocoa products have a higher total flavonol content on a per weight basis than many others. This was the case both for the actual foods and beverages, as well as the powder and extracts of the substances. Cocoa powder (not Dutch processed) and cocoa extracts showed more powerful antioxidant capacity than the extracts of any other flavonol (including green and black tea, red wine, blueberry, garlic, and strawberry).

Chocolate: A Fast-Acting "Drug"

Whenever research scientists look at the effect of foods or medications, they have to look at the issue of absorption and bioavailability; *bioavailability* refers to the degree to which the foods or prescription medications we take can be used or metabolized by our bodies.

Studies show that flavonols and other flavonoid components in chocolate are rapidly absorbed in our bodies (so they have a high level of bioavailability) in what's called a dose-dependent manner. This means the more flavonol-rich food we consume, the more is absorbed (which is not always the case with flavonoids from other foods). And not only do flavonols make it through the GI tract, but research has also shown that the most heart-healthy flavonoid class, the catechins, which are highly concentrated in dark chocolate, can be found in the blood as quickly as only an hour after a person eats cocoa or dark chocolate. Even more remarkable is that researchers have also seen a reduction in the oxidation of LDLs (the bad cholesterol) within two hours after people in the study ate a cocoa product.

The levels of heart-healthy flavonols available to us depend on how the cocoa is handled after it's harvested, as well as how much of the cocoa is added to the final packaged product. If you are looking to buy heart-healthy dark chocolate, read the label and look for a minimum of 60 percent cocoa.

The Case of the Kuna Indians, Blood Pressure, and Cocoa

Off the Atlantic coast of Panama, a chain of more than 360 islands, the San Blas Archipelago, is home to the indigenous Kuna Indians. Some of the Kuna have moved to mainland Panama.

In 1996, Norman Hollenberg, M.D., Ph.D., professor of medicine at Harvard Medical School, began working with volunteers from the Kuna tribe. His first major discovery was that the island-dwelling Kuna have remarkably healthy blood pressure levels, and do not experience the same age-related increase in blood pressure that is typical of the aging process in other parts of the world.

Dr. Hollenberg and his team thought perhaps the Kuna might have a special gene that was passed on to each generation that protected them from heart disease, so the team then examined the Kuna who had moved to the mainland, and found that those tribe members who had left the islands experienced increases in blood pressure. When they discovered such a stark difference, they realized there was something more behind the healthy blood pressure of the island-dwelling Kuna than just genetics.

Dr. Hollenberg and his team reasoned that the difference between the healthy blood pressure of the island-dwelling Kuna versus the worsening blood pressure of the Kuna who had moved to the mainland had to lie in lifestyle factors. These include things over which people have control, like whether or not they smoke, what they eat, how much exercise they get.

As part of his research, Dr. Hollenberg and his team examined death certificates for both the island-dwelling and the mainland-dwelling members of the Kuna tribe. What they found was a real shocker at the time: the Kuna Indians living on the islands had significantly lower rates of heart disease and cancer. They calculated that the relative risk (the measurement of the likelihood of event occurring in one group versus in another) of death from heart disease on the Panama mainland was 1,280 percent higher, and death from cancer was 630 percent higher than on the islands.

When they analyzed the diets of both populations, they found one striking difference. The Kuna Indians still living in San Blas consumed as many as *five cups* a day of different cocoa-based beverages, whereas the mainland-dwelling Kuna drank almost none of the same cocoa-based beverages they used to drink. The scientists wondered if something in the cocoa, which, after all, is a flavonoid (derived from plants), might be what made the difference.

When the team did an analysis of the cocoa powder in the traditional beverages, they found it was a rich source of flavonols, especially one called epicatechin. They concluded that the flavonols in the cocoa drink had to contribute to the lower blood pressure.

In a paper published in the January 24, 2006, *Proceedings of the National Academy of Sciences* (*PNAS*), Dr. Hollenberg and his team wrote that the island-dwelling Kuna Indians had significantly higher levels of flavonols in their bloodstream, as well as higher levels of nitric oxide metabolites in their circulatory systems, compared to the mainland Indians who consume little cocoa. This was the first study to show direct evidence that epicatechin can help improve blood vessel relaxation, which is critical to cardiovascular health.

Dr. Hollenberg's work with the Kuna Indians was one of a five-part study his team undertook to determine whether or not the flavonol epicatechin met certain criteria for being called a compound that directly improves circulation in the human body.

In the four other research projects, the team successfully demonstrated that:

- Levels of nitric oxide in the blood were higher in individuals who drank flavonol-rich cocoa, compared to those who drank cocoa beverages with low flavonol levels.

- Levels of the flavonol epicatechin in the bloodstream were accompanied by improved blood flow.
- In the laboratory, flavonols administered to sample tissue of blood vessels caused the tissue to relax.
- Pure epicatechin consumed by humans had much the same effect as did consumption of flavonol-rich cocoa.

More Support for Chocolate

The scientific literature is filled with articles on the many benefits of dark chocolate. For example, two articles in particular show how the flavonols in chocolate have translated into improved heart health in humans.

A paper published in the peer-reviewed journal *Thrombosis Research* in 2002 appears to support the idea that heart health can be improved by positively affecting the way certain blood components function.

Researchers from both the University of Wisconsin and the University of California, Davis, compared the effects on the cardiovascular system of drinking a cocoa-based beverage and of taking aspirin. As we know, taking aspirin has been associated with a decrease in coronary heart disease.

They found that people who drank the cocoa-based beverage showed a decrease in blood platelet activity, meaning that they were less prone to blood clots just two hours after they drank the cocoa.

The people who took the aspirin showed similar positive effects, but it took six hours for these positive effects to happen. Equally interesting is that the positive effects were even more pronounced in the group that both drank the cocoa beverage and took the aspirin. This was the first time that clinical studies (in people) were done showing the effects of flavonols in comparison to taking aspirin.

In 2003, a paper reviewing the cardiovascular health benefits of cocoa-based products appeared in the *Journal of the American Dietetic Association* (*JADA*). The paper, published in the February 2003 issue, describes the fatty acid makeup, mineral content, and flavonoid composition of chocolate, as well as how these components may work to support cardiovascular health.

As the researchers explain, the fatty acids in chocolate are predominantly saturated (stearic and palmitic) and monounsaturated (oleic, a monounsaturated fat found in olive oil that is believed to lower both total cholesterol and

LDL cholesterol), with the remaining being polyunsaturated linoleic (omega-6 essential fatty acid). Fats, especially saturated fat, had been presumed to be harmful to cardiovascular health. Since chocolate contains saturated fat, it has been considered a food that might be harmful to our overall heart health.

But chocolate contains stearic acid, a fatty acid that does not elevate blood cholesterol as other fats do. In fact, studies have found that diets containing cocoa and chocolate have a neutral effect on blood cholesterol levels in humans.

Cocoa and Additional Heart-Healthy Benefits

It turns out that researchers have discovered more health benefits of chocolate than just its powerful antioxidant abilities. It seems that when studies were done examining the other cardiovascular processes that flavonols affect, the results were fascinating. Researchers found that flavonols can also help prevent inflammation, a process in the body that is a factor in almost all illness, especially heart disease, as well as Alzheimer's disease, autoimmune disease (like rheumatoid arthritis and lupus, among others), asthma and allergies, and even cancer.

Inflammation is the result of hormonal signals secreted by damaged body tissues triggered by an injury or infection. The immune system responds by releasing blood cells to the site of injury to kill any potential bacterial or viral invader that could cause infection. These cells also cause blood cells to clot to stop bleeding. In some cases, a strong immune response is a good thing that can save your life, but not always. For example, when the endothelium, lining of an artery is hurt by exposure to LDL cholesterol, the immune system will send the same powerful disease-fighting cells to what it perceives as an injury. But this time, instead of promoting healing, these cells only aggravate the situation by making it more inflamed.

But researchers looked at what happened when healthy people ate flavonol-rich cocoa liquor (which is unsweetened chocolate, also known as bitter or baking chocolate; it is unadulterated chocolate from pure, ground roasted chocolate beans). What they saw is fairly miraculous, in my opinion. They saw time and again that the cocoa liquor could stimulate the production of nitric oxide and significantly reduce inflammation throughout the body. They also found that cocoa flavonols and procyanidins could positively affect

other inflammatory markers. If proven true, this finding could catapult chocolate into the cardiovascular suites of every hospital or cardiologist's office.

FRUITS AND VEGETABLES

BONUS YEARS RX: *At least 400 grams or 4 cups (measured raw) or five
¾-cup servings daily. (One medium apple, or one handful of grapes
or one cereal-size bowl of salad is equal to one serving. One 8-ounce
glass of unsweetened juice is also equal to one serving, but do not have
more than 1 glass of juice daily. The whole fruit or vegetable is preferred. For more information, see how to get your daily dose of fruits
and vegetables, page 96.)*
BONUS YEARS BENEFIT: *Reduces overall risk of cardiovascular disease by 21 percent*

- Lowers blood pressure by keeping the arteries open, protecting the
  endothelium from injury, and enhancing the production of nitric
  oxide
- Rich in fiber, which has been shown to lower blood pressure

BOOSTER BENEFITS
- A lower risk of cancer and other diseases associated with diets rich
  in fruits and vegetables

Mix It Up!

You may be wondering why we don't make specific recommendations
about which fruits and vegetables you should be eating. The truth is, the
studies that link consumption of fruits and vegetables to bonus years of life
don't differentiate between the different varieties. We do know, however,
that different types of fruits and vegetables offer different benefits. The point
is, you *do* want to mix apples and oranges . . . and carrots and watermelon

and pomegranate. Therefore, to get the full benefit of fruits and vegetables, your best bet is to eat as wide an assortment of fresh fruits and vegetables as you can every day.

There is only one vegetable that does not count toward your Bonus Years foods—the potato. Why? Potatoes tend to be less nutrient dense than other vegetables, meaning they are higher in calories and lower in phytochemicals. Theoretically, sweet potatoes should count toward your Bonus Years foods because they do contain a fair amount of phytochemicals. However, the scientific studies on which we base the Bonus Years Foods Rx do not include any type of potatoes as vegetables, and therefore we don't either.

Why Asian Cuisine Keeps You Slim

I admit that I didn't like vegetables too much when I was growing up, and I certainly didn't think of a piece of fruit as an acceptable dessert.

When I was training as a chef in Asian cuisine, my life really began to change. Now I toss into almost every dish I prepare florets of cauliflower or broccoli, beautiful stalks of celery, bright red cabbage, eggplant, tomatoes, peas . . . whatever I can find that is fresh.

And I learned that fresh fruit is a great dessert or snack. On a recent trip to China, I noticed that the Chinese eat fresh melon slices after dinner for dessert and never eat Western-style high-sugar desserts. Perhaps that is why for the entire two weeks I was in China, I don't think I saw a single overweight person.

The Remarkable Health Benefits of Fruits and Vegetables

Without getting into the advanced chemistry of it, I do want to share with you some of the fascinating discoveries we have made about these miraculous foods. We humans share our environment with plants, and they are exposed to same potentially damaging elements as we are. The UV rays from the sun can damage plant cells just like they can damage skin cells. Viruses, bacteria, and fungi can make plants sick just like they can make humans sick. Oxidation, the natural process that is a result of energy production in plants and humans, can damage plant cells just like it can damage the lining of an artery, which can promote atherosclerosis.

Plants have a natural defense system that protects them from our common enemies. They rely on an arsenal of phytochemicals, naturally occurring disease fighters that help ward off infection, that can help repel or attract insects (whichever is more beneficial for a plant at a particular time), and that provide antioxidants.

Preventing Damage from Oxidation: Plants to the Rescue

Since we know that fruits and vegetables generate antioxidants to protect themselves from potential damage from the sun (and in the process produce their characteristic bright colors), it makes sense that the richest source of antioxidants in fruits and vegetables is found on the skin and in the lining of the fruit. For example, citrus fruits have that spongy lining you see in oranges and lemons; that's where the antioxidants are most concentrated. (Check out some of my recipes that call for orange or lemon zest—created from the skins of the fruits. Those recipes will give you an extra boost of antioxidants because you are actually eating some of the skin.)

More than any other benefit of eating fruits and vegetables, it's the reduction in blood pressure that appears to protect us most from heart disease. Several research studies have provided scientific evidence that flavonoids can restore the normal functions of the endothelium, the lining of blood cells, even when it is effectively disrupted by the effects of oxidation; as we've seen, flavonoids can help open up (dilate) the blood vessels, making blood platelets less sticky, which decreases clotting in blood. These effects make the blood flow more smoothly and easily, creating less pressure on the heart, vessels, and arteries (also known as blood pressure).

Regarding the protective effects, one study looked at the separate effects of eating fruits and vegetables for women and for men. For women, it showed that the more flavonoids women consumed from fruits and vegetables, the lower their risk of overall death from heart disease from clogged arteries. For men, it showed that the higher their intake of flavonoids from fruits and vegetables, the lower their risk of stroke. These are some pretty amazing results from eating produce. Keep in mind that all of these studies

looked at the actual consumption of various fruits and vegetables themselves, and not the use of dietary supplements.

Quercetin—A Special Flavonoid

Scientists have found that quercetin, the most active of the flavonoids, directly stops or slows many initial processes of inflammation, such as the
production and release of histamine and other allergic/inflammatory re-
sponses. And of course it is a potent antioxidant.

Many flavonoids are derived from quercetin, including the citrus
flavonoids rutin, hesperidin, naringin, and tangeritin. Moreover, plants that
have been found to have medicinal properties owe much of their activity to
their high quercetin content.

Citrus fruits, apples, onions (the outermost rings have the highest concentration of the healing compound), broccoli, parsley, tea, and red wine are
the primary dietary sources of quercetin. Olive oil, grapes, dark cherries,
and dark berries, such as blueberries, cherries, blackberries, and raspberries are also high in flavonoids including quercetin.

Phytochemicals

Numerous studies show that phytochemicals promote a healthy immune
system, act directly against bacteria and viruses, and reduce inflammation,
making them tremendously protective against chronic and deadly disease.

Phytochemicals are what create the bright colors in fruits and vegetables.
For example, lutein makes corn yellow, lycopene makes tomatoes red,
carotene makes carrots orange, and anthocyanin makes blueberries blue.

For example, very little comes close to the health benefits (not to mention the delicious taste) of fresh tomato sauce, brimming with lycopene, the
compound responsible for the bright red color of tomatoes and other red
vegetables and fruits. Lycopene is a carotenoid (naturally occurring pig-
ment), and while there are more than six hundred known carotenoids,

lycopene is the most common carotenoid in the human body and is one of the most potent carotenoid antioxidants. Fruits and vegetables that are high in lycopene include not only tomatoes, but watermelon, pink grapefruit, papaya, and rosehip. Unlike other fruits and vegetables, where nutritional content such as vitamin C is diminished upon cooking, processing of tomatoes increases the concentration of lycopene that our bodies can use. Thus cooked tomato products such as tomato juice, paste, soup, sauce, and ketchup contain the highest concentrations of lycopene.

The USDA's List of the Top 20 Antioxidant Foods

Notice that all of the USDA's top twenty antioxidant foods are, of course, Bonus Years foods or Booster foods. Notice, too, that of the twenty, sixteen are fruits, two are nuts, and two are vegetables. As we can see, fruits are the category of foods highest in antioxidants; but vegetables are extremely high in fiber, which is associated with lowered blood pressure. The lowering of blood pressure is considered the benefit of eating fruits and vegetables that is most responsible for the decrease in heart disease.

1. Small red beans
2. Wild blueberries
3. Red kidney beans
4. Pinto beans
5. Cultivated blueberries
6. Cranberries
7. Artichokes
8. Blackberries
9. Prunes
10. Raspberries
11. Strawberries
12. Red Delicious and Granny Smith apples
13. Pecans
14. Sweet cherries
15. Black plums
16. Russet potatoes
17. Black beans
18. Plums
19. Gala apples
20. Walnuts

Is Organic Better?

The scientific studies on fruits and vegetables that earned them a place among the Bonus Years foods did not specify whether the produce consumed by the participants was organic or not. Since only a minority of people buy organic, we have to assume that in most cases, it wasn't. That means that you should get your full Bonus Years whether or not you buy organic fruits and vegetables. However, there are other reasons to buy organic produce if you can afford the additional expense. Pesticides are known to be neurotoxins, which means they can damage nerve cells. Although pesticides are supposed to be safe in low doses, the cumulative effect of a lifetime of exposure may not be so benign. Furthermore, organic farming is more ecological than standard commercial farming. So, if you want to buy organic for all the right reasons, do so.

Why Is Fiber So Important?

Dietary fiber has been shown to reduce cholesterol, which is one of the most important protections against coronary artery disease or heart disease.

There are two primary types of dietary fiber: soluble and insoluble. Insoluble fiber is bulk that changes little as it passes through the body. Soluble fiber, on the other hand, forms a soft gel in solution with water. Most foods provide a mixture of both, but are listed as mostly one or the other. Soluble fiber has been shown to be able to bind bile salts, which may reduce blood cholesterol levels. It also may slow the absorption of glucose from the intestine, thereby requiring less insulin secretion.

Fiber provides bulk to food moving through the digestive tract, and may decrease spasms in the gastrointestinal tract. There are two great advantages to this: by bulking up the digested food (known as the bolus) that moves through the digestive tract, eventually increasing the weight of the stool, it's easier for the digestive system to move it through, and the bulkier stool also tends to retain normal amounts of moisture to make it easier to eliminate with less straining and abrasion.

It appears that a high-fiber diet prevents the absorption of fat and reduces cholesterol levels. High-fiber foods help move waste through the digestive tract faster and easier, so possibly harmful substances do not have as much contact with the gastrointestinal tract and may be more readily excreted by the body.

Soluble fiber is found in many foods, including:

- legumes (peas, soybeans, and other beans)
- oats
- some fruits (particularly apples, bananas, and berries)
- certain vegetables, such as broccoli and carrots
- root vegetables, such as sweet potatoes (the skins are insoluble fiber)
- psyllium seed (only about ⅔ soluble fiber)

Insoluble fiber is found in:

- whole-grain foods
- bran
- nuts and seeds
- vegetables such as green beans, cauliflower, zucchini, celery
- the skins of some fruits, including tomatoes

The Bold and Beautiful Pomegranate

Pomegranates have been native to Iran and the Middle East for thousands of years. The ancient Egyptians were buried with pomegranates, and the Babylonians believed chewing the seeds before battle made them invincible.

This beautiful, ruby-red fruit has recently gained great acclaim because of its exceptionally high level of antioxidant activity. Brimming with polyphenols, anthrocyanins (as in berries), and tannins (as in wine), pomegranates have almost three times the antioxidant power per serving as does wine or tea.

Pomegranate juice has been found to actively improve endothelial function and increase its nitric oxide production; the juice has also been found to reduce blood pressure, and to decrease plaque buildup in arteries. The fresh fruit is available only from September to December, so for most of us the most reliable source is pomegranate juice, which is easily available, although high in sugar content, so it's best not to drink too much at once.

FISH

BONUS YEARS RX: *Three (5-ounce) servings per week (each serving slightly less than the size of two standard decks of cards)*

BONUS YEARS BENEFIT: *Reduces the overall risk of cardiovascular disease by an average of 14 percent*

- Prevents blood clots
- Lowers triglycerides, a fat in the blood
- Prevents fatal heart arrythmias (interruption of normal heart rate, which can be lethal) and sudden death
- Helps prevent inflammation

Fish Tales

When I was a kid I would do anything to avoid eating fish, and I mean anything. I hated it, or at least I hated the way my mom prepared it. It always tasted bland and had a soggy, watery texture. Whenever we had fish for dinner, I would take one bite, start coughing, and complain that I couldn't finish because I must be allergic! If that didn't work, I would try to make myself throw up. I grew up convinced that I had a natural aversion to fish, but I was wrong. As an adult, fish has become one of my favorite foods.

Why the change of heart? First, having studied Asian cooking, I now know countless ways to make fish and seafood dishes that taste *nothing* like my mother's. And I now know that whether you grill it, steam it, poach it, or bake it, if you cook it correctly, fish can be truly delicious. It's all in the cooking technique. I also learned how to enhance the naturally delicate flavor of fish with garlic, wine, vegetables, spices, and even nuts and fruits. I have become such an enthusiastic fish aficionado that I could easily eat it every day. And on some weeks I do, but I watch out for the types of fish I eat and the amounts of certain fish (see "A Word About Mercury Levels in Fish," on page 49).

So, if you're like me, and you grew up thinking that you hate fish, I urge you to give it another chance. In Chapter 7, you will find some wonderful fish recipes that can please the fussiest palates. Even better, they are fairly simple to prepare and don't require a great deal of skill. (I know many people are intimidated by the thought of cooking fish. I devote an entire chapter, "Fear of 'Fishing,'" to this topic.) I eat fish not only because I like it, but also because it offers very specific health benefits. Most important, fatty fish (such as salmon, bluefish, tuna, mackerel, arctic char, herring, and sardines) are a rich source of omega-3 fatty acids, good fats that are essential for health.

And Speaking of Fat . . .

The word *fat* has a negative connotation these days—you don't want to be fat and you don't want to eat too much fat. But the fact is, there are different kinds of fat and not all are bad; in fact, some are good. There's a lot of good fat in fish, which may explain many of its health benefits. But in order to understand why the fat in fish is beneficial, you need to know a bit about fat in general.

There are three primary categories of fat—saturated fat, polyunsaturated fat, and monounsaturated fat. The difference between these fats has to do with their chemical structure, which is too complicated to go into here. But what you do need to know is that each type of fat behaves differently in your body.

Saturated fat is found in beef, lamb, pork, and full-fat dairy products (milk and cheese) and in smaller amounts in poultry and fish. This kind of fat is known to promote atherosclerosis, or plaque formation in your arteries.

Polyunsaturated fat is found primarily in vegetable oils (such as soy, sesame, sunflower, safflower, cottonseed, and peanut) and is the fat used in margarine. Some polyunsaturated fats are good for your heart and others (such as trans-fatty acids and hydrogenated fats) commonly used in processed foods and many brands of margarine can be deadly.

Essential fatty acids are polyunsaturated fats that play an important role in many metabolic processes, and there is compelling evidence to suggest that low levels of essential fatty acids may be a factor in a number of illnesses ranging from heart disease to arthritis to impaired mental performance.

There are two types of essential fatty acids: omega-3 fatty acids and omega-6 fatty acids. Cold-water fatty fish is the best food source of omega-3 fatty acids, which are also found in deep green vegetables, some grains, flaxseed, and pumpkin seeds.

In the body, omega-3 fatty acids are broken down into two other fatty acids, eicosapentanoic acid (EPA) and docosahexaenoic acid (DHA). If you've ever wondered why fish is called "brain food," it's because there are high concentrations of DHA in the brain. In fact, low levels of DHA have been linked to decreased cognitive function, depression, and even Alzheimer's disease.

Omega-6 fatty acids are found primarily in vegetable oils, nuts, most seeds, and cereals. Although they are also considered "essential," typically, we eat more than enough omega-6 fatty acids but do not get enough omega-3s in our diet. This imbalance in fatty acid consumption may promote inflammation and cause serious health problems, including heart disease.

The Eskimo Paradox

You may know that the American Heart Association, as well as numerous other professional health organizations, recommends that you limit your fat intake to less than 30 percent of your total daily calories. Several major population studies have shown a direct link between high consumption of fatty foods—especially those rich in saturated fat—and a higher incidence of heart disease. There was one exception to this rule: Eskimos who typically consume more than half of their daily calories in the form of fat actually have *lower* rates of heart disease than found in countries where less fat is consumed. This phenomenon has been called the Eskimo Paradox.

Researchers noticed a major difference between the typical Eskimo diet and Western diet. Unlike countries like the United States, where most of the fat consumed is either saturated fat from meat and dairy products or polyunsaturated fat from margarine or processed food, the primary fat consumed by Eskimos is omega-3 fatty acids from fish, which is a mainstay of their diet. This clue led scientists to suspect that omega-3 fatty acids may be protective to the heart.

Several large-scale epidemiological studies have confirmed those suspicions:

- The Chicago Western Electric Study, which followed more than two thousand men ages forty to fifty-five for more than thirty years, found that those who consumed 35 grams or more of fish daily compared to those who consumed none had substantially lower rates of death from heart disease and stroke.
- A major study of mortality data from thirty-six countries, "Fish Consumption and Mortality From All Causes, Ischemic Heart Disease, and Stroke: An Ecological Study," published in *Preventive Medicine* (May 1999), concluded that "fish consumption is associated with a reduced risk from all-cause, ischemic heart disease, and stroke mortality at the population level."
- The Nurses Health Study, a major study involving more than 120,000 nurses in the United States, found that those who ate the most fish had the lowest rates of death from heart disease.
- A 2004 meta-analysis of nearly twenty studies on the effect of eating on heart disease published in the *American Journal of Cardiology* concluded that "fish consumption may be an important component of lifestyle modification for the prevention of CHD (coronary heart disease)." The authors noted that the benefit accrued from eating fish and a reduced rate of fatal CHD was more striking in those consuming between two to four servings than their counterparts who reported consuming less than two portions of fish per week.

Omega-3s Get the Official Nod

The studies mentioned above, as well as some others, convinced the U.S. Food and Drug Administration in 2004 to give what they call "qualified health claim" status to DHA and EPA omega-3 fatty acids. The FDA stated that that "supportive but not conclusive research shows that consumption of EPA and DHA omega-3 fatty acids may reduce the risk of coronary heart disease." As you can imagine, it takes quite a lot of persuasive findings to get the FDA to allow even such a qualified claim about food.

Researchers suspect eating omega-3 fatty acids offers additional benefits, including healthful effects on levels of blood triglycerides (the major form of fat that is both produced by the body and comes from the food we eat), blood pressure, blood clotting mechanisms, and on our immune systems. Researchers have even seen a positive effect on the central nervous systems of infants who take in omega-3 fatty acids through breast milk.

What I also find fascinating is that fish have omega-3 fatty acids in their fat cells, and so are able to live and thrive in cold water. It works like this: the cell membranes of the fish tend to become rigid because they are in cold water; but the omega-3 fatty acids give the membranes flexibility through its lipid (fat) layers in a cold environment.

It turns out that the most important proven benefit of eating fish is its drastic lowering of the risk of sudden death in people having coronary ischemia, decreased blood flow to the heart because of blocked or narrowed blood vessels. Why? The omega-3 fatty acids stabilize the cell membrane, as they do in the fish that carry them, and prevent arrhythmias, abnormal, rapid heart rhythms that can be deadly.

In addition to preventing arrhythmias, some of the other mechanisms by which omega-3 fatty acids may reduce risk for heart disease include:

- preventing formation of blood clots, which can cause heart attacks and stroke
- reducing levels of triglycerides
- preventing or staving off the growth of plaque in arteries
- promoting the relaxation of the endothelium via production of nitric oxide
- serving as an anti-inflammatory
- reducing stickiness of the blood

Resolvins—Natural Anti-inflammatories

Resolvins are compounds made by the human body from the omega-3 fatty acids eicosapentanoic acid (EPA) and docosahexanoic acid (DHA). In 2002, researchers from both Harvard Medical School and Brigham and Women's

Hospital identified a new class of fats in the human body, called resolvins, made from omega-3 fatty acids found in oily fish. The researchers showed that resolvins can control inflammation by their effect on cells, preventing the movement of inflammatory cells to places where there is already inflammation, as well as by activating other cells; they are sometimes put in the eicosanoids class. Interestingly, the researchers found that resolvins are particularly effective when working together with aspirin.

Out of Balance

Research has shown that Americans have doubled their consumption of omega-6 from 1940 levels.

When humans were hunter-gatherers thousands of years ago, their diets likely consisted of approximately equal parts of omega-3 and omega-6 essential fatty acids. Studies suggest that the evolutionary human diet, rich in seafood, nuts, and other sources of omega-3, may have provided such a ratio. As I mentioned earlier, cold-water oily fish, such as salmon, herring, mackerel, anchovies, and sardines, are highest in omega-3 fatty acids. The oil from these fish has a profile of around seven times as much omega-3 as omega-6.

Unfortunately, we have seen a steady increase in omega-6 at the expense of omega-3 fat in the human diet, accelerated about fifty years ago when cattle started being fed more and more on grains rather than on grass. Processed foods, such as commercial baked goods, snack foods, and frozen dinners, which have become a staple of the American diet, have high amounts of omega-6 fatty acids. In addition, up until the past decade, nutritionists insisted we eat margarine (polyunsaturated fats) rather than butter (saturated fats). But as it turns out, margarine is not only high in omega-6 fatty acids in general, but many brands are also high in trans-fatty acids, which are *really* bad fats. Fortunately, some of the latest imitation butter spreads don't have trans fats and are rich in healthy monounsaturated fats, and are thus more user-friendly. (See "How to Stay out of the Penalty Box," on page 89.)

Recent research suggests a correlation between diets high in trans fats and diseases like atherosclerosis and coronary heart disease. Thus, the United States National Academy of Sciences recommended in 2002 that dietary intake of trans-fatty acids be totally eliminated.

Nearly every responsible medical group supports adding more omega-3s to our diets, but the trend is going the other way. Unfortunately, the current ratio of omega-6 to omega-3 fatty acids is somewhere between 7 to 1 (7:1) to 10 to 1 (10:1), with some cases of a ratio of 30:1 for people who eat mainly fast food and processed sweets. All indicators point to this imbalance in favor of more omega-6 fatty acids, leading to an incidence of cancer, heart disease, allergies, diabetes, and other disease and illness.

Farm-Raised or Wild?

I'm frequently asked which type of fish is better: wild fish, which may have been exposed to mercury and other pollutants in our oceans and waterways, or farm-raised fish, which theoretically should be raised in a cleaner environment?

First, let me assure you that the benefits of eating fish regardless of where it's been raised far outweigh not eating fish. If you have a choice, however, I recommend that you select wild fish. Why? For one thing, wild fish has nearly three times more omega-3 fatty acids than farm-raised, which gives it a big advantage. Although it's true that wild fish may be more contaminated with mercury than their farm-raised counterparts, farm-raised fish may be given growth hormones, antibiotics, and other chemicals to stimulate growth. They may also be fed grain, which is not what fish eat in the wild (they eat vegetation or other fish) and will alter their omega-3 content. Furthermore, the water farm-raised fish swim in is far from contaminant free. In fact, it could be tainted with pesticides, dioxins, and other chemicals that spill into freshwater supplies.

Recently, I have seen some organically raised farmed fish sold at health food stores. If you can't get wild fish, this is a good alternative.

A Word About Mercury Levels in Fish

The issue of mercury in fish is, unfortunately, a product of our industrialized economy. The good news is that the levels of mercury vary from one species of fish to another. The predatory species (the ones that eat other fish) tend to contain more mercury because they also contain the mercury in the smaller fish they have eaten.

If you're going to eat fish every day, eat smaller portions and vary the types of fish you eat. Don't eat more than one serving per week of the fish with high mercury levels, which include:

Atlantic cod	Ling	Rockfish
Bluefish	Marlin	Sea bass
Barramundi	Orange roughy	Shark (flake)
Bonito	Oysters (Gulf of	Swordfish
Gemfish	Mexico)	Tuna steaks
Grouper, black	Pacific cod	Walleye
Grouper, red	Pike	White croaker
Halibut	Porgy	Yellowtail
Lake trout	Ray	
Largemouth bass	Red snapper	

Here are our recommendations for the safest species:

Blue crab (mid-Atlantic)
Catfish
Croaker
Haddock
Pollock
Salmon (wild Pacific)
Sardines
Summer flounder
Tilapia
Trout
Tuna (canned light)

GARLIC

BONUS YEARS RX: *One clove (cooked or raw) daily*

BONUS YEARS BENEFIT: *Reduces overall risk of cardiovascular disease by an average of 38 percent*

- Inhibits the production of cholesterol by the liver, similar to statin drugs
- Lowers LDL (bad cholesterol) that can burrow into the lining of an artery, beginning a chain of events that can ultimately end with a heart attack or a stroke
- May have a "phyto-HDL effect," meaning that it helps rid the body of bad LDL cholesterol, thus achieving effects similar to those of HDL good cholesterol.

BOOSTER BENEFITS: *Has been used as a natural remedy for thousands of years and well into the twentieth century*

- Some garlic extracts can prevent the growth of bacteria in the gut, including the kind of bacteria (*H. pylori*) that have been shown to cause ulcers and that could lead to gastric cancer
- And may be a natural blood thinner

Not Just to Keep Vampires at Bay

Like chocolate, garlic is a Bonus Years food that has always had an aura of mystery and folklore surrounding it. Garlic is a not just a spice, an herb, or a vegetable, but a combination of all three. It likely evolved thousands of years ago from cultivated *Allium longicupis,* or wild garlic, which grows naturally in central Asia. It is in the allium family along with the other pungent members, onions and leeks.

Garlic Facts

Americans want garlic, whether for the taste, health benefits, or both. The United States produces about 250 million pounds of garlic per year, of which some 50 million pounds are sold as fresh garlic; nearly 90 percent of this is produced in California. The remainder is dehydrated and turned into garlic flakes, salt, and ingredients in packaged foods. In the 1980s and 1990s, Americans consumed an average of 1.3 pounds per person per year; by 1999, the average for each person went up to 3.3 pounds.

When I trained with Chef Tong learning the art and science of Chinese cooking, I could have earned a second Ph.D. in cooking with garlic. As a scientist, I am keenly aware of the many health benefits of garlic. As a chef, I love how garlic enhances the flavor of everything in a recipe. In fact, nearly every Asian sauce has garlic and ginger in it. I have no doubt that the daily consumption of garlic plays a big role in the consistently excellent cardiovascular health that many people in Asian countries enjoy.

You'll notice my recipes have a lot of garlic in them. Try them and use all the garlic called for when you make them. In addition to giving the food a wonderful flavor, you'll be giving your cardiovascular system a real boost.

Garlic's Long History of Health Benefits

Garlic may be a Bonus Years food, but we are not the first to appreciate garlic's potential health benefits. Cultivated garlic was used in ancient Mesopotamia and Egypt from at least 2000 B.C. as both a food and a medicine. To the ancient Greeks and Romans, garlic was their version of a performance-enhancing drug—they believed that it increased the strength and endurance of those who ate it. Before the discovery of antibiotics, garlic was used on wounds to prevent infection. Legend has it that medieval monks chewed on garlic to protect themselves against plague. And it may surprise you to learn that well into the twentieth century, during World War II, garlic was still used on battle wounds to prevent gangrene when penicillin and sulfa drugs were hard to come by.

One garlic clove is a virtual pharmacy of beneficial chemicals. Modern researchers have shown evidence that one of garlic's most potent compounds, sulfur, has displayed the ability to function as an antibiotic, an antioxidant, and as a substance that can help reduce cholesterol and blood pressure levels. Sulfur is a highly volatile compound and changes chemically depending on the way in which the garlic is prepared (fresh, dried, crushed, or cooked).

As we have seen with fruits and vegetables, the plants that are rich in tannins, terpenoids, alkaloids, flavonoids, and sulfur compounds have particularly powerful antibacterial abilities. In fact, researchers found that *Helicobacter pylori* (or *H. pylori*), the bacteria associated with gastric ulcers (and potentially gastric cancer), is affected by some forms of garlic, specifically garlic extracts, which were shown to prevent the bacteria from reproducing inside the intestine. Many cultures still use garlic to treat intestinal parasites.

Interestingly, the healing qualities of garlic are affected by the way in which it is prepared. When the clove is either cut or crushed, an enzyme contained within the plant cells combines with an amino acid to create allicin, one of the most potent compounds in garlic. Research has shown that allicin can kill twenty-three types of bacteria, including salmonella and staphylococcus.

Garlic may do lots of other things, but its strongest scientifically proven benefit, which earns it a place in the Bonus Years foods, is its ability to reduce cholesterol, more specifically, to improve the ratio between good and bad cholesterol. Similar to statin drugs used to lower cholesterol, garlic inhibits the production of cholesterol by the liver, which also lowers total cholesterol levels, but probably through a mechanism other than that of statins. It also appears that garlic has blood-thinning properties, which, of course, are helpful in preventing heart attacks and strokes.

The Cardiovascular Benefits of Garlic

Much of the modern research on garlic has focused on its cardiovascular disease–preventing abilities. In the first half of the twentieth century, several research papers hinted at garlic's possible properties to aid circulation. By the late 1960s, there was enough information to begin to see and understand how garlic is of benefit to the cardiovascular system. What scientists found was a complex set of biochemical and pharmacological mechanisms, all of them well researched. They found that the mechanisms all work together to produce the rather remarkable effects on circulation that we get from this somewhat mythical, mystical bulb.

One study that appeared in the *Annals of Internal Medicine* in 2000—the bible of primary-care physicians—reported on a review of thirteen existing studies. In what is called a meta-analysis, a statistical method of combining the results of many studies to come to a stronger conclusion than any one study, the authors found clear scientific evidence across the board that garlic does, in fact, reduce total cholesterol levels. This is the pivotal study that earned garlic a place among the Bonus Years foods.

To me, one of the most amazing properties of garlic is that it not only lowers low-density lipoprotein (LDL, the bad cholesterol) in the blood, but it also moves the ratio of LDL in favor of high-density lipoprotein (HDL, the good cholesterol). HDL helps to deliver fats to the liver to be metabolized, rather than allow them to be deposited in tissue. All this from an herb that is delicious in any dish.

Garlic has also been shown to protect blood vessels from the effects of free radicals. This activity has also been linked to its blood cholesterol-lowering action and its ability to decrease deposits of cholesterol on the walls of blood vessels. By lowering lipids in the blood (such as cholesterol and triglycerides), it benefits the heart.

In addition, garlic may reduce the stickiness of blood platelets and their ability to aggregate, or produce blockage, called thrombocyte adhesiveness and aggregation. It also enhances a process known as fibrinolysis, a normal body process that occurs continuously to keep naturally occurring blood clots from growing and causing problems. So, fibrinolysis helps to speed up the process of moving blood throughout the blood vessels smoothly, breaking down plaque, or clots.

We are now seeing increasing evidence that garlic may also have the ability to alter blood pressure and cause the arterial walls to relax, which is a huge benefit to the cardiovascular system. We usually see a stiffening of the artery walls together with high systolic (the top number) blood pressure;

factors such as age, gender, hormones, and genetics can influence the stiffening. The latest studies have shown that garlic appears to have an ongoing effect in keeping blood pressure down, in part, because of its effect on helping the arterial walls relax and remain more flexible.

While we continue to perform scientific studies on the health effects of garlic, clearly there is a reason why, over thousands of years, humankind has reported benefits of everything from protection against vampires to, more recently, cardiovascular benefits, antimicrobial properties (working like antibiotics), blood-thinning properties (much in the same way fish oils do), and even anticarcinogenic (protection against cancer) abilities.

Do We Have to Smell Like Garlic to Reap Its Benefits?

The biggest problem with garlic from a social as well as a manufacturing perspective is the characteristic odor that garlic leaves on the breath. While large amounts of raw garlic can be irritating to the digestive tract, by far the largest complaint about garlic is its "fragrant odor." Many people avoid garlic for fear of offending others.

A good way to dispel some of the odor of garlic is by chewing fennel seeds or parsley after eating it.

What causes garlic breath? The intestines themselves produce another type of garlic odor. In the intestines, the allicin in garlic preparations can be transformed into a highly odoriferous compound called allyl mercaptan, some of which is absorbed into the bloodstream and makes its way to the lungs, producing garlic breath. Among the odor-affecting manufacturing procedures are the addition of various types of extracts and aging, which can also produce less fragrant products.

NUTS

BONUS YEARS RX: *Two ounces daily (almonds, walnuts, pecans, macadamias, and other varieties, including seeds, such as pumpkin and sunflower)*

BONUS YEARS BENEFIT: *Reduces overall risk of cardiovascular disease by 12.5 percent*

- As part of a moderate-fat diet, nuts produced a 14 percent drop in LDL cholesterol and a 13 percent drop in triglyceride levels after one month in people with normal blood cholesterol levels.
- Pistachio nuts and sunflower seeds contain the highest amounts of phytosterols among the commonly eaten nuts and seeds (only wheat germ and sesame seeds have higher levels); phytosterols have specifically been associated with lowering blood cholesterol levels.

BOOSTER BENEFITS
- Walnuts have been shown to reduce levels of C-reactive protein (CRP), a marker of inflammation that is strongly associated with atherosclerosis and heart disease; the fat in walnuts contains omega-3 fatty acids, which reduce the stickiness of blood cells (platelets), thus lowering the risk of heart attacks (myocardial infarction).

The Perfect Bonus Years Food

"Sweets for the sweet. Here, have some nuts!" I remember that incantation from when I was a kid. Who knew that the "nuttiest" among us would have reaped such lasting health benefits? And while I'm at it (being corny), notice the first three letters in the word *nutrition*.

Of all the Bonus Years foods, I would say that nuts are just about perfect because they contain all three of the major nutrients our bodies need: protein, carbohydrate, and fat. They're portable and are rich in polyunsaturated and monounsaturated fatty acids (ranging from 13 grams of fat in cashews to 22 grams of fat in macadamia nuts), which is one of the reasons they are protective against heart disease. Polyunsaturated and monounsaturated fats are derived from plant sources, and are thus rich in phytochemicals, including phytosterols, which have specifically been associated with lowering serum cholesterol. And the good fat in nuts makes them satisfying, because eating fats make us feel full. It's true that nuts are high in calories—approximately 190 calories per ounce—but these are calories that are packed with essential nutrients, so we get excellent nutritive value for the calories consumed.

People from the Mediterranean countries (including the Middle East) have been depending on the nutritive value of nuts for thousands of years. There are two types of nuts: tree nuts, which come from a one-seeded fruit in a hard shell, and peanuts, which are actually members of the legume family.

Unfortunately, Americans typically eat less than an ounce of nuts and nut butters each day, and nuts make up only about 2.5 percent of our total fat intake. By contrast, people in Mediterranean countries eat about twice the level of nuts as Americans do.

On average, nuts also contain about 170 mg of potassium and 60 mg of magnesium per ounce, both of which help lower blood pressure. Most types of nuts also have substantial amounts of zinc, copper, and protective phytochemicals, including flavonoids.

The Health Benefits of Eating Nuts

By 1990, researchers were already seeing evidence that consumption of nuts was directly correlated with lowering total blood cholesterol. Since then, study after study points to the reduction of risk for heart disease in people who consume nuts on a regular and frequent basis.

In one example, the Adventist Health Study, conducted at Loma Linda University (called this because it was looking at dietary habits and risk for heart disease in populations of Seventh-day Adventists), for those people who ate nuts (mostly walnuts and almonds, with some peanuts) between one and four times per week, results showed they had a 24 percent reduction in their risk of heart disease. Most astounding for the researchers was that people who ate nuts five or more times a week experienced a 50 percent reduction in their risk of heart disease, even when the researchers made allowances for known risk factors for heart disease. That's some pretty convincing evidence.

In another ongoing study in Iowa, the Women's Health Study researchers found a clear association between the consumption of nuts and decreased risk of heart disease.

At the University of Nevada, Reno, scientists carrying out the Heart Study discovered that people who eat nuts frequently tend to have lower body weights, and showed more of an awareness of their own health and health habits than those who didn't eat nuts.

It is clear why the FDA finally had to allow producers of nuts to make health claims about their products. One after another, clinical trials examining the ability of nuts to lower total cholesterol levels have shown that diets rich in almonds and walnuts in particular have consistently lowered blood cholesterol by 10 to 15 percent.

In 2001, researchers from Loma Linda University published in the *Journal of Nutrition* results of their study that found that a diet in which 20 percent of the calories came from walnuts (3 ounces a day) produced a 16 percent decrease in LDL cholesterol levels after four weeks compared with a similar diet not containing the nuts. Walnuts are different from most other nuts in that they contain a high amount of linolenic acid (omega-3 fat).

One study, called the Multiple Risk Factor Intervention Trial (MRFIT), offers evidence that higher levels of linolenic acid in the blood are associated with lower risk of stroke in the middle-aged men at high risk for heart and circulatory (cardiovascular) disease.

When the FDA Went Nuts

As a physician, scientist, and chef, I am always fascinated, as well as frustrated, by our food choices and preferences in America.

In 1990, the Food and Drug Administration (FDA) passed the Nutrition Labeling and Education Act that requires all packaged foods to bear nutrition labeling and all health claims for foods to be consistent with terms defined by the secretary of Health and Human Services. This federal law preempted any state requirements about food standards and nutrition labeling and for the first time authorized companies to make some health claims for foods, although many of those claims have since been refuted and banned. But the FDA standardized the food ingredient panel, serving sizes, and terms such as "low fat" and "light." The act required labeling for most prepared foods, such as breads, cereals, canned and frozen foods, snacks, desserts, and drinks. Nutrition labeling for raw produce (fruits and vegetables) and fish is voluntary. To me, this is one of the ironies of our culture—if only we insisted on labeling fruits, vegetables, and nuts I suspect we could do quite a lot for our collective improved health as a nation.

It wasn't until 2003 that the FDA allowed producers of nut products to advertise that a handful a day of most nuts may be enough to lower the risk of heart disease. But scientists had been studying the effects of nuts on serum cholesterol for years. In fact, the *American Journal of Clinical Nutrition* published a study in May 1994 showing that the replacement of saturated fatty acids with almonds or walnuts lowered not only the bad cholesterol (LDL), but that they also lowered total blood cholesterol. Still, it took another nine full years before the FDA would allow the labeling of nuts as protective for heart disease.

Beginning in July 2003, the FDA said that almonds, hazelnuts, pecans, pistachios, walnuts, and peanuts could bear this labeling: "Scientific evidence suggests but does not prove that eating 1.5 ounces per day of most nuts, as part of a diet low in saturated fat and cholesterol, may reduce the risk of heart disease."

The government's National Cholesterol Education Program notes that for every 1 percent reduction in LDL (the bad) cholesterol, there is a 1.5 percent reduction in the incidence of coronary heart disease.

In addition, nut protein is high in the amino acid arginine and has a high arginine-lysine ratio. Recent studies have shown that arginine is a precursor of nitric oxide, which has been proven to dilate (open up) blood vessels and enable blood to flow more smoothly and with less pressure (reduced blood pressure). Nitric oxide is an endothelium-derived relaxing factor (EDRF), which has demonstrated the abilities to relax the vascular smooth muscle, inhibit blood clotting, and reduce the stickiness of blood (thus preventing the buildup of plaque on artery walls). Moreover, scientists believe that the low ratio of lysine to arginine in dietary proteins is both an effective way of reducing overall cholesterol levels in blood as well as serving as protective against an artery-clogging buildup of plaque.

CHAPTER 4

The Booster Foods

Booster foods are known to have special health benefits but, as of yet, not quite the same scientific backing as Bonus Years foods.

This is not to say that the science on Booster foods is scant—there's a growing body of research supporting these foods. I have no doubt, however, that at some point in the future, one or more of these Booster foods are going to end up in the Bonus Years column.

I don't recommend daily doses of Booster foods as I do with Bonus Years foods—but I do urge you to incorporate them into your daily diet. I make use of Booster foods in the suggested menus and recipes starting in Chapter 7.

Booster foods complement Bonus Compatible foods—acceptable foods that can be added to the diet for variety but do not offer any particular health benefits. (For more on Bonus Compatible foods, see pages 86–89.)

The Booster Foods

The right oils: olive, grapeseed, and canola
Tea
Flaxseed
Legumes
Soy
Whole grains

The Right Oils: Olive, Grapeseed, and Canola

For years, we've known that people who adhere to a Mediterranean-style diet have much lower rates of heart disease than those who follow the standard Western diet. One reason is that the Mediterranean diet is rich in monounsaturated fats, which, unlike the saturated fats and trans fats that dominate the American diet, are actually *good* for your heart. Olive oil is the predominant fat used in Mediterranean cooking, but there are two other monounsaturated fats that are growing in popularity and are also heart healthy—grapeseed and canola oils.

OLIVE OIL

Olive oil is rich in oleic acid, a heart-healthy fatty acid that prevents the oxidation of bad LDL cholesterol, which can damage the artery lining. (When LDLs are oxidized, they can promote the development of plaque on the arteries, and a stiffening of the arteries as well.) Olive oil is also a good source of polyphenols, the family of plant chemicals that includes flavonoids.

Olive oil (as well as the other monunsaturated fats) increases the production of nitric oxide, which helps regulate the muscle tone of blood vessels, keeping the muscles smooth and functioning at their highest levels.

Generally, we get olive oil by extracting the oil after pressing or crushing the olives. Olive oil comes in different varieties, depending on the amount of processing involved. Varieties include:

Extra-virgin: It is considered to be the best, as it comes from the first pressing of the olives. Of all the types of olive oil, extra-virgin contains the most beneficial polyphenols.

Virgin: Since it comes from the second pressing, it is not as desirable as extra-virgin.

Pure: This variety undergoes some processing, such as filtering and refining.

Extra-light: It undergoes considerable processing and only retains a very mild olive flavor.

Olive oil may offer a number of other health benefits, including reduced risk of some cancers (such as breast cancer), reduced risk of diabetes, and possibly, a delayed onset of complications in established diabetes.

While olive oil is wonderful in salads and on pasta, breads, and fish, it is not always a good oil to cook with. So it's important to get a good balance of other monounsaturated oils as well.

Grapeseed Oil

Grapeseed oil (also called grape oil) is a vegetable oil pressed from the seeds of various varieties of *Vitis vinifera* grapes, an abundant by-product of wine making.

Italy is the largest producer of grapeseed oil, but other countries, including France, Spain, and Switzerland also produce it. Although known to Europeans for centuries, grapeseed oil was not produced or used on a large scale until the twentieth century, mostly because grapeseeds contain a lower percentage of oil as compared to other oil-producing seeds, nuts, and beans.

Grapeseed oil is used for salad dressings, marinades, deep frying, flavored oils, baking, massage oil, sunburn-repair lotion, hair products, body hygiene creams, lip balm, and hand creams.

Studies have shown that grapeseed oil is full of antioxidants, such as vitamins C and E, as well as beta-carotene, and that it has heart-healthy benefits. Scientists suspect, but have not proven, that grapeseed oil also contains vitamin D.

The *Journal of the American College of Cardiology* published an article in 1993 showing a sample group of fifty-six men and women using up to 1.5 ounces (43 g) per day of grapeseed oil, which is a perfect amount to cook with. In this study, it appears that grapeseed oil had the ability to raise HDL (good cholesterol) levels by 13 percent and reduce LDL levels by 7 percent in just three weeks. Results also showed among the people in the sample group: their total cholesterol/HDL ratio was reduced 15.6 percent, and their total LDL/HDL ratio was reduced by 15.3 percent. These are significant results, especially for people at high risk for having a heart attack.

I use grapeseed oil when I cook because of its excellent nutritional benefits and clean, light, almost nutlike taste. I also use it in salad dressings or as a base for infusing or flavoring with garlic, rosemary, or other herbs or spices.

Grapeseed oil has the added benefit of a pretty high smoke point (approximately 420° F.; 216° C.), so you can also cook with it at high temperatures. You can be creative and use it for vegetable stir-fries, sautéing, and dark chocolate fondue.

CANOLA OIL

When I first heard of canola oil, I wondered where it came from. In all my training as a physician, I had never heard of a canola plant. Well, as it turns out, the word *canola* is a contraction of "Canadian oil, low acid"; the oil was initially introduced in Canada in the 1970s.

Canola oil comes from rapeseed, a member of the mustard family, and is higher in both omega-3 fatty acids, the polyunsaturated fat that can lower cholesterol and triglycerides, and omega-9 monosaturated fatty acids, the cholesterol-balancing monounsaturated fat, than any oil except olive oil.

Canola oil has the lowest concentration of saturated fatty acids of any of the cooking oils. It has a neutral taste, but is good for cooking and in salad dressings.

There was concern about canola oil because it comes from rapeseed, which contains the toxin eruric acid. However, seeds used for canola oil are carefully selected, so they contain almost no eruric acid. Canola is thus also known as LEAR oil (for low eruric acid rapeseed).

The popularity of canola oil is rising fast in the United States, probably because it's been discovered to be lower in saturated fat (about 6 percent) than any other oil. This compares to the saturated fat content of peanut oil (about 18 percent) and palm oil (at a shockingly high 79 percent). Canola has evolved into a major North American cash crop from its start as a specialty crop in Canada. Canada and the United States produce between 7 and 10 million metric tons of canola seed per year. The United States is a net consumer of canola oil, which means that we use more than we produce.

MONOUNSATURATED FATS AND YOUR SHAPE

Monounsaturated fats offer yet another very important health benefit: studies suggest that although they have same calorie content as other fats, it may be more difficult to put on weight from monounsaturated fats. Researchers compared the weight loss results from one group of people following a diet of large amounts of fish, olive oil, vegetables, and fruits to another group of people who were sticking to low-fat and high-carbohydrate diets. They found that those following the fish/olive oil/vegetables and fruit diet shed excess pounds from both the upper and lower body, but the other group mainly lost fat from the lower body. People who store their body fat around the waist and abdomen (apple-shaped) have a higher risk of heart disease than those people who carry their weight at the hips and thighs (pear-shaped) because fat stored around the waist is more likely to affect lipids in the blood and clog up arteries than fat stored around the thighs and hips.

Why is this important? According to a recent study reported in *The Lancet*, your waist-to-hip ratio, or WHR (which you can find by dividing your waist measurement by your hip measurement), is three times more effective at predicting cardiovascular risk than using body mass index, or BMI, the commonly used ratio of weight to height.

Furthermore, if obesity is redefined using WHR instead of BMI, the proportion of "abdominally obese" people at risk of heart attack increases by threefold, according to the researchers.

The Three Types of Dietary Fats

There are three types of fat: saturated, polyunsaturated, and monounsaturated. These terms describe the type of chemical bonding between the atoms. Each type consists of fatty acids (which are actually chains of carbon and hydrogen atoms) in different combinations.

Saturated fat is found primarily in food of animal origin, such as meat and dairy products. It can promote the oxidation of bad LDL cholesterol, which increases the risk for heart attack, so therefore you want to strictly limit your intake of saturated fat. Both polyunsaturated and monounsaturated fats can lower blood cholesterol levels. Foods containing mostly monounsaturated fats include olive oil, avocadoes, canola oil, and peanuts.

Tea

Black, oolong, white, and green—but not herbal—teas are all made from an infusion of the leaves of the *Camellia sinensis* plant. The types differ in the amount of time they are fermented before being heated, with black tea undergoing the greatest fermentation, and green the least. The oxidation process changes the phytochemical composition of the individual teas, so that black teas and green teas are very different chemically.

All teas are high in flavonoids, the powerful antioxidants that are also found in many of the Bonus Years foods. There is some evidence that green tea and white teas, which are the least processed, may pack a stronger antioxidant punch than other teas. White tea is harvested when the leaves and buds of the plant are still young and covered by fine white hair—which is how it got its name.

For years, researchers have studied records and interviewed people on the connection between those who drink tea daily and their overall heart health. More recently, scientists have done clinical (involving direct observation of the participants) studies about tea drinking and heart health. Both population and clinical studies clearly show that drinking tea daily is associated with better heart and cardiovascular health.

In fact, the American College of Cardiology revealed findings of two studies about the cardiovascular health benefits as early as 2001, at its 50th Annual Scientific Session.

In an analysis of thirteen published studies, researchers found that study participants who drank three or more cups of tea per day suffered an average of 11 percent fewer heart attacks than did those participants who drank fewer than three cups per day. Taking the results a step further, researchers from the University of North Carolina at Chapel Hill said that drinking three or more cups of tea per day could translate into preventing heart attacks in some 100,000 to 110,000 people, based on the average number of heart attacks per year in the United States, reported to be 1.1 million.

In another study looking at the effects of black tea specifically, researchers at the Boston University School of Medicine worked with a group of people already diagnosed with coronary artery disease (CAD). Their findings were extremely dramatic: participants with CAD who drank four cups of black tea daily showed measurable improvement in their blood vessel function, thus reducing a major risk factor for a fatal heart attack. These results suggest that drinking tea may improve an important underlying abnormality of blood vessel function that may be related to coronary artery disease.

In yet another major study, researchers found that heart attack victims who drank the most tea were the least likely to die in the several years following a heart attack.

Flavonoids: The Key to Tea's Heart-Healthy Benefits

Researchers (whose study was funded by the National Heart, Lung, and Blood Institute) on staff at Harvard Medical School believe that the key to the heart-healthy protection that tea drinking offers lies in the plentiful flavonoids in tea.

The types and amount of flavonoids found in a particular tea depend on several factors: the variety of the leaf that's being used for the tea, the environment in which the tea leaves are grown, how they are processed and manufactured, as well as the particle size of the ground tea leaves. For example, green teas contain more of the simple flavonoids called catechins, while the oxidization of the leaves that is needed to make black tea converts these simple flavonoids into the more complex kind, called theaflavins and thearubigins. The longer the tea is left to brew, the higher the concentration of flavonoids.

How Tea Appears to Help the Circulatory System

There are several studies showing how tea can have an important role in keeping the endothelium, the layer of cells lining various blood vessels in our bodies, working smoothly. One study of people with existing heart disease (coronary artery disease) demonstrated that for people who drank 900 ml (about four cups) of black tea daily, their endothelial function improved. In addition, another study looking at the effects of tea drinking on people with cholesterol levels that were moderately high showed that when they drank five cups of black tea a day for five weeks, their arteries were more open and blood could flow through more efficiently.

Flaxseed

The shiny brownish-red seeds of the flax plant are packed with omega-3 fatty acid power. Although walnuts and grapeseed oil also provide a good source of omega-3s, nothing in the nuts/seeds/legumes class really compares to the richness of flaxseed in omega-3 essential fatty acids.

The omega-3 fatty acids derived from flaxseed, like those from fish, have the ability to protect the heart from life-threatening arrhythmias and prevent the blood (platelets) from sticking to the artery walls.

You can buy flaxseed—either whole or ground—at health food stores. But remember to keep it refrigerated. Because flaxseed is so high in omega-3 essential fatty acids, it can easily become rancid. A good idea is to buy flaxseed whole and then grind it as needed (and store both the whole and the ground seed in the refrigerator). If you buy ground flaxseed, make sure it is either refrigerated or vacuum sealed to protect from spoilage. While whole flaxseed features a soft crunch, the nutrients in ground seed are more easily absorbed. To make sure I get the maximum nutritive value from meals, I sometimes sprinkle flaxseed on cereals and on cooked vegetables; I also add it to shakes and baked products.

Flaxseed is high in fiber, so if you choose to take flaxseed in its oil form, you get all of its benefits except for the fiber.

RICH IN LIFESAVING FIBER

The omega-3 fats in flaxseed are far from all this exceptional food has to offer. Both flaxseed meal and flour provide very good source of fiber, which can lower cholesterol levels in people with atherosclerosis and diabetic heart disease, reduce the exposure of colon cells to cancer-causing chemicals, relieve the constipation or diarrhea of irritable bowel syndrome sufferers, and help stabilize blood sugar levels in diabetic patients. Flaxseed is also a good source of magnesium, which helps to reduce the severity of asthma by keeping airways relaxed and open, lowers high blood pressure, and reduces the risk of heart attack and stroke in people with atherosclerosis and diabetic heart disease. In addition, it prevents the blood vessel spasm that leads to migraine attacks, and generally promotes relaxation and restores normal sleep patterns.

A study published in the September 8, 2003, issue of the *Archives of Internal Medicine* confirms that eating high-fiber foods such as flaxseed helps prevent heart disease. Almost ten thousand American adults participated in this study and were followed for nineteen years, during which time there were 1,843 cases of coronary heart disease (CHD) or atherosclerosis and 3,762 cases of cardiovascular disease (CVD), which also includes stroke and all other diseases of the cardiovascular system. People eating the most fiber, 21 grams per day, had 12 percent less CHD and 11 percent less CVD compared with those eating the least fiber, 5 grams daily. Those eating the most water-soluble dietary fiber fared even better, with a 15 percent reduction in risk of CHD and a 10 percent risk reduction in CVD.

FLAXSEED OIL

Flaxseed oil is rich in alpha linolenic acid (ALA), an omega-3 fat that is similar to the form of that found in fish oils (called eicosapentanoic acid, or EPA). ALA, in addition to providing several beneficial effects of its own, can be converted in the body to EPA, thus providing EPA's beneficial effects. For this conversion to readily take place, however, depends on your having a specific enzyme (called delta-6-destaurase), which, in some people, is less available or less active than in others. Moreover, in diabetics and in people whose diets include a lot of saturated fat and alcohol, the enzyme is hardly active. So diabetics and people with poor diets need to consume more flaxseed oil to get the optimal benefits of the omega-3 fats in it.

Anti-inflammatory Benefits of Flaxseed

The body uses omega-3 fatty acids to produce hormone-like substances that can help reduce inflammation. Over the past decade, researchers have found that inflammation is at the core of many diseases and conditions, including asthma, osteoarthritis, rheumatoid arthritis, migraine headaches, and even cardiovascular (heart and circulatory) disease.

And regarding cardiovascular disease: the body makes use of omega-3 fats to make the blood less sticky, which reduces the risk of blood clots, heart attack, and stroke, especially in people who have atherosclerosis or diabetic heart disease.

Lignans: The Compounds Women Need to Know About

Flaxseed is particularly rich in lignans, special compounds also found in other seeds, grains, and legumes. The main dietary sources of lignans are oilseeds (which include flaxseed, rapeseed, pumpkin, poppy, mustard, safflower, and sunflower seeds), broccoli, and fruit (especially berries). They are also found in whole grains (rye, oats, and barley), bran (wheat, oats, and rye), and vegetables.

Studies have shown that lignans protect a woman's cognitive performance, the heart, and the cardiovascular system, especially after menopause.

Over the past several years, researchers have consistently found flaxseed meal and flour to have important health effects for women.

In a community-based survey of 394 postmenopausal women, Dr. Oscar Franco and his colleagues from the Netherlands studied the relationship between eating plant-based foods, including flaxseed, and cognitive function, the women's abilities to use their brains efficiently for short- and longer-term memory tests. What Dr. Franco found is rather remarkable: it seems that women who ate foods rich in lignans consistently scored higher on the test. The results were especially clear in women who had gone through menopause some twenty to thirty years earlier.

In another study (double-blind and randomized), flaxseed reduced total cholesterol levels in the blood of postmenopausal women who were not on hormone replacement therapy by an average of 6 percent.

The lower GI tract converts lignans into two hormone-like substances, enterolactone and enterodiol, that demonstrate a number of protective effects against breast cancer and are believed to be one reason a vegetarian diet is associated with a lower risk for breast cancer. Studies show that women with breast cancer and women who regularly consume meat and other fatty proteins have much lower levels of lignans in their urine than women who are vegetarian and who don't have breast cancer. Lignan-rich fiber has also been shown to decrease insulin resistance, which, in turn, reduces the estrogen available for postmenopausal women, which also lessens breast cancer risk. And, as insulin resistance is an early warning sign for type 2 diabetes, flaxseed may also provide protection against this disease.

In other studies looking to evaluate the effect of lignans, supplementing a high-fat diet with flaxseed flour reduced early markers for breast (in rats, mammary) cancer in rats by more than 55 percent.

And here are some more interesting findings. In a study published in the February 2004 issue of the *American Journal of Clinical Nutrition,* postmenopausal women ate a daily muffin for sixteen weeks containing either 25 grams (a little less than 1 ounce) of soy protein, or 25 grams of ground flaxseed, or a placebo muffin containing neither soy nor flaxseed, and researchers found that the estrogen metabolism of the women eating flaxseed (but not soy and not the placebo muffin with neither substance) was altered in several important protective ways:

- Levels of a less biologically active estrogen metabolite thought to be protective against breast cancer (2-hydroxyestrone) increased significantly.
- The ratio of 2-hydroxyestrone (the protective estrogen metabolite) to an estrogen metabolite thought to promote cancer (16-alpha-hydroxyestrone) increased.
- The blood levels of various types of estrogen present in small amounts (estradiol, estrone, and estrone sulfate) did not change significantly; this is important, since estradiol helps in maintaining bone mass and preventing osteoporosis.

So what does all of this mean for women? It means that if women who have reached and passed menopause eat about an ounce of ground flaxseed each day, it appears that the flaxseed's nutrients will be protective against breast cancer but will not interfere with estrogen's role in normal bone maintenance. That's a pretty astounding capability.

Lignans Are Beneficial for Men as Well

In a prospective cohort study (an observational study in which a group of people—known as a cohort—are interviewed or tested for risk factors, such as nutrient intake, and then followed up at specific intervals to determine their status with respect to a disease or health outcome) of 1,889 Finnish men followed for an average of twelve years, those men whose blood indicated the highest levels of lignans showed a significant reduction in deaths from coronary heart disease or disease of the heart and circulatory systems than those with the lowest levels in their blood.

Add Flaxseed to Your Diet

- Sprinkle ground flaxseed onto hot or cold cereal.
- If adding ground flaxseed to a cooked cereal or grain dish, do so at the end of cooking since the fiber in the flaxseed can thicken liquids if left too long.

- Add flaxseed to a homemade muffin, cookie, or bread recipe.
- Add ground flaxseed to a breakfast shake to give it a terrific nutritional boost.
- Sprinkle ground flaxseed on top of cooked vegetables for a nutlike taste.

Legumes

As is true for many of the Booster foods, legumes are among the most versatile and nutritious foods available. Legumes are a class of vegetables that includes beans (like navy beans, lima beans, and garbanzo beans, which are also known as chickpeas), lentils, and peas. They are plants that have pods with tidy rows of seeds inside, are typically low in fat, contain no cholesterol, and are high in protein, folate (a B vitamin), potassium, iron, and magnesium.

Legumes are a good source of fiber, which delays the emptying of food from the stomach. The more slowly food empties out of the stomach, the more slowly carbohydrates are absorbed, which helps to keep blood glucose and insulin levels in check. Legumes also bind to bile in the digestive tract, lowering the absorption of cholesterol. Like fruits and vegetables, they are loaded with health-promoting plant-based compounds (phytochemicals), which research has shown can be protective against both chronic cardiovascular disease and cancer.

Studies have confirmed that people who eat legumes on a regular basis have a lower incidence of heart disease than do people who either eat them less frequently or don't eat them at all.

Soybeans are the only members of the legume family that contain all of the amino acids needed to make up a complete protein, just like any animal protein (such as meat or fish or chicken). Soybeans and the products made from them (tofu, soymilk, tempeh) contain isoflavones, plant-based compounds that may reduce the risk of some types of cancer (see the following section on soy, a Booster food in its own right).

Peanuts grow underground and, despite their name, are also a member of the legume family. They contain more fat and fewer carbohydrates than other legumes. Peanuts are a good source of protein, fiber, iron, magnesium, phosphorus, zinc, copper, niacin, and folate. Although the fat content of peanuts is relatively high, most of the fat is monounsaturated—the healthier type of fat (versus trans fat, the artery-clogging kind).

PROTEIN COMPLEMENTATION

Protein, which our bodies need to function properly, is made up of amino acids, often referred to as building blocks, as we need to consume amino acids to build new proteins in the body. Our bodies can make some amino acids from the protein we eat, but not others; the ones the body cannot make are considered essential amino acids because we need to get them either from foods (preferably) or in the form of supplements.

Since grains, fruits, and vegetables lack at least one of the essential amino acids, they don't provide complete protein.

When we combine nonmeat or nondairy (plant) sources of protein, such as legumes, seeds, and whole grains, which separately offer some protein but eaten together offer complete protein, we consider them complementary proteins; this means they only offer complete protein when eaten together.

Although we should eat legumes, seeds, and whole grains in combination and during the same day, we don't necessarily have to eat them during the same meal to get the complementary protein, as we once thought.

Some examples of plant-based dishes that eaten together contain complete protein, which means all the essential amino acids, include: brown rice and beans; peanut butter and whole-wheat bread; cornbread and pinto beans; and refried beans with wheat or corn tortillas. You can also add dairy products—preferably the low-fat variety—to a meatless dish to enhance the protein content of a meal, such as low-fat cheese melted on top of refried beans with wheat or corn tortillas.

If you experiment with various kinds of legumes, you will find the ones you like best; then you can include them in your meals and snacks for variety and extra nutrition.

Soy

Soybeans are probably the most versatile food on the planet. You can steam them to eat as a snack. You can grind soybeans into a custardlike curd called tofu; ferment them to create tempeh, which has a meaty texture; or turn them into soymilk or a bean paste called miso. In Asia, where soy is a staple, people do all of the above and more with this amazing legume. Soy deserves its own place among the Booster foods because it is the only legume that contains isoflavones, plant-based compounds that research suggests may reduce the risk of both heart disease and some cancers.

I love to cook with tofu because you can do practically anything to it and it takes on whatever flavors you add to it. I use whipped tofu for fruit smoothies and both tofu and miso as a base for salad dressing. In China, where soy is known as "meat without bones," tofu is commonly used as a meat substitute in stir-fry dishes.

Soy protein appears to stop the oxidation of LDL cholesterol, the kind that can inflict damage to the endothelium, the cells that protect the lining of the artery wall. In test tubes, a compound in soybeans called genistein has been found to inhibit the growth of cells that form artery-clogging plaque.

While people in Asian cultures have used soy extensively for centuries, Americans have been slow to adopt soy as part of our mainstream food staples. In the United States, soybean is a huge cash crop, but the product is used largely as livestock feed.

However, with the increased emphasis on healthy diets, especially among the 76 million baby boomers, that may be changing. Sales of soy products are up and are projected to increase, due in part, say industry officials, to the FDA-approved health claim.

Because soy protein can be added to a variety of foods, it is possible for consumers to eat dishes containing soy protein at all three meals and for snacks.

Soy and Fiber

Research has shown time and again that a fiber-rich diet is important in reducing the risk of certain types of cancer and heart disease. In fact, the National Cancer Institute (NCI) has issued a formal recommendation that Americans consume 25 to 30 grams of fiber a day. However, most people don't eat anywhere near that amount.

Enter the all-purpose soybean: in addition to being a complete protein, soybeans and some soy foods are excellent sources of fiber. In fact, just one-quarter cup of soybeans provides 8 grams of fiber, nearly a third of the NCI recommended daily amount.

Foods made from the whole soybean, such as soy flour, textured soy protein, and tempeh, are also fiber rich. But some soy foods lose their fiber in processing: the soy products tofu and soymilk contain very little fiber but still offer all the other nutrients we find in soy products.

SOY AND ISOFLAVONES

Soybeans contain a variety of phytochemicals (plant-based compounds). But soybeans are the only food source with significant amounts of one important phytochemical called isoflavones. In various experiments, isoflavones directly or indirectly have been found to lower cholesterol, inhibit bone resorption (the process by which calcium is released into circulation, helping to regulate calcium balance), relieve menopause symptoms, and even set in motion anticancer activity. Some research shows that just one daily serving of soy foods—one cup of soymilk or half cup of tofu—is enough to provide some of these benefits.

Isoflavones are chemically similar to the hormone estrogen in structure; in fact, isoflavones are classified as weak estrogens, and scientists will sometimes refer to them as phytoestrogens.

Raw, dry soybeans contain between two and four milligrams of isoflavones per gram. Most traditional soyfoods, such as tofu, soymilk, tempeh, and miso, are rich sources of isoflavones, providing about 30 to 40 milligrams per serving. Only two soy products, soy sauce and soybean oil, do not contain isoflavones.

Soy foods that are based on soy, but which have many other ingredients, are sometimes referred to as "second-generation products" (such as soy hot dogs and soy-based ice cream); these have much lower amounts of isoflavones, because of all the nonsoy ingredients they contain.

THE FDA-APPROVED HEALTH CLAIM ABOUT SOY PROTEINS AND HEART HEALTH

Approximately 40 million Americans have blood cholesterol levels that are too high. But many studies have shown that among such people, soy protein can reduce high blood cholesterol levels by 10 to 15 percent—enough to cut the chances of a heart attack by up to 30 percent.

On October 26, 1999, the FDA authorized the use of health claims about the role of soy protein in reducing the risk of coronary heart disease (CHD) on labeling of foods containing soy protein, based on the FDA's conclusion that people following a diet low in saturated fat and cholesterol who include foods containing soy protein may lower their overall cholesterol levels, thus reducing their risk of heart disease.

Only foods that contain at least 6.25 grams of soy protein per serving and fit other criteria, such as being low in fat, cholesterol, and sodium are covered by the FDA health claim.

The FDA approved other claims, even before soy proteins, including claims for the cholesterol-lowering effects of soluble fiber in oat bran and psyllium seeds.

Based on findings in research, the FDA determined that diets with four daily soy servings can reduce levels of low-density lipoproteins (LDLs), the so-called bad cholesterol that builds up in blood vessels, by as much as 10 percent. This number is significant because heart experts generally agree that a 1 percent drop in total cholesterol can equal a 2 percent drop in heart disease risk.

Studies suggest that as little as 25 grams of soy protein per day may be enough to lower cholesterol levels, and greater amounts—25 to 50 grams per day—may well decrease cholesterol levels even more. One cup of cooked soybeans, tempeh, or roasted soy nuts contains the higher amount—some 25 to 50 grams per day. To me, that sounds like a pretty great way to reduce my cholesterol levels.

One study, conducted over nine weeks at Wake Forest University Baptist Medical Center and reported in the *Archives of Internal Medicine* in 1999, found that soy protein can reduce total and LDL cholesterol but does not negatively affect levels of HDL, or good cholesterol.

Another often-quoted study, published in the *New England Journal of Medicine* in 1995, looked at thirty-eight separate studies and concluded that soy protein can prompt "significant reductions" not only in total and LDL cholesterol, but also in triglycerides, other fats linked to heart and circulatory problems when present at high levels.

How to Get More Soy on Your Plate

While not every form of soy foods will qualify for the FDA health claim, these are some of the most common sources of soy protein:

Tofu is made from cooked puréed soybeans processed into a custardlike cake. It has a neutral flavor and can be stir-fried, mixed into smoothies, or blended into a cream cheese texture for use in dips or as a cheese substitute. It comes in firm, soft, and silken textures.

Soymilk is produced by grinding hulled soybeans and mixing them with water to form a milklike liquid. It can be consumed as a beverage or used in recipes as a substitute for cow's milk. Soymilk, sometimes fortified with calcium, comes plain or in flavors such as vanilla, chocolate, and coffee. For lactose-intolerant individuals, it can be a good replacement for dairy products.

Soy flour, made by grinding roasted soybeans into a fine powder, adds protein to baked goods, and, because it adds moisture, it can be used as an egg substitute in these products. It also can be found in cereals, pancake mixes, frozen desserts, and other common foods.

Textured soy protein is made from defatted soy flour, which is compressed and dehydrated. It can be used as a meat substitute or as filler in dishes such as meat loaf.

Tempeh is made from whole, cooked soybeans formed into a chewy cake and used as a meat substitute.

Miso is a fermented soybean paste used for seasoning and in soup stock.

There are other products that manufacturers have created to look like meat products, such as soy sausages, burgers, franks, and cold cuts, as well as soy yogurts and cheese, all of which are intended as substitutes for animal-based foods with the same names.

Since not all foods that contain soy ingredients meet the FDA health claim, be sure to read the labels. Make sure the products contain enough soy protein to make a meaningful contribution to the total daily diet without being high in saturated fat and other unhealthy substances.

Some typical counts of grams of soy protein for certain foods

---

FOOD	NUMBER OF GRAMS OF SOY PROTEIN
4 ounces of firm tofu	13
1 soy "sausage" link	6
1 soy "burger"	10 to 12
8-oz. glass of plain soymilk	10
1 soy protein bar	14
½ cup tempeh	19.5
¼ cup roasted soy nuts	19

The American Dietetic Association recommends introducing soy slowly by adding small amounts to the daily diet or mixing into existing foods. Then, once the taste and texture have become familiar, add more.

Because many soy protein products have a mild or even neutral flavor, you can add them to dishes with barely any effect on the taste. Use soy flour to thicken sauces and gravies; add soymilk to baked goods and desserts. Tofu takes on the flavor of whatever it is cooked in, so you can use it in stews and stir-fries.

A good way to introduce yourself or family members to the pleasures of eating soy proteins is to go to a restaurant that specializes in vegetarian/soy dishes.

Whole Grains

Whole grains include wheat, corn, rice, oats, barley, quinoa, sorghum, spelt, and rye. Whole wheat flour, bulgur (cracked wheat), rolled oats, whole cornmeal, and brown rice are some of the whole grains that are familiar to us. These are found in some breakfast cereals, some dark breads, popcorn, cooked oatmeal, and wheat germ, to name a few.

Whole grain means the entire seed of the plant, as opposed to processed grains that have been stripped of most of their beneficial fiber and nutrients. All grain seeds contain an outer husk covering that we remove because it's just not digestible, like the outer husks on corn. Inside the husk is the bran, which surrounds and protects the germ and the endosperm. Whole grains contain all three parts of the kernel—the bran, germ, and endosperm.

The bran is the multilayered outer skin of the kernel that contains key antioxidants, B vitamins, and fiber. The bran is tough enough to protect the other two parts of the kernel from the harsh effects of sunlight, insects or other pests, water, and disease.

The germ is the embryo of the kernel. When it is fertilized by pollen, it grows into a new plant. The germ part of the kernel contains many B vitamins, some protein, minerals, and healthy fats. Wheat germ has become popular and widely available, as it offers an excellent way to get the benefits of the germ of the wheat berry.

Refining normally removes the bran and the germ, leaving only the endosperm, which is high in starchy carbohydrates. Without the bran and germ, about 25 percent of a grain's protein is lost, along with at least seventeen key nutrients, including vitamin E, magnesium, and fiber.

Research has shown that whole grains have been associated with potential health benefits, including a lowered risk for metabolic syndrome, a cluster of conditions that often occur together, including obesity, high blood sugar, high blood pressure, and high triglycerides (a type of blood fat), each and all of which can lead to cardiovascular disease.

Our risk of developing metabolic syndrome increases when we eat a lot of sugar and are significantly overweight (more than twenty pounds over our ideal weight). Higher levels of both blood glucose and body weight increase the risk of developing metabolic syndrome, which increases the risk of both heart disease and diabetes in people of all ages, including children if they are obese.

A 2006 study conducted by the USDA Jean Mayer Human Nutrition Research Center on Aging found that people who ate about 2.5 or more servings of whole grains a day compared with those who ate less than one serving daily were half as likely to have metabolic syndrome. That is a pretty powerful argument for including whole grains in the diet. The same researchers found that people who ate 2.5 or more servings of whole grains compared with those who ate less than one serving a day of whole grains had half as many deaths from heart disease. But if they ate refined grains, it had no effect on their risk of developing metabolic syndrome or of dying of heart disease. These statistics offer a strong argument for eating three ounces or more of whole-grain products per day. I've included some very tasty, easy-to-make dishes in the recipes section of the book that include whole grains as well as many other key nutrients. If you haven't yet discovered that nutritious, heart-healthy foods can also be delicious, then you're in for a great surprise when you see the recipes I've included for you.

Another recent study showed that eating whole-grain (but not refined-grain) cereals for breakfast both prolonged life and reduced deaths from heart disease. Moreover, researchers have shown that substituting whole-grain for refined-grain products lowers a woman's risk both of developing type 2 (adult-onset) diabetes and of developing heart disease.

Moreover, in 1982, researchers at Harvard Medical School began a study of 86,190 male physicians in the United States, ages forty to eighty-four, who had no heart disease or cancer when the study began. Over five and a half years, results showed that for the men who ate whole-grain breakfast cereal, they lived longer and had less heart disease than those men who did not eat whole-grain breakfast cereals. These results were consistently true despite age, weight, body mass index (BMI), alcohol consumption, high blood pressure, high cholesterol, physical activity, and even smoking.

Other, similar studies have supported these findings—which is certainly a compelling reason to make sure we're getting whole grains in our diets.

The United States Department of Agriculture's Center for Nutrition Policy and Promotion houses the famous Food Pyramid (see http://www.mypyramid.gov), which has undergone many changes over the years as our knowledge of nutrition becomes more sophisticated. The current food pyramid is designed to be tailored to each person depending on age, gender, and level of normal daily activity, and includes a high ratio of whole grains as part of its recommendations.

How to Add More Whole Grains to Your Diet

We have a lot of options for getting more whole grains into our diets. Here are some suggestions:

- Substitute a whole-grain product for a refined product—choose whole wheat bread instead of white bread; brown rice instead of white rice. It's important to substitute the whole-grain product for the refined one, rather than adding the whole-grain product.

- Try brown rice or whole wheat pasta. For example, use brown rice stuffing in baked green peppers or tomatoes and whole wheat macaroni in macaroni and cheese.
- Add whole grains to soups, stews, and vegetables. For example, use barley in vegetable soup or stews and bulgur wheat in casseroles or stir-fries.
- Create a whole-grain pilaf with a mixture of barley, wild rice, brown rice, broth, and spices. To add more flavor and nutritional value, stir in toasted nuts or chopped dried fruit.
- Experiment by substituting whole wheat or oat flour for up to half of the flour in pancake, waffle, muffin, or other flour-based recipes. See some of the recipes I've included; you'll notice the foods made with the whole-grain flour may need a bit more leavening.
- Use whole-grain bread or cracker crumbs in meat loaf.
- If you're making baked chicken, fish, veal, or eggplant, use rolled oats or a crushed, unsweetened whole-grain cereal as breading.
- With salads and soups, try whole-grain ready-to-eat cereal as croutons or instead of crackers.
- Choose ready-to-eat whole-grain cereals (such as toasted oats) for breakfast or as snack food.
- If you're making cookies or other baked goods, add whole grains such as wheat or oat flour; make oatmeal-raisin cookies with whole oats.
- Try a whole-grain snack chip, such as baked tortilla chips.
- Serve popcorn, a whole grain and a healthy snack, with little or no added salt and butter.

What Exactly Are Steel-Cut Oats?

Steel-cut oats are whole-grain groats (the inner portion of the oat kernel) that have been cut into only two or three pieces; they look like mini rice particles.

Steel-cut oats are high in B vitamins, calcium, protein, and fiber, while low in salt and unsaturated fat. One cup of cooked steel-cut oatmeal contains more fiber than a bran muffin and twice as much fiber as Cream of Wheat.

Oatmeal is the only food that naturally contains GLA (gamma linolenic acid), an essential fatty acid critical to the body's production of the favorable eicosanoids (PGE1 prostaglandins). Eating steel-cut oats four times a week provides a good supply of GLA.

In August 1999, the Food and Drug Administration (FDA) authorized a new claim allowing companies to state in advertisements and on product labels that diets rich in whole grains, such as oats, may reduce the risk of heart disease and cancers.

What to Look for on the Food Label

No matter if the packaging says "old-fashioned" or "homemade taste," you should still look for the words "whole grains." For example, "rolled oats" sounds good, but rolled oats are actually flakes of oats that have been steamed, rolled, resteamed, and toasted, reducing their nutritional value each time they are processed.

Foods labeled with the words "multigrain," "stone-ground," "100% wheat," "cracked wheat," "seven-grain," or "bran" are usually not whole-grain products.

Color is not an indication of a whole grain. Bread can be brown because of molasses or other added ingredients. Read the ingredient list to see if it is a whole-grain product.

Use the Nutrition Facts label and choose products with a higher % Daily Value (%DV) for fiber—the %DV (percentage of the daily value) for fiber is a good indication of the amount of whole grain in the product.

Read the food label's ingredient list. Look for words that indicate added sugars (sucrose, high-fructose corn syrup, honey, molasses) and oils (partially hydrogenated vegetable oils) that add extra calories. Choose foods with the fewest added sugars, fats, and oils.

Choose foods that name one of the following whole-grain ingredients first on the label's ingredient list:

- brown rice
- bulgur
- graham flour
- oats
- whole-grain corn
- whole oats
- whole rye
- whole wheat
- wild rice

CHAPTER 5

How to Get Your Bonus Years

By now, you're probably eager to get started on the Bonus Years Foods Rx. So here are the basics:

- Get your full dose of Bonus Years foods daily.
- Plan your meals around Bonus Years foods, Booster foods, and Bonus Compatible foods.
- Avoid foods that are in the Penalty Box.

Bonus Years Foods: The Stars

At the core of the Bonus Years Foods Rx are the Bonus Years foods, the seven special foods that when properly dosed, earn you the Bonus Years. These include wine, chocolate, fruits and vegetables, fish, garlic, and nuts. (See Chapter 6, "Getting Your Daily Dose of Bonus Years Foods.")

Booster Foods: The Supporting Cast

The seven Booster foods offer special health benefits of their own and bring variety into your diet. I have included them in many of the Bonus Years recipes. Use them liberally with your Bonus Years foods.

Bonus Compatible Foods: The Extras

Bonus Compatible foods, which are discussed later in this chapter, complement the Bonus Years foods. Although they don't have the same proven medicinal benefits, they aren't bad for you either. Compatible foods have been included to afford a richly diverse culinary palate that has been carefully vetted so you don't have to worry that you might be introducing foods that will undercut the efficacy of your Bonus Years foods. (For a list of Bonus Compatible foods, see pages 87–88.)

The Penalty Box: Off-limits

Foods that have the dubious distinction of being in the Penalty Box are those that can undermine the positive health impact of the Bonus Years foods. Clearly, the Penalty Box is a place that you want to avoid. See pages 89–92 for information about which foods you should eat rarely, if at all.

Cooking Up the Bonus Years Foods

In Chapter 7, you will find thirty days' worth of sample menus to show you how easy it is to incorporate Bonus Years foods into your daily diet. In addition to providing you with great meal ideas, the menus are also a useful tool for teaching how to get these foods every day. To help you keep track of your daily intake of Bonus Years foods, I have devised a simple system called Bonus Points (see Chapter 7).

I also offer numerous recipes to accompany the menus. I know that some people may be intimidated by the mere thought of cooking. You don't think you have the skill—or the time, for that matter—to cook anything from scratch. I completely understand your feelings. I may be a chef, but I'm also a practicing physician with a hectic schedule, so I understand the need for recipes to be simple and quick. In most cases, the recipes in this book are easy enough for the novice cook to follow.

To make it really easy for you, I have provided simple instructions on basic cooking skills that can help you create restaurant-quality food in a matter of minutes. I strongly recommend that you read Chapter 9, Bonus Years

Cooking Techniques, before you try out the recipes. You will find that knowing a few simple cooking tricks will make a huge difference in your confidence level, as well as the quality of your cooking.

What Foods Are Bonus Compatible?

Bonus Compatible foods are foods that are neutral in that they don't have scientifically proven health benefits but are not harmful. This is not to suggest that these foods are not wholesome or even good for you—merely that they have not undergone the same level of scientific investigation as bona fide Bonus Years foods or Booster foods.

Compatible Proteins

Compatible proteins are relatively low in heart-clogging saturated fat. If you don't see a cut of meat that you like on the list (for example, brisket of beef or New York strip steak, high in saturated fat but admittedly delicious), it doesn't mean that you should never eat it. I do recommend that you indulge in these foods on special occasions only and most of the time stick to leaner proteins.

POULTRY
Chicken, white meat, skin removed
Cornish hen, skin removed
Turkey, white meat, skin removed
Ground turkey
Ground chicken
Chicken or turkey sausage, no nitrates

BEEF
Beef tenderloin
Filet mignon
Flank steak
Roast beef (top round or rump)
Sirloin steak

GAME
Buffalo burgers
Duck (well drained, no skin)
Ostrich
Venison
Rabbit

PORK
Canadian bacon (no nitrates, if possible)
Lean ham
Loin chop
Pork tenderloin

LAMB
Chop
Roast
Leg

DAIRY
Cheese (5 grams of fat or less per slice)
Cottage cheese (1% or no-fat)
Eggs with yolks (okay if your cholesterol is within normal limits)
Egg whites
Egg substitutes
Milk (1% or no-fat)
Ricotta cheese (low-fat or no-fat)
Yogurt (1% or no-fat)

Compatible Beverages

Coffee
Seltzer
Water

Compatible Starches

I'm not against carbohydrates, nor do I insist that you always eat whole wheat breads and pastas. Although whole grains are Booster foods, I understand that if you're out at a great Italian restaurant, and you want to order the linguine with white clam sauce, you will feel deprived if you can't. And if I was in your shoes, I would too.

Some forms of carbohydrates are really bad for you, and you should steer clear of them. These include sugary and/or processed starches such as chips, crackers, and presweetened cereals. These foods are in the Penalty Box (see box on pages 91–92) for a reason. They cause a rapid rise in blood sugar that sends insulin levels soaring, which over time can lead to prediabetes and diabetes. Eat these foods rarely, if at all.

So feel free to enjoy a piece of bread, a plate of pasta or French toast on a Sunday morning—I do! If possible, eat whole grains. Try to buy bread that contains at least 3 grams of fiber per slice, and start the day with whole-grain cereal for breakfast.

Fortunately, you don't have to go to a health food store anymore to find good whole-grain products. They are now sold in most supermarkets and they taste better than ever.

A word about pasta: I used to turn my nose up at whole-grain pasta, but the fact is, the new whole-grain pastas, especially those imported from Italy, have a wonderful texture and flavor. They are substantially higher in fiber than pasta made with white flour, which means that they are digested more slowly and don't cause the precipitous spike in blood sugar.

How to Stay out of the Penalty Box

All food isn't created equal. There are some that can counteract the good things that the Bonus Years foods are doing for you. Therefore, they should be eaten only in limited quantities, if at all. There are not that many foods that fall into the Penalty Box, and frankly, the worst offenders don't really taste that good, anyway. Furthermore, there are so many other foods outside the Penalty Box for you to choose from, you really shouldn't feel deprived.

So make an effort to stay out of the Penalty Box by avoiding the foods listed below.

Trans Fats (Trans-fatty Acids)

Many brands of margarine and polyunsaturated oils undergo a chemical process called hydrogenation to make them easier to use in baking and to retard spoilage. The problem is, trans fats (trans-fatty acids) are bad for your heart and just about every other part of your body. Trans fats can raise levels of LDL (bad cholesterol) and lower levels of HDL (good cholesterol). Another reason to avoid trans fats is, like other fats, they can get incorporated into your cell membranes, making them hard and rigid, affecting their ability to make energy, get adequate nutrition, or communicate with other cells. Trans fats do the opposite of what good omega-3 fats do: when good omega-3 fats get into the cell membranes, they make them more flexible and actually *improve* the function of the cell. But when trans fats are around, they crowd out the good fats, getting into the cell membranes first. Therefore, you need to avoid eating food with trans fats as much as possible. Don't use margarine unless the label clearly states no trans fats. There are some new spreads on the market such as Smart Balance that contain only good fats, and are vastly preferable to the old-style margarines in flavor.

Although tiny amounts of trans fats occur naturally in various meat and dairy products, it's the trans fats from processed and fried foods that pose the greatest health threat. The primary sources of trans fats in the diet include commercial baked goods, fried foods (yes, even French fries from your favorite fast-food restaurant), cookies, chips, pies, and doughnuts.

Your best defense against trans fats is to read package labels very carefully. As of January 2006, the FDA is requiring food manufacturers to list the trans fat content on nutrition labels along with saturated fat and total cholesterol. Even so, some food companies have gotten the FDA to grant them an extension so they don't have to comply with the ruling until a later date. And here's the kicker: if foods contain less than 1 gram of trans fat per serving, they are not required to list it on the label. So the package will say 0 trans fats even if it contains slightly under 1 gram. If you eat several servings of processed food or fried food daily, it's possible to consume a substantial amount of trans fat and not even know it. So you have to do some detective work on your own. Be sure to read food ingredient labels, and don't buy the product if its label includes the words *shortening, hydrogenated vegetable oil,* or *partially hydrogenated oil.* These ingredients are the tip-off that the product contain trans fats. And do avoid fried food, especially from fast-food restaurants, unless the restaurant specifies that it uses oil that does not contain trans fats.

Try to cook with Booster food oils—olive, grapeseed, and canola oils. These oils not only taste better than oils laden with trans fats, but are good for your heart.

Saturated Fat

Saturated fat is found primarily in full-fat dairy products such as cheese, cream, butter, and fatty cuts of meat, organ meats, veal, most cuts of lamb, and certain cuts of pork. Saturated fat is very atherogenic—it stimulates the production of LDL cholesterol by the liver and encourages plaque formation in your arteries. Although current American Heart Association guidelines suggest that you limit saturated fat to less than 10 percent of your daily caloric intake, many Americans eat a lot more saturated fat than they should. Maybe that's why we have such a high rate of heart disease in the United States.

Processed meats such as hot dogs, luncheon meats, and pastrami not only are very high in saturated fat, but are cured with nitrates and nitrites, preservatives that prevent spoilage but form a powerful cancer-causing chemical, nitrosamine, in your stomach. I'm not telling you to pass up hot dogs at the ball park, but if you crave these foods, save them for special occasions.

If you choose your food selections from Bonus Years foods, Bonus Compatible foods, and Booster foods, you will easily be able to keep your intake of saturated fat down to safe levels.

A Word About Processed "Junk"

Many of the highly processed convenience goods so readily available at the supermarket are packed with sugar, bad fat, and lots of calories. These foods (and I use the word loosely) include chips, dips, crackers, salad dressings, breads, frozen foods, and processed desserts. Anything that comes in a box, plastic bag, or a wrapper is suspect. Your only defense is to read nutrition labels. Pay particular attention to calories per serving. You will be shocked to see how a snack of chips and dip, for example, can easily add up to 500-plus calories and dozens of fat grams (mostly bad fat) at one sitting—that's about 25 percent of the usual recommended caloric daily intake.

Avoid eating processed grain, which has been stripped of fiber and nutrients. Whole grains are included in Booster foods because they are so vital for good health. Look for bread that contains at least 3 grams of fiber per slice and cereal that contains 5 or more grams of fiber per serving.

Liquid Candy

Finally, avoid presweetened drinks such as colas, commercial iced tea, and fruit drinks. They are loaded with excess calories that quickly accumulate into extra pounds.

Instead of reaching for a sweetened drink, try making your own iced tea. You get the benefit of the flavonoids from the home-brewed tea, and you can sweeten it lightly with a teaspoon or two of sugar and flavor it with a splash of lemon, which adds about 40 calories. When you compare this to the 120 calories or more in the prepackaged iced tea, you're still way ahead of the game. You can also use an artificial sweetener such as Sucrilose if you prefer. Diet soda is fine for people who need to cut back on calories.

SUGAR SUBSTITUTES

I am often asked about using sugar substitutes for cooking or as a sweetener. I'm not a big fan of processed sugar. Unlike fruit, which is naturally sweet, sugar supplies empty calories, meaning it doesn't contain any nutrients. My advice is to limit the use of sugar whenever possible. Nevertheless, there are times when some sugar must be added to make a dish taste right. When that is the case, I try to do it with moderation. If you are trying to lose weight, feel free to use whatever sugar substitute you like best.

The Cholesterol Question

People often ask me how the cholesterol in the food we eat affects our blood cholesterol levels. You would think that the answer would be pretty obvious: the more cholesterol you eat, the higher your cholesterol level. But it's not that simple. While some people are very sensitive to cholesterol from food, others, for reasons we don't understand, can eat lots of high-cholesterol food with no negative consequences.

We get cholesterol from two sources: from the food that we eat and the cholesterol that is produced by our bodies. Our bodies use cholesterol to make steroid hormones such as testosterone and estrogen and it is also a structural component of every cell membrane. There is no dietary requirement for cholesterol because our body makes all the cholesterol that we need. Both saturated fat and trans fat stimulate the liver to produce more cholesterol.

Cholesterol is found only in animal foods such as meat, seafood, eggs, and dairy products. Some foods are higher in cholesterol than others—3.5 ounces of lean beef has about 60 mg of cholesterol (and most people eat twice as much as that at one sitting), the same amount of skinless chicken breast has 58 mg of cholesterol, and salmon, 74 mg. One egg yolk has 215 mg of cholesterol and 3.5 ounces of shrimp has about 150 mg. The American Heart Association recommends limiting cholesterol intake to about 300 mg daily, which I think is sound advice that I follow myself, but you can see, given the cholesterol content of many foods, that could be hard to do.

At one time the American Heart Association advised everyone to stringently limit consumption of egg yolks. Today that warning is extended only to people with high cholesterol levels or other risk factors for heart disease. Why the switch? Some studies suggest that the cholesterol in egg yolks is different from the cholesterol in beef or other high-cholesterol foods, and is actually harmless for most people. However, I tend to err on the side of caution. I often recommend using egg whites instead of whole eggs whenever possible, or commercial egg substitutes which taste just like the real thing. If you have high cholesterol (usually defined as over 200 mg/dl) you definitely should limit consumption of egg yolks.

The bottom line, we don't know who is going to be affected by eating cholesterol-rich foods and who is immune. To me, it just makes sense to keep an eye on your cholesterol intake. The amount of cholesterol in packaged food products is listed on the nutrition label along with trans fats and saturated fat. Since so many high-cholesterol foods also contain saturated fat, if you are already watching your saturated fat intake, you will naturally reduce your intake of cholesterol.

CHAPTER 6

Getting Your Daily Dose of Bonus Years Foods

E ating should never be a chore, and I don't want to make it hard for you to get your daily dose of Bonus Years foods. And it won't be, as long as you do a little planning ahead. In Chapter 7, you will find thirty days' worth of sample menus and recipes showing you how to get your full dose of Bonus Years foods every day. These menus are not meant to be followed rigidly; rather, they are to be used as guidelines. Once you understand how to include Bonus Years foods in your daily diet, it will be easy to create your own meals to suit your likes and dislikes.

Snacks count, too! A handful of nuts, fruit, or a piece of dark chocolate as an afternoon pick-me-up as a useful way to fill your Bonus Years Foods Rx.

Below are some easy suggestions to get more Bonus Foods into your life.

WINE

Bonus Years Foods Rx: 1 (5-ounce) glass daily

This is as easy as it gets. Sip one glass of wine (preferably red) with dinner every night or before dinner as a cocktail. That way, you get your full dose of wine in one sitting. For suggestions on which wines go well with which food, look at my sample menus.

DARK CHOCOLATE

Bonus Years Foods Rx: 2 ounces daily

Did you ever think that you'd *have* to eat chocolate every day, doctor's orders? Getting your daily dose of chocolate is what makes the Bonus Years Foods Rx a real pleasure. Some of you may want to enjoy your dose of chocolate in one sitting, and that's fine. Dark chocolate is very rich, however, so you may want to divide your dose (and spread the joy) over two meals or snacks. I sometimes start the day with homemade hot chocolate (see recipe, page 109), which gives me 1 ounce of dark chocolate. That leaves 1 more ounce of chocolate to have later as a snack during the day or for dessert. Buy only dark chocolate that contains at least 60 percent cocoa solids (70 percent is better), to make sure that you are getting enough heart-healthy flavonoids, or else you're just eating a candy bar.

FRUITS AND VEGETABLES

Bonus Years Foods Rx: 4 cups or 5 (¾ cups) servings

Consume at least five servings of fruits and vegetables daily, each serving about ¾ of a cup. The reality is, unless you are following one of my recipes, where the vegetables and fruits are carefully "dosed," cup measurements don't work. Most people probably eat a whole apple or banana rather than slicing it up and measuring it. Others may eat celery or cut-up vegetables as a snack by the handful. I've made it easier for you by providing a list of what constitutes one serving of a representative group of fruits and vegetables.

One Bonus Years Food serving =

1 pear
1 apple
1 orange
2 small plums or 1 standard-size plum

1 ear of corn
1 banana
1 cereal bowl of mixed salad
7 medium strawberries
3 whole dried apricots
1 handful of grapes, cherries, or small berries
1 carrot, whole or sliced
1 cereal bowl of mixed fruit
2–3 broccoli stalks with florets
¼ cantaloupe

Fruits and vegetables make great snacks and are a terrific way to quell hunger pains, especially if you are interested in slimming down. I incorporate a lot of fruits and vegetables in my meals, as you will see from my recipes.

FISH

Bonus Years Foods Rx: Three 5-ounce servings a week
(each serving about the size of two decks of cards)

Of all the Bonus Years foods, fish is the one that gives most people pause. Not that they don't like it, but they feel that buying and cooking fish is so much trouble, that they can't commit to having it three times a week. Actually, following the fish Rx is very simple if you have a strategy. First, if you absolutely can't get to the store to buy fresh fish, canned fish is fine. Stock your pantry with canned salmon, light tuna (white tuna contains too much mercury), and sardines, all of which are high in beneficial omega-3 fatty acids. When you need to fill your fish Rx, all you do is open a can, add a salad, and you have a quick meal. Second, if you're afraid to cook fish, the information in Chapter 10 will help ease your fears. Once you know the proper technique, fish is actually fairly simple for even the most inexperienced of cooks. And finally, when you eat out, order the fish entrée. It's a safe bet for getting heart-healthy benefits.

GARLIC

Bonus Years Foods Rx: 1 cooked or raw clove daily

Garlic is one of my favorite herbs, and I use it liberally in my cooking. For suggestions on how to cook with garlic, review the Bonus Years recipes starting in Chapter 7. Stir-fry vegetables with a few garlic cloves, sauté broccoli in olive oil with some garlic and serve it over pasta, or take a bunch of garlic cloves and roast them in the oven. Keep some fresh parsley on hand to get rid of garlic breath and you're good to go.

NUTS

Bonus Years Foods Rx: 2 ounces daily

The suggested dose of nuts is given in terms of ounces, and it's very difficult to know how many of each type of nut are in two ounces, unless you carry a mini scale around with you. So I researched the question and here are my answers. Two ounces is approximately:

- 93 shelled pistachios
- 56 peanuts
- 48 almonds
- 40 pecan halves
- 40 hazelnuts
- 28 walnut halves

Because they are portable, filling, and nutritious, nuts make a wonderful snack. Commercially prepared nuts can be very salty, so try to eat unsalted nuts whenever possible. Dry-roasted and raw nuts are your best choices because they are minimally processed and do not contain a lot of extra fat.

Lightening Up the Bonus Years

Following the basic Bonus Years Foods Rx will help you maintain a normal, healthy weight. Although the prescription is not a weight-loss diet, eating a minimum of five fruits and vegetables a day and three fish meals a week is a vast improvement over how most people eat. And although nuts and chocolate are fairly high in calories, they have enough beneficial nutrients to make them worth the splurge if you don't have a weight problem. Not to mention the fact that they are very satisfying and fill you up quickly.

If you have to take off ten or more pounds, you may have to make some adjustments in the Bonus Years Foods Rx. Below are simple ways to cut back on calories without losing the benefits of the Bonus Years.

Cut your dose of chocolate and nuts. You don't have to eliminate chocolate and nuts from your daily diet, but you can cut your dose for both in half. So instead of eating 2 ounces of chocolate and 2 ounces of nuts, eat 1 ounce of chocolate and 1 ounce of nuts. That will save you about 325 calories a day. But you'll still get nearly all the heart-healthy benefits of each food as well as the enjoyment that comes from eating them.

Increase your daily servings of fruits and vegetables. A recent study recorded in the July 18, 2006, *Journal of the American Dietetic Association* showed that people who eat the most fruit and fiber (which is abundant in fruit, vegetables, legumes, and whole grains) stay the slimmest. According to the study, compared with normal-weight people, overweight people eat one less fruit serving daily. Make a conscious effort to eat more fruit, salads, and other high-fiber foods.

Use low-fat cooking techniques. Review the section on Bonus Years cooking techniques starting in Chapter 9. It will provide you with a wealth of information on how to prepare great food using little or no fat, which can add lots of calories to your meal.

Speak up at restaurants. When you eat out, give very specific instructions to the waitstaff as to how you want your meal prepared or your fish may emerge from the kitchen swimming in butter and your salad drenched in a high-fat dressing. Ask for the entrée to be baked or broiled in lemon juice, wine, or broth. Order the salad with dressing on the side, or even better, ask for olive oil and vinegar and make your own heart-healthy dressing. Pass on the bread basket, and order fresh fruit for dessert. But don't forget to order a glass of red wine—it's only about 106 calories or so, and chock-full of flavonoids.

Eat at home whenever you can. The reality is, the only way to have total control over how food is prepared is to do it yourself. If you are serious about shedding some excess pounds, try to eat at home as often as possible.

Increase your activity level. Weight loss is the interaction between burning calories and cutting calories. The only way to burn more calories is to be physically active. That means trying to get some form of regular exercise every day, whether it's walking briskly, working out at the gym, or taking a Pilates class. Of course, check with your doctor before beginning any new exercise program if you are over forty or have been sedentary.

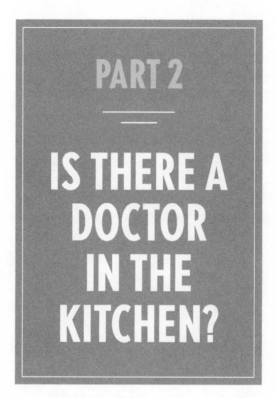

PART 2

IS THERE A DOCTOR IN THE KITCHEN?

CHAPTER 7

30 Days on the
Bonus Years Diet

I love to eat. In fact, I love almost everything about food. Just looking at fresh produce or seafood at the market excites me. Fortunately, good food and good health are not a contradiction in terms. I have learned that you don't have to sacrifice taste or variety to achieve your full Bonus Years. And I believe that once you have sampled the more than four weeks' of suggested menus and recipes below, you will agree with me.

In the pages that follow, you will find thirty days' worth of meals and snacks on the Bonus Years Diet. These menus are not meant to be followed rigidly; rather, they are intended as guidelines. Feel free to design your own menus to suit your likes and dislikes. You can add other side dishes, servings of bread products, or light desserts if you want to round out some of the menus to suit your taste. You can have lunch for dinner or dinner for lunch, depending on your schedule, as long as you eat the prescribed amount of Bonus Point foods each day.

In the recipes, I often refer to specific cooking techniques that enable even the most inexperienced of cooks to create great-tasting Bonus Years meals. If you are interested in trying some of the recipes, review the Bonus Years cooking techniques, beginning on page 361, where I provide step-by-step instructions on food preparation.

To make sure that you always have the right ingredients on hand, I have provided a list of foods to stock in your pantry, beginning on page 353.

Getting Your Bonus Points

You will notice that on each of the recipes (plus for any single items such as a pear or side without an actual recipe), I list the daily Bonus Points for each Bonus Years food. Bonus Points are a useful tool for learning how to track your daily dose of Bonus Years foods. Within a few days of following the program, you will probably be able to keep a running tally in your head without having to count up Bonus Points. But in the beginning, it's a good idea to use the Bonus Points system until you are familiar with the food prescription.

How do Bonus Points work? The goal is to consume 100 Bonus Points for EACH of the Bonus Years foods every day. By the end of the day, you must accrue 100 percent of your Bonus Points *for each food*. Some Bonus Years foods are easier to track than others. For example, wine is really simple because you can get your full 5-ounce dose of wine, about one glass (or 100 Bonus Points), in one sitting. Fruits and vegetables, however, can be a bit trickier because you will probably divide your daily dose of five (usually ¾ cup raw) servings over several meals. In this case, one serving of fruits or vegetables would count as 20 Bonus Points. At the end of the day, when you have had your five servings, you will have earned your 100 Bonus Points for fruits and vegetables. As you review the daily menus, you will easily see how the Bonus Points system works.

About the Nutritional Analysis

All recipes and snacks were analyzed using the Food Processor, Version 8.1. Ingredients that are to taste, such as salt, or are optional are not included in the analysis. If there is a choice of two or more ingredients in a recipe, the first ingredient has been used in the analysis. Because nuts vary in the number of calories and amounts of fat and other ingredients, unsalted, dry-roasted mixed nuts for the snacks were used for analysis. If a specific nut, such as almonds, is called for in a recipe, then the nutritional information for almonds has been used. Dark chocolate can vary by brand, but usually by only a few calories per ounce, so a generic dark chocolate was used in the recipes and for the snacks.

DAY 1: SUNDAY

Breakfast

Stuffed French Toast with
Strawberry-Rhubarb Compote
Hot Chocolate
BONUS YEARS POINTS: CHOCOLATE 50%; FRUITS
AND VEGETABLES 25%; NUTS 25%
CALORIES: 653

Lunch

Italian Bean and Mushroom
Ragout
Mixed Baby Greens
with Roasted Garlic Vinaigrette
BONUS YEARS POINTS: FRUITS AND VEGETABLES 70%;
GARLIC 150%
CALORIES: 499

Dinner

Pan-Roasted Pork Tenderloin
with Apple
Mashed Sweet Potatoes
½ cup steamed spinach
BONUS YEARS POINTS: FRUITS AND VEGETABLES 50%
CALORIES: 418

5 ounces red wine
BONUS YEARS POINTS: WINE 100%
CALORIES: 108

Snacks

1 ounce dark chocolate
BONUS YEARS POINTS: CHOCOLATE 50%
CALORIES: 151

1½ ounces unsalted dry-roasted
or natural nuts
BONUS YEARS POINTS: NUTS 75%
CALORIES: 253

DAY'S TOTAL BONUS YEARS POINTS: WINE 100%; CHOCOLATE 100%;
FRUITS AND VEGETABLES 145%; GARLIC 150%; NUTS 100%
TOTAL CALORIES: 2,080

Stuffed French Toast with Strawberry-Rhubarb Compote

MAKES 4 SERVINGS

Strawberry-Rhubarb Compote (recipe follows)
¾ cup egg substitute, or 3 large eggs, lightly beaten
⅔ cup low-fat buttermilk
1 teaspoon vanilla extract
4 tablespoons low-fat cream cheese
8 (½-inch-thick) slices bread with an open crumb, such as
   challah or Italian ciabatta or pugliese, left out overnight to
   dry out
4 tablespoons strawberry jam or orange marmalade
8 tablespoons sliced almonds

Prepare the compote and let cool to room temperature. (The compote can be made the night before and refrigerated in a tightly covered glass bowl. Bring to room temperature before serving.)

Preheat the oven to 400 degrees. Mix the egg substitute, buttermilk, and vanilla in a shallow bowl. Spread 1 tablespoon of the cream cheese on one slice of bread, and 1 tablespoon of the strawberry jam on another slice. Place the 2 slices together to form a sandwich. Repeat with the remaining bread, cream cheese, and jam to make a total of 4 sandwiches. Soak the sandwiches in the egg batter for 1 minute on each side, then drain off any excess and let the sandwiches rest for another minute or so.

Spray a nonstick skillet generously with cooking spray. Heat over medium heat until the cooking spray has just begun to liquefy. Add the sandwiches, one at a time, and cook until the sandwich is golden brown on each side, about 3 minutes per side. Transfer the sandwiches to a nonstick baking sheet and bake for 5 minutes. Transfer the sandwiches to four plates and top each one with one-fourth of the compote and 2 tablespoons of the almonds.

BONUS YEARS DAILY PERCENTAGES

Per serving with compote: Fruits and vegetables 25%; Nuts 25%

NUTRITIONAL ANALYSIS

Per serving (without compote): Calories 318, Protein 14g, Total fat 12g, Sat fat 3g, Trans fat 0g, Cholesterol 10mg, Carbohydrate 38g, Dietary fiber 2g, Sodium 396mg

Strawberry-Rhubarb Compote

MAKES 4 SERVINGS

___

Steeping fruit in a simple syrup of sugar and water is a classic way to prepare fruit sauces (see also Blackberry Coulis, page 171). The mild tartness of the lemon juice adds a crispness to the sauce, which intensifies the fruitiness of the strawberries and rhubarb.

1½ cups peeled, diced fresh rhubarb (6 ounces)
⅓ cup sugar
½ cup water
2 cups ripe fresh strawberries, hulled and diced (8 ounces)
1½ tablespoons freshly squeezed lemon juice
1 teaspoon vanilla extract

Add the rhubarb, sugar, and water to a saucepan. Bring to a low simmer over medium heat. Reduce the heat, and simmer, covered, until the rhubarb is tender, about 10 minutes, stirring occasionally.

Add the strawberries, and cook, uncovered, for 5 minutes. Remove from the heat and stir in the lemon juice and vanilla. Let the sauce cool.

NUTRITIONAL ANALYSIS

Per serving: Calories 102, Protein 1g, Total fat 0g, Sat fat 0g, Trans fat 0g, Cholesterol 0mg, Carbohydrate 25g, Dietary fiber 3g, Sodium 3mg

Hot Chocolate

MAKES 4 SERVINGS

The higher the percentage of cocoa solids in the chocolate, the more antioxidants it contains, and the better it is for you.

4 ounces dark chocolate (greater than 60% cocoa solids),
    finely chopped
½ cup water
4 cups fat-free milk
1 teaspoon ground cinnamon
2 teaspoons vanilla extract, or to taste
1 tablespoon sugar, to taste

Combine the chocolate and water in a heavy saucepan over medium heat, stirring, until the chocolate starts to melt. Remove from heat and stir the chocolate until melted. Return to the heat and slowly whisk in the milk. Whisk in the cinnamon, vanilla, and sugar and heat until the mixture is frothy and the milk is hot. Pour into cups.

BONUS YEARS DAILY PERCENTAGES
Per serving: Chocolate 50%

NUTRITIONAL ANALYSIS
Per serving: Calories 233, Protein 10g, Total fat 12g, Sat fat 6g, Trans fat 0g, Cholesterol 5mg, Carbohydrate 27g, Dietary fiber 2g, Sodium 127mg

Variations

Thicker Hot Chocolate: Mix 1 tablespoon cornstarch with 2 tablespoons cold water. Stir into the hot chocolate and cook, stirring, until thickened.

Southwest Hot Chocolate: Add about ¼ teaspoon ground medium-hot chilies, or to taste.

Italian Bean
and Mushroom Ragout

MAKES 8 CUPS

Serve a Chianti Classico with this hearty Italian dish, keeping the food and wine in the same region.

2 tablespoons extra-virgin olive oil
2 medium onions (about 12 ounces total), thinly sliced (about
   3 cups)
8 cloves garlic, thinly sliced
1½ pounds cremini or button mushrooms, stems removed
   and caps quartered (about 9 cups)
1 tablespoon Italian seasoning
2 (14.5-ounce) cans diced tomatoes, preferably Italian
¼ cup freshly squeezed lemon juice (juice of 1 large lemon)
1 tablespoon sugar
1½ cups dried cannellini beans (see Dr. Chef's Note below), or
   4½ cups cooked or canned cannellini beans, drained
kosher salt and freshly ground black pepper, to taste

Heat the oil in a 12-inch skillet over medium heat. Add the onions and garlic and sauté for about 3 minutes. Add the mushrooms and sauté for 3 minutes. Add the Italian seasoning and sauté until the mushrooms release almost all of their liquid. Add the tomatoes and their juices, lemon juice, and sugar and bring to a very low simmer. Simmer for 10 minutes. Add the beans, mix thoroughly, season with salt and pepper, and heat until the beans are hot.

Ladle 1½ cups of the ragout onto each of four plates. Refrigerate the remaining 2 cups and use for two 1-cup servings for lunch.

BONUS YEARS DAILY PERCENTAGES

Per 1½-cup serving: Fruits and vegetables 35%; Garlic 150%

Per 1-cup serving: Fruits and vegetables 20%; Garlic 100%

NUTRITIONAL ANALYSIS

Per 1½-cup serving: Calories 385, Protein 21g, Total fat 6g, Sat fat 1g, Trans fat 0g, Cholesterol 0mg, Carbohydrate 64g, Dietary fiber 13g, Sodium 505mg

Per 1-cup serving: Calories 257, Protein 14g, Total fat 4g, Sat fat 0g, Trans fat 0g, Cholesterol 0mg, Carbohydrate 43g, Dietary fiber 9g, Sodium 337mg

Dr. Chef's Note

Canned beans work well in this recipe, but if you have the time, soak 1½ cups of dried beans in cold water overnight. The next day, drain them, rinse them off, and place them in a pot of cold water. Simmer for about 45 minutes; they should be al dente, with some firmness to the bite. The freshly cooked beans have a crunch and a crispness in flavor not found in the canned variety.

Mixed Baby Greens
with Roasted Garlic Vinaigrette

MAKES 4 SERVINGS

½ large red onion (about 4 ounces), thinly sliced

1 cup small plum tomatoes (about 6 ounces), preferably a
combination of red and yellow tomatoes, halved

¾ cup coarsely chopped pitted olives of your choice (3 ounces)

6 ounces mixed baby or garden salad green (8 cups), rinsed
and spun dry

½ to ¾ cup Roasted Garlic Vinaigrette (recipe follows) or
other low-fat Italian dressing

kosher salt and freshly ground black pepper, to taste

Soak the onion in cold water for at least 30 minutes; drain well. Combine the onion, tomatoes, olives, and greens in a large bowl.

Add the dressing, and toss to combine. Season with salt and pepper. Divide among four plates.

BONUS YEARS DAILY PERCENTAGES

Per serving: Fruits and vegetables 35%

NUTRITIONAL ANALYSIS

Per serving: Calories 114, Protein 3g, Total fat 8g, Sat fat 0g, Trans fat 0g,
Cholesterol 0mg, Carbohydrate 11g, Dietary fiber 3g, Sodium 536mg

Roasted Garlic Vinaigrette

6 tablespoons thickened low-sodium chicken broth
 (see Dr. Chef's Note below)
2 tablespoons extra-virgin olive oil
3 tablespoons tomato juice
6 cloves garlic, roasted (see page 373)
3 tablespoons cider vinegar
2 tablespoons unsweetened apple juice
½ teaspoon kosher salt
¼ teaspoon sugar
¼ teaspoon ground white pepper
1 teaspoon dried oregano
½ teaspoon dry mustard
1 tablespoon chopped fresh flat-leaf parsley

Combine the broth, olive oil, tomato juice, and garlic in a blender;
blend until the garlic is pureed. Pour into a bowl and thoroughly
whisk in the remaining ingredients.

NUTRITIONAL ANALYSIS

Per 2 tablespoons: Calories 43, Protein 0g, Total fat 4g, Sat fat 0g, Trans fat 0g,
Cholesterol 0mg, Carbohydrate 2g, Dietary fiber 0g, Sodium 144mg

Dr. Chef's Note

To thicken chicken broth to make a lower-fat salad dressing, whisk ½
cup low-sodium chicken broth with 1 teaspoon arrowroot. Cook over
low heat, whisking, until slightly thickened.

Pan-Roasted Pork Tenderloin
with Apple

MAKES 4 SERVINGS

———
———

The texture of a Pinot Noir works great with pork, but certainly a Chardonnay would be in keeping with the apples if you prefer a white wine for a change of pace.

1¼ pounds pork tenderloin, trimmed of fat and silverskin,
     preferably brined (see page 376) for 2 hours
freshly ground black pepper, to taste
1 tablespoon extra-virgin olive oil
2 medium shallots, minced
½ cup low-sodium chicken broth
½ cup unsweetened apple juice
⅔ cup diced unpeeled Golden Delicious apple (1 medium)
1 teaspoon Dijon mustard
1 to 2 teaspoons sugar
1 tablespoon freshly squeezed lemon juice
¼ cup Calvados (apple brandy)
1 teaspoon arrowroot dissolved in 2 teaspoons cold water
kosher salt and freshly ground black pepper, to taste

Rinse the pork under cold water and pat dry.
     Let stand at room temperature about 30 minutes. Season with pepper.

Preheat the oven to 375 degrees. Heat the oil in an ovenproof skillet over medium heat. Brown the pork tenderloin about 5 minutes, turning frequently. Transfer to the oven and cook about 15 minutes, or until an instant-read thermometer registers 140 degrees. Transfer the tenderloin to a plate, cover, and keep warm.

Place the skillet over medium heat, add the shallots, and sauté for about 2 minutes. Add the broth and juice, and stir, scraping the browned bits at the bottom of the skillet and incorporating them into the liquid. Add the apple. Simmer until reduced to about ¾ cup. Stir in the mustard and heat for 1 minute. Add the sugar, lemon juice, and Calvados, then whisk in the dissolved arrowroot and season with salt and pepper. Simmer, stirring, until the desired thickness of the sauce is achieved.

Cut the tenderloin into thin slices and serve with the sauce.

BONUS YEARS DAILY PERCENTAGES

Per serving: Fruits and vegetables 10%

NUTRITIONAL ANALYSIS

Per serving (without brining): Calories 282, Protein 31g, Total fat 9g, Sat fat 2g, Trans fat 0g, Cholesterol 97mg, Carbohydrate 11g, Dietary fiber 0g, Sodium 115mg

Dr. Chef's Note

Because pork tenderloin is very low in fat, a short brine (see page 376) helps to ensure tender and moist meat. Don't overcook the tenderloin; take the meat out of the oven at about 140 degrees. Use an instant-read thermometer to check the internal temperature of the meat; it should be slightly pink in the middle.

Mashed Sweet Potatoes

MAKES 4 SERVINGS

Use the orange-colored sweet potatoes, not the white variety. The orange ones are sweeter and make a more flavorful dish. They are sometimes mislabeled as yams in the supermarket. True yams are a Caribbean vegetable, not readily available in the United States.

1½ pounds sweet potatoes, peeled and quartered
¾ to 1 cup low-fat buttermilk
1 tablespoon minced green onion (green part only)
2 teaspoons prepared horseradish
kosher salt and freshly ground black pepper, to taste

Place the sweet potatoes in a pot and cover with cold water. Bring to a low boil. Reduce the heat; simmer, covered, until the potatoes are tender when pierced with the tip of a sharp knife, 15 to 20 minutes.

For the best texture, force the potatoes through a ricer, or mash with a potato masher. Add the buttermilk slowly and mix into the sweet potatoes. Stir in the green onion and horseradish and season with salt and pepper.

BONUS YEARS DAILY PERCENTAGES
Per serving: Fruits and vegetables 20%

NUTRITIONAL ANALYSIS
Per serving: Calories 125, Protein 3g, Total fat 0g, Sat fat 0g, Trans fat 0g, Cholesterol 2mg, Carbohydrate 27g, Dietary fiber 3g, Sodium 59mg

Variation

Mashed Sweet Potatoes with Garlic: Prepare as above but fold in half of a roasted garlic bulb. To roast the garlic, cut off the top of a whole unpeeled garlic bulb. Lightly spray with cooking spray or drizzle with olive oil. Wrap in aluminum foil or place in a small covered baking dish and roast in a preheated 350-degree oven for 40 minutes. Squeeze garlic cloves out of their skins.

STEAMED SPINACH

BONUS YEARS DAILY PERCENTAGES

Per ½-cup serving: Fruits and vegetables 20%

NUTRITIONAL ANALYSIS

Per ½-cup serving: Calories 11, Protein 1g, Total fat 0g, Sat fat 0g, Trans fat 0g, Cholesterol 0mg, Carbohydrate 2g, Dietary fiber 1g, Sodium 96mg

RED WINE

NUTRITIONAL ANALYSIS

Per 5 ounces: Calories 106, Protein 0g, Total fat 0g, Sat fat 0g, Trans fat 0g, Cholesterol 0mg, Carbohydrate 2g, Dietary fiber 0g, Sodium 7mg

DARK CHOCOLATE

NUTRITIONAL ANALYSIS

Per 1 ounce: Calories 151, Protein 1g, Total fat 8g, Sat fat 5g, Trans fat 0g, Cholesterol 0mg, Carbohydrate 18g, Dietary fiber 1g, Sodium 5mg

NUTS

NUTRITIONAL ANALYSIS

Per 1½ ounces: Calories 253, Protein 7g, Total fat 22g, Sat fat 3g, Trans fat 0g, Cholesterol 0mg, Carbohydrate 11g, Dietary fiber 4g, Sodium 5mg

DAY 2: MONDAY

Breakfast

Almond-Berry Breakfast Parfait

BONUS YEARS POINTS: FRUITS AND VEGETABLES 35%;
NUTS 25%

CALORIES: 481

Lunch

Asian Salad with
Tangy Miso Dressing

BONUS YEARS POINTS: FRUITS AND VEGETABLES 60%

CALORIES: 196

Dinner

Salsa Snapper
½ cup steamed brown rice

BONUS YEARS POINTS: FRUITS AND VEGETABLES 45%;
FISH 100%; GARLIC 100%

CALORIES: 366

5 ounces red wine

BONUS YEARS POINTS: WINE 100%

CALORIES: 106

Snacks

2 ounces dark chocolate

BONUS YEARS POINTS: CHOCOLATE 100%

CALORIES: 302

1½ ounces unsalted dry-roasted
or natural nuts

BONUS YEARS POINTS: NUTS 75%

CALORIES: 253

DAY'S TOTAL BONUS YEARS POINTS: WINE 100%; CHOCOLATE 100%;
FRUITS AND VEGETABLES 140%; FISH 100%; GARLIC 100%; NUTS 100%
TOTAL CALORIES: 1,704

Almond-Berry Breakfast Parfait

¾ cup vanilla low-fat yogurt
1 small banana, sliced (about ⅔ cup)
½ cup mixed fresh berries
¼ cup low-fat granola or low-fat high-fiber cereal
2 tablespoons slivered almonds

Place half of the yogurt in the bottom of a small bowl or tall glass. Top with half of the banana, berries, and granola. Repeat layers, starting with yogurt and ending with granola. Sprinkle with the almonds.

BONUS YEARS DAILY PERCENTAGES
Per serving: Fruits and vegetables 35%; Nuts 25%
NUTRITIONAL ANALYSIS
Per serving: Calories 481, Protein 17g, Total fat 13g, Sat fat 3g, Trans fat 0g, Cholesterol 9mg, Carbohydrate 78g, Dietary fiber 7g, Sodium 150mg

Asian Salad with Tangy Miso Dressing

MAKES 4 SERVINGS

This light, spicy salad is perfect for a hot summer's day.

⅓ pound snow peas, ends removed
½ cup fresh bean sprouts
½ pound Napa cabbage, shredded (about 3 cups)
½ pound red cabbage, shredded (about 3 cups)
½ cup thinly sliced green onions
    (white and green parts)
12 ounces extra-firm tofu, cut into ½-inch dice,
    or 12 ounces cooked chicken breast, cut into
    bite-size pieces
Tangy Miso Salad Dressing (recipe follows)

Bring a large pot of water to a boil. Prepare a large bowl of ice and water. Add the snow peas and bean sprouts to the boiling water and drain after 30 seconds. Immediately transfer them to the ice water to stop the cooking. Drain the vegetables and reserve them.

Toss together the snow peas, bean sprouts, cabbages, green onions, and tofu. Add the dressing, toss to combine, and divide the salad among four plates and serve.

To Make Ahead: Toss the vegetables and tofu together in a bowl. Prepare the dressing. Cover and refrigerate separately. Toss with the dressing just before serving.

BONUS YEARS DAILY PERCENTAGES

Per serving: Fruits and vegetables 60% (prepared with tofu);
40% (prepared with chicken)

NUTRITIONAL ANALYSIS

Per serving: Calories 196, Protein 13g, Total fat 7g, Sat fat 1g, Trans fat 0g,
Cholesterol 0mg, Carbohydrate 22g, Dietary fiber 4g, Sodium 394mg

Tangy Miso Salad Dressing

Miso, or Japanese soybean paste, available in Asian markets, adds a unique flavor to this dressing. Be sure to use the milder (yellow or white) shiro miso, not the more powerful red or dark miso for this recipe.

2 tablespoons unseasoned rice vinegar

2 tablespoons mild miso (shiro)

2 tablespoons freshly squeezed orange juice

3 tablespoons mirin (rice wine)

1 tablespoon ketchup

½ tablespoon sugar

½ teaspoon Asian sesame oil

¼ teaspoon Asian chili paste

Thoroughly whisk all the ingredients in a bowl until combined.

NUTRITIONAL ANALYSIS

Per 2 tablespoons: Calories 43, Protein 1g, Total fat 1g, Sat fat 0g, Trans fat 0g, Cholesterol 0mg, Carbohydrate 7g, Dietary fiber 0g, Sodium 245mg

Salsa Snapper

MAKES 4 SERVINGS

This is an easy basic recipe, which when mastered can serve as a springboard for endless variations using different tomato-based sauces and fish fillets. For example, prepare a tomato sauce with okra, bell peppers, onions, and Creole seasoning over catfish and you will have a great Cajun dinner. In the summer, substitute fresh ripe tomatoes for the canned variety.

1 tablespoon extra-virgin olive oil

2 cups thinly sliced onions (8 ounces)

4 cloves garlic, thinly sliced

1 small green bell pepper (4 ounces), cut into ¼-inch-thick
   strips

½ cup dry red wine

1 (14.5-ounce) can Mexican-style tomatoes

1 to 2 tablespoons moderately hot salsa, use your favorite
   commercial brand or make your own

1½ tablespoons freshly squeezed lime juice

3 tablespoons chopped fresh cilantro

4 (5- to 6-ounce) snapper fillets

Preheat the oven to 375 degrees. Heat the oil in a 12-inch ovenproof skillet over medium heat. Add the onions and garlic and sauté for about 3 minutes, stirring occasionally. Add the bell pepper and sauté for 2 to 3 minutes, stirring occasionally. Add the wine and simmer until most of the wine evaporates.

Add the tomatoes and their juices, salsa, and lime juice and simmer for about 3 minutes. Stir in the cilantro. Add the fish fillets, spooning the sauce over the fish. Transfer to the oven and cook for 15 to 20 minutes, or until the fish is opaque.

To serve: Place a fish fillet on each plate and spoon the sauce over the fish.

BONUS YEARS DAILY PERCENTAGES

Per serving: Fruits and vegetables 45%; Fish 100%; Garlic 100%

NUTRITIONAL ANALYSIS

Per serving: Calories 258, Protein 31g, Total fat 5g, Sat fat 1g, Trans fat 0g, Cholesterol 52mg, Carbohydrate 16g, Dietary fiber 13g, Sodium 438mg

STEAMED BROWN RICE

NUTRITIONAL ANALYSIS

Per H-cup serving: Calories 108, Protein 2g, Total fat 0g, Sat fat 0g, Trans fat 0g, Cholesterol 0mg, Carbohydrate 22g, Dietary fiber 2g, Sodium 5mg

RED WINE

NUTRITIONAL ANALYSIS

Per 5 ounces: Calories 106, Protein 0g, Total fat 0g, Sat fat 0g, Trans fat 0g, Cholesterol 0mg, Carbohydrate 2g, Dietary fiber 0g, Sodium 7mg

DARK CHOCOLATE

NUTRITIONAL ANALYSIS

Per 2 ounces: Calories 302, Protein 3g, Total fat 16g, Sat fat 10g, Trans fat 0g, Cholesterol 0mg, Carbohydrate 36g, Dietary fiber 2g, Sodium 9mg

NUTS

NUTRITIONAL ANALYSIS

Per 1½ ounces: Calories 253, Protein 7g, Total fat 22g, Sat fat 3g, Trans fat 0g, Cholesterol 0mg, Carbohydrate 11g, Dietary fiber 4g, Sodium 5mg

DAY 3: TUESDAY

Breakfast

Apple Buckwheat Cereal
BONUS YEARS POINTS: FRUITS AND VEGETABLES 20%;
NUTS 25%
CALORIES: 384

Lunch

Italian Bean and Mushroom Ragout (left over from Sunday, page 110)
1 apple
BONUS YEARS POINTS: FRUITS AND VEGETABLES 40%;
GARLIC 100%
CALORIES: 337

Dinner

Toasted Almond and Cumin-Crusted Chicken Breasts
½ cup steamed carrots
Strawberry-Spinach Salad
BONUS YEARS POINTS: FRUITS AND VEGETABLES 40%;
NUTS 50%
CALORIES: 644

5 ounces red wine
BONUS YEARS POINTS: WINE 100%
CALORIES: 106

Snacks

2 ounces dark chocolate
BONUS YEARS POINTS: CHOCOLATE 100%
CALORIES: 302

½ ounce unsalted dry-roasted or natural nuts
BONUS YEARS POINTS: NUTS 25%
CALORIES: 84

DAY'S TOTAL BONUS YEARS POINTS: WINE **100%**; CHOCOLATE **100%**;
FRUITS AND VEGETABLES **100%**; GARLIC **100%**; NUTS **100%**
TOTAL CALORIES: **1,857**

Apple Buckwheat Cereal

MAKES 2 SERVINGS

1 cup unsweetened apple juice

1 tablespoon apple preserves (optional)

¼ teaspoon ground nutmeg

¼ teaspoon ground cinnamon

½ cup kasha (roasted buckwheat), available in the kosher or
cereal section of your local supermarket

1 large apple (about 8 ounces), peeled, cored, cut into ¼-inch
dice (about 1½ cups), ¼ cup reserved, for garnish

4 teaspoons light brown sugar (optional)

4 tablespoons slivered almonds

Place the apple juice and apple preserves (if using) in a saucepan and bring to a low simmer. Add the nutmeg, cinnamon, kasha, and apple. Cover the pan, reduce the heat to low, and simmer for about 10 minutes. Uncover the pan, fluff the cereal, and divide the kasha among two plates. Top each plate with 2 teaspoons of the sugar (if using), 2 tablespoons of the reserved apple, and 2 tablespoons of the almonds.

BONUS YEARS DAILY PERCENTAGES
Per serving: Fruits and vegetables 20%; Nuts 25%

NUTRITIONAL ANALYSIS
Per serving: Calories 384, Protein 9g, Total fat 13g, Sat fat 2g, Trans fat 0g,
Cholesterol 0mg, Carbohydrate 62g, Dietary fiber 15g, Sodium 11mg

APPLE

BONUS YEARS DAILY PERCENTAGES

Per apple: Fruits and vegetables 20%

NUTRITIONAL ANALYSIS

Per serving: Calories 80, Protein 0g, Total fat 0g, Sat fat 0g, Trans fat 0g, Cholesterol 0mg, Carbohydrate 22g, Dietary fiber 5g, Sodium 0mg

Toasted Almond and Cumin-Crusted Chicken Breasts

MAKES 4 SERVINGS

———

There are two ways to cook the chicken breasts: oven frying or pan roasting. For pan roasting, the chicken is first browned in oil before transferring to the oven; this results in a crisper crust.

To reduce the preparation time, use a rub or spice mixture with similar flavors and skip roasting and grinding the whole spices.

½ tablespoon cumin seed
½ tablespoon fennel seed
½ tablespoon coriander seed
½ tablespoon black peppercorns
4 ounces whole blanched almonds
5 slices good-quality homemade-style bread
½ teaspoon kosher salt
1 large egg white
⅓ cup low-fat buttermilk
4 boneless, skinless chicken breast halves, preferably brined
  (see page 376) for 1 hour
4 tablespoons canola oil (optional, for pan roasting)

Heat a small heavy skillet over medium-low heat. Add the cumin, fennel, and coriander seeds and the peppercorns and toast for about 3 minutes, constantly stirring the spices to prevent burning. When some wisps of smoke begin to appear, take them out of the skillet and cool slightly. Place in a small spice grinder or food processor and quickly grind into a powder. Add the almonds to the hot skillet, and toast, stirring occasionally, until they just begin to brown; be careful not to burn them. Transfer to a food processor or spice grinder, and process until the almonds are granular in appearance; do not turn into a paste. Toast the bread, remove the crust, and process into crumbs in a food processor. Thoroughly mix the spices, almonds, bread crumbs, and salt together.

Whisk together the egg white and buttermilk in a shallow bowl. Dip each of the chicken breasts in the egg white mixture, then coat both sides with the spice mixture; it will be necessary to pat the mixture onto the chicken breasts to get it to stick. Refrigerate the coated chicken for about 15 minutes so that the coating will set.

To oven-fry: Preheat the oven to 400 degrees. Spray the chicken with cooking spray. Place on a nonstick baking sheet. Transfer to the oven and cook the chicken for 20 to 25 minutes, depending on the thickness, or until the chicken is cooked through. (I often like to place a rack in the baking pan and place the chicken on it so it receives heat from both above and below.)

To pan-roast: Preheat the oven to 400 degrees. Heat the oil in a large heavy-bottomed skillet. Place the chicken in the skillet, skin side down, and cook for 1½ to 2 minutes; watch carefully because the nuts in the coating burn easily. Turn over and cook on the other side. Drain off the excess oil. Turn the chicken, skin side down, in the skillet and transfer to the oven. Roast the chicken for 15 to 20 minutes, depending on the thickness, or until the chicken is cooked through.

BONUS YEARS DAILY PERCENTAGES
Per serving: Nuts 50%

NUTRITIONAL ANALYSIS
Per serving: Calories 474, Protein 39g, Total fat 19g, Sat fat 2g, Trans fat 1g, Cholesterol 66mg, Carbohydrate 37g, Dietary fiber 8g, Sodium 545mg

STEAMED CARROTS

BONUS YEARS DAILY PERCENTAGES
Per ½-cup serving: Fruits and vegetables 20%

NUTRITIONAL ANALYSIS
Per ½-cup serving: Calories 35, Protein 1g, Total fat g, Sat fat 0g, Trans fat 0g, Cholesterol 0g, Carbohydrate 8g, Dietary fiber 2g, Sodium 20mg

Strawberry-Spinach Salad

6 ounces fresh spinach (about 5 cups loosely packed)
1 cup fresh strawberries
1 tablespoon toasted sesame seeds
3 tablespoons canola oil
1½ tablespoons balsamic vinegar
1 tablespoon minced green onion (green part only)
1 tablespoon sugar
generous pinch hot paprika
kosher salt and freshly ground black pepper, to taste

Rinse and thoroughly dry the spinach and tear into bite-size pieces. Hull and halve the strawberries. Combine the spinach, strawberries, and sesame seeds in a salad bowl.

Thoroughly mix the oil, vinegar, onion, sugar, paprika, salt, and pepper in a small bowl until the sugar dissolves. Pour the dressing over the salad and toss to combine. Divide among four salad plates.

To Make Ahead: Toss the spinach, strawberries, and sesame seeds in a bowl. Prepare the dressing. Cover and refrigerate separately. Toss with the dressing just before serving.

BONUS YEARS DAILY PERCENTAGES

Per serving: Fruits and vegetables 20%

NUTRITIONAL ANALYSIS

Per serving: Calories 135, Protein 1g, Total fat 12g, Saturated fat 1g, Cholesterol 0mg, Carbohydrate 8g, Dietary Fiber 2g, Sodium 57mg

RED WINE

NUTRITIONAL ANALYSIS

Per 5 ounces: Calories 106, Protein 0g, Total fat 0g, Sat fat 0g, Trans fat 0g, Cholesterol 0mg, Carbohydrate 2g, Dietary fiber 0g, Sodium 7mg

DARK CHOCOLATE

NUTRITIONAL ANALYSIS

Per 2 ounces: Calories 302, Protein 3g, Total fat 16g, Sat fat 10g, Trans fat 0g, Cholesterol 0mg, Carbohydrate 36g, Dietary fiber 2g, Sodium 9mg

NUTS

NUTRITIONAL ANALYSIS

Per ½ ounce: Calories 84, Protein 2g, Total fat 7g, Sat fat 1g, Trans fat 0g, Cholesterol 0mg, Carbohydrate 3g, Dietary fiber 1g, Sodium 2mg

DAY 4: WEDNESDAY

Breakfast

Peach-Raspberry Smoothie
BONUS YEARS POINTS: FRUITS AND VEGETABLES 15%
CALORIES: 155

Lunch

Smoked Ham Sandwich with
Apple-Apricot Chutney
BONUS YEARS POINTS: FRUITS AND VEGETABLES 45%;
GARLIC 50%
CALORIES: 573

Dinner

Pan-Grilled Salmon
with Frisée Salad Lyonnaise
Chocolate Mousse
BONUS YEARS POINTS: CHOCOLATE 25%; FRUITS AND
VEGETABLES 50%; FISH 100%; GARLIC 50%; NUTS 25%
CALORIES: 852

5 ounces red wine
BONUS YEARS POINTS: WINE 100%
CALORIES: 106

Snacks

1½ ounces dark chocolate
BONUS YEARS POINTS: CHOCOLATE 75%
CALORIES: 227

1½ ounces unsalted dry-roasted
or natural nuts
BONUS YEARS POINTS: NUTS 75%
CALORIES: 253

DAY'S TOTAL BONUS YEARS POINTS: WINE 100%; CHOCOLATE 100%;
FRUITS AND VEGETABLES 110%; FISH 100%; GARLIC 100%; NUTS 100%
TOTAL CALORIES: 2,166

Peach-Raspberry Smoothie

MAKES 2 SERVINGS

Using frozen fruit saves time and money plus it makes a thicker smoothie.

½ cup frozen sliced unsweetened peaches (about 4 ounces),
   coarsely chopped
½ cup frozen unsweetened raspberries (about 4 ounces)
1 cup plain fat-free yogurt
1 cup fat-free milk
1 tablespoon sugar, or to taste
1 teaspoon vanilla extract

Combine the peaches, raspberries, yogurt, and ½ cup of the milk in a blender. Blend until smooth. Add the remaining milk, sugar, and vanilla and blend until combined. Pour into glasses and serve.

BONUS YEARS DAILY PERCENTAGES
Per serving: Fruits and vegetables 15%

NUTRITIONAL ANALYSIS
Per serving: Calories 155, Protein 10g, Total fat 0g, Sat fat 0g, Trans fat 0g, Cholesterol 5mg, Carbohydrate 30g, Dietary fiber 3g, Sodium 131mg

Smoked Ham Sandwich
with Apple-Apricot Chutney

MAKES 4 SERVINGS

Serve the sandwich with the Apple-Apricot Chutney on the side (recipe follows). Note that the chutney needs to be chilled over-night to allow the flavors to blend.

8 slices hearty rye bread
whole-grain mustard of your choice
8 slices tomato
12 ounces sliced low-fat, lower-sodium ham
8 slices lettuce

Spread one side of each slice of the bread with mustard. Top half of the bread slices with one slice of the tomato, then three slices ham, then another tomato slice and finally 2 lettuce slices. Top with the remaining slices of bread.

BONUS YEARS DAILY PERCENTAGES
Per serving: Fruits and vegetables 15%

NUTRITIONAL ANALYSIS
Per serving: Calories 266, Protein 20g, Total fat 5g, Sat fat 1g, Trans fat 0g, Cholesterol 36mg, Carbohydrate 35g, Dietary fiber 4g, Sodium 1,133mg

Apple-Apricot Chutney

MAKES 4 (½-CUP) SERVINGS

2 Granny Smith apples (about 12 ounces total), cored, peeled, and diced
¾ cup chopped dried apricots (3 ounces)
¾ cup white wine vinegar
½ cup packed light brown sugar
1 tablespoon freshly squeezed lemon juice
2 teaspoons minced fresh ginger
2 cloves garlic, minced
½ cup golden raisins
½ teaspoon salt
½ teaspoon ground cumin
⅛ teaspoon cayenne pepper

Combine all the ingredients in a small saucepan. Simmer, stirring occasionally, until thickened, about 25 minutes. Cool to room temperature. Cover and refrigerate overnight before serving.

BONUS YEARS DAILY PERCENTAGES
Per ½-cup serving: Fruits and vegetables 30%; Garlic 50%

NUTRITIONAL ANALYSIS
Per ½-cup serving: Calories 307, Protein g, Total fat 0g, Sat fat 0g, Trans fat 0g, Cholesterol 0mg, Carbohydrate 76g, Dietary fiber 4g, Sodium 250mg

Pan-Grilled Salmon
with Frisée Salad Lyonnaise

MAKES 4 SERVINGS

---

*This is one of my favorite recipes for salmon, the bitterness of
the frisée perfectly cuts the richness of the salmon. Traditionally, poached eggs are used to top this salad in Lyon, but I
found grilled salmon is even better. It's healthier, too. The
sautéed bacon or lardons often used in France are replaced by
the meaty earthiness of the roasted mushrooms.*

*Serve a light earthy red wine, such as a French red Bur-
gundy or European Pinot Noir.*

Roasted Mushrooms with Onions (recipe follows)
4 5- to 6-ounce salmon fillets
9 ounces frisée (about 3 small bunches), cut into 1-inch-long
    pieces
10 ounces pear tomatoes (about 45, use a mixture of red and
    yellow tomatoes if available), sliced in half
4 ounces croutons (about 40 croutons), cut into ½-inch cubes
⅔ cup Roasted Garlic Vinaigrette (page 113) or other low-fat
    Italian vinaigrette

Preheat the oven to 350 degrees. Prepare the mushrooms and
onions and leave the oven on.

Spray a ridged stovetop grill pan with nonstick cooking spray,
and heat over medium-high heat. Add the salmon, flesh side down,
and grill for 3 minutes. Place the pan with the salmon in the oven and
roast for 6 to 8 minutes, or until the salmon is just slightly opaque.

Meanwhile, mix the frisée with the roasted mushrooms and
onions, tomatoes, and croutons in a large bowl. Toss the mixture with
the vinaigrette.

Arrange one-fourth of the salad on each of four plates and top with a piece of the salmon.

BONUS YEARS DAILY PERCENTAGES

Per serving: Fruits and vegetables 50%; Fish 100%; Garlic 50%

NUTRITIONAL ANALYSIS

Per serving: Calories 577, Protein 40g, Total fat 28g, Sat fat 6g, Trans fat 0g, Cholesterol 94mg, Carbohydrate 35g, Dietary fiber 7g, Sodium 408mg

Roasted Mushrooms with Onions

About 20 ounces mushrooms, such as a combination of
   cremini, button, and shiitake, cleaned, stems removed, and
   caps coarsely chopped
1½ cups coarsely chopped onions
1 cup low-sodium chicken broth
1 tablespoon extra-virgin olive oil
kosher salt and freshly ground black pepper, to taste

Preheat the oven to 350 degrees. Combine all the ingredients in a medium baking dish and cover. Bake for 35 minutes. Remove from the oven and let the vegetables cool. Remove the mushrooms and the onions from the liquid with a slotted spoon. (Reserve the liquid for uses in sauces and dressings.)

Chocolate Mousse

Make this a day ahead, cover, and refrigerate. Chilling the mousse mixture allows the flavors to blend.

1 cup (8 ounces) soft silken tofu

½ cup (4 ounces) light cream cheese

2 tablespoons unsweetened cocoa powder (not Dutch processed)

¼ cup dark honey or maple syrup

1 tablespoon vanilla extract

8 tablespoons chopped almonds, hazelnuts, or pecans

Add the tofu and cream cheese to a blender or small food processor. Process until smooth. Add the cocoa powder and process until combined. Add the honey and vanilla and process until smooth.

Spoon into four small dessert dishes. Sprinkle with the nuts, cover, and refrigerate until chilled, or overnight.

BONUS YEARS DAILY PERCENTAGES

Per serving: Chocolate 25%; Nuts 25%

NUTRITIONAL ANALYSIS

Per serving: Calories 275, Protein 11g, Total fat 15g, Sat fat 3g, Trans fat 0g, Cholesterol 10mg, Carbohydrate 25g, Dietary fiber 3g, Sodium 156mg

RED WINE

NUTRITIONAL ANALYSIS

Per 5 ounces: Calories 106, Protein 0g, Total fat 0g, Sat fat 0g, Trans fat 0g, Cholesterol 0mg, Carbohydrate 2g, Dietary fiber 0g, Sodium 7mg

DARK CHOCOLATE

NUTRITIONAL ANALYSIS

Per 1½ ounces: Calories 227, Protein 2g, Total fat 12g, Sat fat 7g, Trans fat 0g, Cholesterol 0mg, Carbohydrate 27g, Dietary fiber 2g, Sodium 7mg

NUTS

NUTRITIONAL ANALYSIS

Per 1½ ounces: Calories 253, Protein 7g, Total fat 22g, Sat fat 3g, Trans fat 0g, Cholesterol 0mg, Carbohydrate 11g, Dietary fiber 4g, Sodium 5mg

DAY 5: THURSDAY

Breakfast

Cantaloupe with
Berries and Ricotta
1 whole wheat English muffin,
toasted
1 tablespoon nut butter
BONUS YEARS POINTS: FRUITS AND VEGETABLES 25%;
NUTS 50%
CALORIES: 531

Lunch

Crab Salad with Creamy Dressing
BONUS YEARS POINTS: FRUITS AND VEGETABLES 65%;
FISH 60%
CALORIES: 243

Dinner

Pan-Grilled
Shiitake Chicken Breasts
½ cup cooked orzo or other small
pasta, preferably good-quality
whole grain
BONUS YEARS POINTS: FRUITS AND VEGETABLES 25%;
GARLIC 100%
CALORIES: 337

5 ounces red wine
BONUS YEARS POINTS: WINE 100%
CALORIES: 106

Snacks

2 ounces dark chocolate
BONUS YEARS POINTS: CHOCOLATE 100%
CALORIES: 302

1 ounce unsalted dry-roasted
or natural nuts
BONUS YEARS POINTS: NUTS 50%
CALORIES: 168

DAY'S TOTAL BONUS YEARS POINTS: WINE 100%; CHOCOLATE 100%;
FRUITS AND VEGETABLES 115%; FISH 60%; GARLIC 100%; NUTS 100%
TOTAL CALORIES: 1,687

Cantaloupe with Berries and Ricotta

MAKES 1 SERVING

½-inch-thick ring cantaloupe, peeled and seeds removed
½ cup part-skim ricotta cheese
½ cup fresh blueberries, or other fresh berries of your choice
2 tablespoons slivered almonds (½ ounce)

Place the ring of cantaloupe on a plate, put the ricotta cheese in the center of the ring, and top with the berries and almonds.

BONUS YEARS DAILY PERCENTAGES

Per serving: Fruits and vegetables 25%; Nuts 25%

NUTRITIONAL ANALYSIS

Per serving: Calories 302, Protein 17g, Total fat 16g, Sat fat 6g, Trans fat 0g, Cholesterol 38mg, Carbohydrate 23g, Dietary fiber 4g, Sodium 164mg

WHOLE WHEAT ENGLISH MUFFIN

NUTRITIONAL ANALYSIS

Per muffin: Calories 134, Protein 6g, Total fat 1g, Sat fat 0g, Trans fat 0g, Cholesterol 0mg, Carbohydrate 26g, Dietary fiber 4g, Sodium 420mg

NUT BUTTER (SUCH AS ALMOND OR PEANUT)

BONUS YEARS DAILY PERCENTAGES

Per tablespoon: Nuts 25%

NUTRITIONAL ANALYSIS

Per tablespoon: Calories 95, Protein 4g, Total fat 8g, Sat fat 1g, Trans fat 0g, Cholesterol 0mg, Carbohydrate 3g, Dietary fiber 1g, Sodium 74mg

Crab Salad with Creamy Dressing

Pasteurized canned crabmeat available in the refrigerated section of the supermarket is excellent for this salad. Or if fresh crabs are available in your area, you can buy cooked crabs or cook your own live crabs and pick out the meat.

4 ounces thin asparagus, woody ends snapped off, cut into
   1-inch-long pieces (about ¾ cup)
12 ounces good-quality, cooked lump crabmeat, coarsely
   flaked and picked over
½ cup cooked fresh or frozen corn kernels (2 ounces)
½ cup roughly chopped celery (2 ounces)
¾ cup prepared low-fat ranch dressing mixed with 1½
   tablespoons freshly squeezed lemon juice and 1½
   tablespoons chopped fresh tarragon
8 cups loosely packed mixed salad greens, such as radicchio
   and spinach, or greens of your choice (6 ounces)
4 medium tomatoes (about 6 ounces each), cored, each cut
   into 8 wedges, and seasoned with kosher salt and freshly
   ground black pepper, to taste
4 lemon wedges

Bring a pot of water to a boil. Prepare a bowl of ice and water. Add the asparagus to the boiling water and drain after 1 minute. Immediately transfer the asparagus to the ice water to stop the cooking. Drain the asparagus.

Gently mix the crabmeat with the corn, celery, asparagus, and dressing in a large bowl.

Take 2 cups of the salad greens and decoratively place them in the center of each of four plates. Arrange 8 tomato wedges around the edge of each plate. Squeeze the juice of 1 lemon wedge over each salad and also on the tomato wedges, to taste.

Scoop one-fourth of the crab salad (a little over 1 cup) into the center of each of the plates.

To Make Ahead: Combine the crabmeat, corn, celery, and asparagus in a bowl. Prepare the dressing. Cover and refrigerate separately. Toss the crabmeat mixture with the dressing just before serving. Serve with the salad greens, tomatoes, and lemon wedges.

BONUS YEARS DAILY PERCENTAGES

Per serving: Fruits and vegetables 65%; Fish 60%

NUTRITIONAL ANALYSIS

Per serving: Calories 243, Protein 23g, Total fat 7g, Sat fat 2g, Trans fat 0g, Cholesterol 92mg, Carbohydrate 22g, Dietary fiber 5g, Sodium 616mg

Pan-Grilled
Shiitake Chicken Breasts

———

The simple vegetable ragout turns a plain grilled chicken breast into a Provençal delight.

Serve an earthy red wine with dry herb characteristics, such as a French Cabernet or southern Rhône wine.

1 tablespoon extra-virgin olive oil

1 medium onion (6 ounces), cut into thin rings

1 medium carrot (about 3 ounces), peeled and roughly diced

1 stalk celery, roughly diced

10 ounces fresh shiitake mushrooms (other fresh mushrooms, such as portobello or button, can also be used), stems removed and caps cut into thin slices

4 cloves garlic, minced

2 tablespoons freshly chopped thyme, or 1½ teaspoons dried thyme

1 teaspoon Italian seasoning

¾ cup dry white wine

freshly ground black pepper, to taste

4 boneless, skinless chicken breast halves, preferably brined (see page 376) for 1 to 2 hours

kosher salt, to taste

½ cup low-sodium chicken broth

Preheat the oven to 375 degrees. Heat the olive oil in a 12-inch non-stick skillet over medium heat. Add the onion, carrot, and celery and sauté for about 3 minutes. Add the mushrooms and sauté for 5 minutes. Add the garlic, thyme, and Italian seasoning and sauté for 2 to 3 minutes. Add the wine and simmer until most of the wine has evaporated, about 10 minutes.

Meanwhile, spray a ridged stovetop grill pan with nonstick cooking spray, and heat over medium-high heat. Season the chicken with pepper and place on the grill pan. Cook the chicken on the grill pan for 3 minutes on each side, rotating a quarter turn after 1½ minutes on a side to give grill markings.

Place the chicken in the pan with the vegetables, spooning the vegetables over the chicken. Add the broth, cover, and transfer to the oven. Bake for 8 minutes, or until the chicken is cooked through.

Remove the chicken from the skillet, season the vegetables and broth with salt and pepper, and divide the chicken and mushroom mixture among four plates.

BONUS YEARS DAILY PERCENTAGES

Per serving: Fruits and vegetables 25%; Garlic 100%

NUTRITIONAL ANALYSIS

Per serving: Calories 256, Protein 30g, Total fat 5g, Sat fat 1g, Trans fat 0g, Cholesterol 69mg, Carbohydrate 12g, Dietary fiber 2g, Sodium 133mg

WHOLE WHEAT PASTA

NUTRITIONAL ANALYSIS

Per ½ cup cooked: Calories 81, Protein 3g, Total fat 0g, Sat fat 0g, Trans fat 0g, Cholesterol 0mg, Carbohydrate 16g, Dietary fiber 3g, Sodium 1mg

RED WINE

NUTRITIONAL ANALYSIS

Per 5 ounces: Calories 106, Protein 0g, Total fat 0g, Sat fat 0g, Trans fat 0g,
Cholesterol 0mg, Carbohydrate 2g, Dietary fiber 0g, Sodium 7mg

DARK CHOCOLATE

NUTRITIONAL ANALYSIS

Per 2 ounces: Calories 302, Protein 3g, Total fat 16g, Sat fat 10g, Trans fat 0g,
Cholesterol 0mg, Carbohydrate 36g, Dietary fiber 2g, Sodium 9mg

NUTS

NUTRITIONAL ANALYSIS

Per 1 ounce: Calories 168, Protein 5g, Total fat 14g, Sat fat 2g, Trans fat 0g,
Cholesterol 0mg, Carbohydrate 7g, Dietary fiber 2g, Sodium 3mg

DAY 6: FRIDAY

Breakfast

Banana-Bran Muffin
BONUS YEARS POINTS: FRUITS AND VEGETABLES 25%
CALORIES: 224

Lunch

Mexican Pinto-Bean Soup
BONUS YEARS POINTS: FRUITS AND VEGETABLES 55%;
GARLIC 100%
CALORIES: 234

Dinner

Sautéed Halibut with Roasted
Brussels Sprouts and Mushrooms
in Red Wine Pan Sauce
Oven-Roasted Fingerling Potatoes
Mixed Baby Greens with Roasted
Garlic Vinaigrette (page 112)
BONUS YEARS POINTS: FRUITS AND VEGETABLES 20%;
FISH 100%; GARLIC 25%
CALORIES: 589

5 ounces red wine
BONUS YEARS POINTS: WINE 100%
CALORIES: 106

Snacks

2 ounces dark chocolate
BONUS YEARS POINTS: CHOCOLATE 100%
CALORIES: 302

2 ounces unsalted dry-roasted
or natural nuts
BONUS YEARS POINTS: NUTS 100%
CALORIES: 337

DAY'S TOTAL BONUS YEARS POINTS: WINE 100%; CHOCOLATE 100%;
FRUITS AND VEGETABLES 100%; FISH 100%; GARLIC 125%; NUTS 100%
TOTAL CALORIES: 1,792

Banana-Bran Muffins

MAKES 12 MUFFINS

These moist muffins will keep, covered, at room temperature for 2 days. They can be frozen for up to 3 months. Thaw in the microwave on low.

2 cups high-fiber cereal, such as low-carb All-Bran
2 cups fat-free milk, heated until hot
¾ cup unbleached all-purpose flour
1 cup white whole wheat or regular whole wheat flour
2½ teaspoons baking powder
¼ teaspoon baking soda
2 teaspoons ground cinnamon
¼ teaspoon freshly ground nutmeg
pinch kosher salt
¼ cup molasses
¼ cup egg substitute, or 1 egg, lightly beaten
¼ cup canola oil
1 teaspoon vanilla extract
2 medium bananas, mashed (about 1 cup)
¾ cup dried Zante currants

Preheat the oven to 375 degrees. Spray 12 2½- to 3-inch nonstick muffin cups with cooking spray. Or line the muffin cups with paper cup liners.

Combine the cereal and milk in a large bowl; let stand, stirring occasionally, about 15 minutes. Combine the flours, baking powder, baking soda, spices, and salt in a medium bowl. Add the molasses, egg substitute, oil, vanilla, and bananas to the cereal mixture. Add the cereal mixture to the dry ingredients and stir just until the dry ingredients are moistened (batter will be lumpy). Stir in the currants.

Spoon the batter into the prepared muffin cups. Bake for about 30 minutes, or until tops spring back when pressed. Remove from the pan and place on a wire cooling rack. Serve warm or at room temperature.

BONUS YEARS DAILY PERCENTAGES

Per serving: Fruits and vegetables 25%

NUTRITIONAL ANALYSIS

Per serving: Calories 224, Protein 6g, Total fat 5g, Sat fat 0g, Trans fat 0g, Cholesterol 0mg, Carbohydrate 41g, Dietary fiber 6g, Sodium 156mg

Mexican Pinto-Bean Soup

MAKES 4 (1-CUP) SERVINGS

Bean soups are an easy and flavorful way to add fiber to your diet. Pureeing a bit of the cooked soup adds lots of flavor and some extra body. This is a great make-ahead lunch. After a night in the refrigerator, the flavors will meld and you won't be able to put down your spoon.

¾ cup dried pinto beans, or 2 cups canned beans, drained
1 tablespoon extra-virgin olive oil
1 large onion (8 ounces), coarsely chopped
1 poblano chili (4 ounces), seeds removed and coarsely
    chopped
4 cloves garlic, thinly sliced
1 tablespoon ground, toasted cumin seed (see page 378)
1 to 1½ tablespoons medium-hot chili powder
3 cups low-sodium chicken broth
2 medium to large Roma tomatoes (about 8 ounces total),
    seeds removed and coarsely chopped
1 teaspoon freshly squeezed lime juice
kosher salt, to taste
sprigs of cilantro, for garnish

If using dried pinto beans, pick over the beans and rinse. Soak the pinto beans overnight in enough cold water to cover. Place the beans in a pot with about 2 cups water and bring to a low boil. Reduce the heat, cover, and simmer until the beans are just soft, about 1 hour. Drain the beans and set aside.

Heat the oil in a heavy-bottomed, 4-quart pot over medium heat. Add the onion and chili and sauté for about 5 minutes. Add the garlic, cumin, and chili powder and sauté for 2 to 3 minutes. Don't burn the garlic.

Add the broth, tomatoes, and beans. Bring to a low simmer, partially cover the pot, and cook for about 45 minutes. Remove 1 cup of the soup, puree in a blender, and stir into the soup in the pot. Stir in the lime juice and season with salt.

Ladle into four bowls and top with cilantro.

To Make Ahead: Prepare as directed above. Transfer to a large heatproof bowl, cover, and refrigerate for up to 3 days or freeze in individual servings for up to 1 month. If frozen thaw in the refrigerator or microwave. Reheat and top with cilantro before serving.

BONUS YEARS DAILY PERCENTAGES

Per serving: Fruits and vegetables 55%; Garlic 100%

NUTRITIONAL ANALYSIS

Per serving: Calories 234, Protein 12g, Total fat 6g, Sat fat 1g, Trans fat 0g, Cholesterol 3mg, Carbohydrate 36g, Dietary fiber 12g, Sodium 114mg

Sautéed Halibut with Roasted Brussels Sprouts and Mushrooms in Red Wine Pan Sauce

MAKES 4 SERVINGS

This is an elegant but easy recipe, so don't be fooled by its length. The sauce can be cooking on the stovetop while the vegetables are roasting in the oven; it really doesn't take that long. Simply roasting vegetables and fish and then surrounding them with flavorful sauce is how four-star restaurants often present their dishes; here is the Bonus Years version.

Serve an earthy Rhône wine, either a Syrah or a Grenache.

3 cups low-sodium chicken broth
1½ cups dry red wine
2 teaspoons red wine vinegar
2 ounces pancetta or Canadian bacon, cut into small dice
11 medium Brussels sprouts, trimmed and quartered
8 ounces button or cremini mushrooms, stems removed
pinch freshly ground nutmeg (optional)
kosher salt and freshly ground black pepper, to taste
4 (5- to 6-ounce) halibut fillets with skin
1 tablespoon extra-virgin olive oil
1 large shallot, minced
1 clove garlic, minced
1 tablespoon unsalted butter, or 1 teaspoon arrowroot
   dissolved in 2 teaspoons water

Simmer the broth, wine, and vinegar in a small pan over medium heat until the mixture is reduced to 1¼ cups, about 25 minutes. Set aside.

Preheat the oven to 375 degrees. Spray an ovenproof skillet large enough to hold the Brussels sprouts and mushrooms in one layer with nonstick cooking spray. Add the pancetta to the skillet and sauté the pancetta until lightly browned, about 5 minutes. Stir in the Brussels sprouts and mushrooms, season with nutmeg (if using), salt, and pepper. Roast the vegetables for 25 minutes. Remove from the oven and reserve; leave the oven on.

After the vegetables have been roasting for about 15 minutes, season the fish fillets with salt and pepper and make shallow cuts in the skin to keep it from curling during sautéing. Heat a 10-inch nonstick skillet over medium-high heat, add the olive oil, and heat to just below smoking. Add the fish fillets, skin side down, and put pressure on them with a spatula for 15 to 30 seconds to help prevent curling. Cook until the skin is golden brown, 2 to 3 minutes. Transfer the fish to a nonstick baking pan and place in the oven for 6 to 7 minutes, or until the fish is opaque.

Meanwhile, add the shallot to the skillet, and cook for about 2 minutes. Add the garlic, and cook for 1 minute. Add the reduced broth mixture and cook over medium-high heat until the liquid is reduced to ¾ to 1 cup, about 10 minutes. Season the sauce with salt and pepper. Whisk in the butter to thicken and enrich the sauce.

To serve, divide the roasted vegetables and pancetta among four plates. Top each serving with one piece of the fish. Drizzle the reduced wine sauce over the fish and around the vegetables.

BONUS YEARS DAILY PERCENTAGES

Per serving: Fruits and vegetables 20%; Fish 100%; Garlic 25%

NUTRITIONAL ANALYSIS

Per serving: Calories 365, Protein 39g, Total fat 12g, Sat fat 3g, Trans fat 0g, Cholesterol 63mg, Carbohydrate 11g, Dietary fiber 2g, Sodium 376mg

Dr. Chef's Note

Pancetta is unsmoked, salted Italian bacon. It is available in well-stocked supermarkets and specialty stores. Leaner Canadian bacon can be substituted but the flavor is not quite the same.

Oven-Roasted Fingerling Potatoes

MAKES 4 SERVINGS

1 pound fingerling potatoes, cut in half lengthwise
1 tablespoon extra-virgin olive oil
2 teaspoons dried rosemary, or 3 small sprigs fresh rosemary
kosher salt and freshly ground black pepper, to taste

Preheat the oven to 375 degrees. In a small baking dish, combine the potatoes, olive oil, rosemary, salt, and pepper. Mix thoroughly. Turn the potatoes, cut side down, and roast for 20 minutes, or until tender.

NUTRITIONAL ANALYSIS

Per serving: Calories 110, Protein 3g, Total fat 3g, Sat fat 0g, Trans fat 0g, Cholesterol 0mg, Carbohydrate 20g, Dietary fiber 2g, Sodium 30mg

Dr. Chef's Note

If fingerling potatoes are not available, use small red-skin potatoes.

RED WINE
NUTRITIONAL ANALYSIS
Per 5 ounces: Calories 106, Protein 0g, Total fat 0g, Sat fat 0g, Trans fat 0g, Cholesterol 0mg, Carbohydrate 2g, Dietary fiber 0g, Sodium 7mg

DARK CHOCOLATE
NUTRITIONAL ANALYSIS
Per 2 ounces: Calories 302, Protein 3g, Total fat 16g, Sat fat 10g, Trans fat 0g, Cholesterol 0mg, Carbohydrate 36g, Dietary fiber 2g, Sodium 9mg

NUTS
NUTRITIONAL ANALYSIS
Per 2 ounces: Calories 337, Protein 10g, Total fat 29g, Sat fat 4g, Trans fat 0g, Cholesterol 0mg, Carbohydrate 14g, Dietary fiber 5g, Sodium 7mg

DAY 7: SATURDAY

Breakfast

Pecan Pancakes
Apple-Maple Syrup
BONUS YEARS POINTS: NUTS 50%
CALORIES: 595

Lunch

Warm Asian-Style Shrimp Salad
BONUS YEARS POINTS: FRUITS AND VEGETABLES 35%;
FISH 20%; GARLIC 100%
CALORIES: 249

Dinner

Sonoran Turkey Cutlets
in Tequila-Lime Sauce
Southwestern
Potato-Vegetable Hash
Pears Poached in Red Wine
with Chocolate
BONUS YEARS POINTS: CHOCOLATE 60%; FRUITS AND
VEGETABLES 75%; GARLIC 100%; NUTS 25%
TOTAL CALORIES: 1,004

5 ounces wine
BONUS YEARS POINTS: WINE 100%
CALORIES: 106

Snacks

.8 ounce dark chocolate
BONUS YEARS POINTS: CHOCOLATE 40%
CALORIES: 120

½ ounce unsalted dry-roasted
or natural nuts
BONUS YEARS POINTS: NUTS 25%
CALORIES: 84

DAY'S TOTAL BONUS YEARS POINTS: WINE 100%; CHOCOLATE 100%;
FRUITS AND VEGETABLES 110%; FISH 20%; GARLIC 200%; NUTS 100%
TOTAL CALORIES: 2,158

Pecan Pancakes

---

1 cup unbleached all-purpose flour

⅓ cup white whole wheat or regular whole wheat flour

¼ cup old-fashioned rolled oats

1¼ teaspoons baking powder

½ teaspoon baking soda

⅛ teaspoon kosher salt

1 teaspoon ground cinnamon

1½ cups low-fat buttermilk

¼ cup egg substitute, or 1 egg, beaten

2 tablespoons canola oil

1 tablespoon honey

1 teaspoon vanilla extract

1 cup chopped pecans, toasted (see Dr. Chef's note below)

Apple-Maple Syrup (recipe follows)

Combine the flours, oats, baking powder, baking soda, salt, and cinnamon in a medium bowl. In another bowl, combine the buttermilk, egg substitute, oil, honey, and vanilla. Stir the milk mixture into the flour mixture until just combined. Gently stir in the toasted pecans.

Spray a nonstick griddle with cooking spray and place over medium heat. Using about ⅓ cup batter for each pancake, cook pancakes on hot griddle until bubbles form. Turn the pancakes and cook until lightly browned on the undersides, about 2 minutes. Place 2 pancakes on each of four plates. Serve with syrup.

BONUS YEARS DAILY PERCENTAGES

Per serving: Nuts 50%

NUTRITIONAL ANALYSIS

Per serving (without syrup): Calories 508, Protein 13g, Total fat 31g, Sat fat 3g, Trans fat 0g, Cholesterol 4mg, Carbohydrate 49g, Dietary fiber 6g, Sodium 489mg

Dr. Chef's Note

To toast chopped or small nuts in the oven: Preheat the oven to 350 degrees. Spread the nuts in a single layer on an ungreased light-colored baking sheet. Bake until lightly golden, about 5 minutes, stirring halfway through the cooking time. Immediately remove from the baking sheet and set aside briefly to cool. To toast on the stovetop: Heat a small skillet over medium heat. Add the nuts and cook, stirring constantly, until lightly golden, 3 to 5 minutes. Immediately remove from the skillet and set aside briefly to cool. For larger whole nuts and nut pieces, increase the cooking time by a few minutes.

Apple-Maple Syrup

MAKES ABOUT 1¼ CUPS; 4 SERVINGS

———

1 cup apple juice
2 teaspoons cornstarch
¼ cup maple syrup
¼ teaspoon ground allspice
⅛ teaspoon freshly grated nutmeg

Whisk ¼ cup of the apple juice with the cornstarch in a small saucepan. Whisk in the remaining apple juice, maple syrup, allspice, and nutmeg. Cook over medium heat, stirring, until slightly thickened.

NUTRITIONAL ANALYSIS

Per serving: Calories 87, Protein 0g, Total fat 0g, Sat fat 0g, Trans fat 0g, Cholesterol 0mg, Carbohydrate 22g, Dietary fiber 0g, Sodium 4mg

Warm Asian-Style Shrimp Salad

MAKES 4 SERVINGS

5 ounces sugar snap peas, strings removed

1 tablespoon canola or grapeseed oil

10 ounces shiitake or brown mushrooms, stems removed and
  caps sliced

1 cup thinly sliced red onion (4 ounces)

1 small red bell pepper (4 ounces), cut into matchstick-size
  pieces

4 cloves garlic, minced

12 ounces shrimp (21 to 25 size), shelled and deveined

3 tablespoons hoisin sauce

1½ tablespoons oyster sauce

¼ cup low-sodium chicken broth

½ tablespoon fish sauce

⅛ teaspoon Asian chili paste

1 tablespoon sugar

1 tablespoon freshly squeezed lime juice

8 cups mixed baby greens (6 ounces), washed and spun dry

3 tablespoons chopped cilantro

Bring a pot of water to a boil. Prepare a bowl of ice and water. Add the peas to the boiling water and drain after 1 minute. Immediately transfer the peas to the ice water to stop the cooking. Drain the peas, cut diagonally in half, and reserve them.

Heat the oil in a large nonstick skillet over medium heat. Add the mushrooms, onion, and bell pepper and sauté for 3 minutes. Add the garlic and shrimp and cook until the shrimp turn pink, about 2 minutes. Add the hoisin sauce, oyster sauce, broth, fish sauce, chili paste, and sugar, and bring to a low simmer. Add the peas, mix thoroughly; heat until hot. Drizzle in the lime juice and mix to combine.

Divide the baby greens among four bowls. With a large slotted spoon or Chinese strainer, remove the cooked ingredients from the skillet and place them on top of the greens. Top each serving with one-fourth of the chopped cilantro.

BONUS YEARS DAILY PERCENTAGES

Per serving: Fruits and vegetables 35%; Fish 20%; Garlic 100%

NUTRITIONAL ANALYSIS

Per serving: Calories 249, Protein 23g, Total fat 6g, Sat fat 1g, Trans fat 0g, Cholesterol 130mg, Carbohydrate 25g, Dietary fiber 6g, Sodium 595mg

Sonoran Turkey Cutlets in Tequila-Lime Sauce

MAKES 4 SERVINGS

Turkey breast is lower in fat and calories than any other meat or poultry, which helps to explain why Americans are eating turkey products like never before. Turkey cutlets are now widely available in supermarkets. They make a healthy but elegant alternative to veal and pork. The turkey cutlets can tend to be a bit tough; brining them magically tenderizes them and makes them succulent when quickly panfried.

8 (about 3-ounce) turkey cutlets, preferably brined (see page 376) for 1½ to 2 hours
sweet paprika
1 (12-ounce) can papaya nectar or pear nectar (1½ cups)
3 tablespoons tequila
3 tablespoons freshly squeezed lime juice
2 tablespoons light brown sugar
2 tablespoons jalapeño jelly or other spicy jelly of your choice
4 cloves garlic, mashed
¾ teaspoon kosher salt

Rinse the turkey under cold water. Pat dry with paper towels. Lightly sprinkle the turkey with the paprika.

Place the nectar, tequila, lime juice, sugar, jelly, garlic, and salt in a small saucepan and heat over low heat, stirring, until the jelly and the brown sugar are dissolved. Mix all the ingredients well and simmer for 10 minutes.

Spray a 12-inch nonstick skillet with cooking spray and heat over medium-high heat. Add the turkey, in batches, and cook until lightly browned, 2 to 3 minutes per side. Remove the turkey from the skillet, cover, and keep warm. Repeat until all the turkey is cooked.

Layer the turkey in the skillet, spooning the tequila sauce around the cutlets, and simmer until the cutlets are reheated, 3 to 5 minutes.

To serve, place two cutlets and one-fourth of the sauce on each of four plates.

BONUS YEARS DAILY PERCENTAGES

Per serving: Fruits and vegetables 10%; Garlic 100%

NUTRITIONAL ANALYSIS

Per serving (without brining): Calories 317, Protein 42g, Total fat 1g, Sat fat 0g, Trans fat 0g, Cholesterol 67mg, Carbohydrate 29g, Dietary fiber 0g, Sodium 161mg

Southwestern Potato-Vegetable Hash

MAKES 4 (1-CUP) SERVINGS

1 (1-pound) package frozen hash brown or O'Brien potatoes

2½ tablespoons grapeseed or canola oil

1 large onion (7 ounces), diced

1 small red bell pepper (4 ounces), cut into ½-inch dice

1 medium zucchini (about 6 ounces), cut into ½-inch dice

1 medium large yellow squash (5 to 6 ounces), cut into
    ½-inch dice

1 poblano chili, seeded, stemmed, and diced

½ teaspoon mild chili powder

1 teaspoon ground toasted cumin seed (see page 378)

2 teaspoons Mexican oregano, or 1 teaspoon dried thyme and
    1 teaspoon regular dried oregano

2 medium plum tomatoes (about 5 ounces), coarsely chopped

1½ tablespoons freshly squeezed lime juice

kosher salt and freshly ground black pepper, to taste

If the frozen potatoes are matted together, first crumble them to separate them into pieces. Heat 1½ tablespoons of the oil in a heavy nonstick skillet over medium heat to shimmering. Add the potatoes, and cook until nicely browned, 10 to 15 minutes, stirring frequently to avoid burning. Remove the potatoes and reserve.

Heat the remaining 1 tablespoon of oil in the skillet. Add the onion, bell pepper, zucchini, yellow squash, and chili and sauté for about 4 minutes. Add the chili powder, cumin, and oregano and sauté until the vegetables are softened, about 2 minutes. Add the tomatoes and lime juice and sauté until the tomatoes soften, about 3 minutes.

Add the reserved potatoes and mix thoroughly. Reheat and season with salt and pepper. Divide among four plates.

BONUS YEARS DAILY PERCENTAGES

Per serving: Fruits and vegetables 55%

NUTRITIONAL ANALYSIS

Per serving: Calories 208, Protein 3g, Total fat 9g, Sat fat 1g, Trans fat 0g, Cholesterol 0mg, Carbohydrate 29g, Dietary fiber 6g, Sodium 50mg

Pears Poached in
Red Wine with Chocolate

MAKES 4 SERVINGS

This dessert was a favorite of my cooking-class students at Kitchen Classics in Phoenix. Don't pass it by.

2 cups dry red wine
¼ cup packed light brown sugar
¼ teaspoon ground cinnamon
⅛ teaspoon ground nutmeg
2 whole cloves
2 firm pears (such as Bartlett), peeled, halved, and cored
⅔ cup semisweet chocolate morsels (about 5 ounces)
2 ounces slivered almonds (½ cup)

Place the wine, sugar, cinnamon, nutmeg, and cloves in a shallow saucepan. Cook, stirring, over medium heat until the sugar dissolves. Simmer until the mixture is reduced by half. Add the pears, cover, and simmer until the pears are crisp-tender when pierced with a thin knife tip, 20 to 25 minutes. Remove the pears from the wine and let them cool. Meanwhile, simmer the wine until reduced to a thick glaze. Discard the whole cloves.

Place the chocolate in a bowl over gently simmering water, stirring, until melted. Place a pear half on each of four plates and drizzle the reduced wine over and around each of the pear halves and then top each with one-fourth of the melted chocolate and one-fourth of the almonds.

BONUS YEARS DAILY PERCENTAGES

Per serving: Chocolate 60%; Fruits and vegetables 10%; Nuts 25%

NUTRITIONAL ANALYSIS

Per serving: Calories 479, Protein 8g, Total fat 25g, Sat fat 7g, Trans fat 0g, Cholesterol 0mg, Carbohydrate 55g, Dietary fiber 7g, Sodium 18mg

RED WINE
NUTRITIONAL ANALYSIS

Per 5 ounces: Calories 106, Protein 0g, Total fat 0g, Sat fat 0g, Trans fat 0g, Cholesterol 0mg, Carbohydrate 2g, Dietary fiber 0g, Sodium 7mg

DARK CHOCOLATE
NUTRITIONAL ANALYSIS

Per .8 ounce: Calories 120, Protein 1g, Total fat 6g, Sat fat 4g, Trans fat 0g, Cholesterol 0mg, Carbohydrate 14g, Dietary fiber 1g, Sodium 4mg

NUTS
NUTRITIONAL ANALYSIS

Per ½ ounce: Calories 84, Protein 2g, Total fat 7g, Sat fat 1g, Trans fat 0g, Cholesterol 0mg, Carbohydrate 3g, Dietary fiber 1g, Sodium 2mg

DAY 8: SUNDAY

Breakfast

Cheese Blintzes
with Blackberry Coulis
BONUS YEARS POINTS: FRUITS AND VEGETABLES 25%;
NUTS 25%
CALORIES: 729

Lunch

Turkey Breast
Cranberry-Apple Relish (optional)
Roasted Root-Vegetable Puree
with Horseradish
½ cup steamed broccoli
BONUS YEARS POINTS: FRUITS AND VEGETABLES 80%;
NUTS 25%
CALORIES: 435

Dinner

Roasted Peppers, Fennel, and
Artichokes with Baked Polenta
BONUS YEARS POINTS: FRUITS AND VEGETABLES 65%;
GARLIC 150%
CALORIES: 412

5 ounces wine
BONUS YEARS POINTS: WINE 100%
CALORIES: 106

Snacks

2 ounces dark chocolate
BONUS YEARS POINTS: CHOCOLATE 100%
CALORIES: 302

1 ounce (1½ ounces if omitting
relish) unsalted dry-roasted
or natural nuts
BONUS YEARS POINTS: NUTS 50% (75%)
CALORIES: 168 (252)

DAY'S TOTAL BONUS YEARS POINTS: WINE 100%; CHOCOLATE 100%;
FRUITS AND VEGETABLES 170%; GARLIC 150%; NUTS 100%
TOTAL CALORIES: 2,236

Cheese Blintzes
with Blackberry Coulis

MAKES 4 SERVINGS

———

1 cup part-skim ricotta cheese
¼ cup blackberry preserves or jam
grated fresh zest of 1 large lemon
8 purchased crepes (available in the refrigerated section of the
   supermarket)
2 cups fresh blackberries
Blackberry Coulis (recipe follows)
½ cup chopped almonds or hazelnuts (2 ounces)

Preheat the oven to 400 degrees. Spray a large baking dish with cooking spray.

Mix the cheese with the blackberry preserves and lemon zest. For each blintz, place 2 tablespoons of the cheese filling on the bottom third of the crepe, roll the crepe over the filling, fold in the sides, and roll up. Place the crepes, seam sides down, in the prepared baking dish. Coat the blintzes with cooking spray and bake for 15 minutes, or until heated through.

For each serving, place 2 blintzes on a plate and top with ½ cup of the blackberries, ¼ cup of the coulis, and 2 tablespoons of the nuts.

BONUS YEARS DAILY PERCENTAGES

Per serving with coulis: Fruits and vegetables 25%; Nuts 25%

NUTRITIONAL ANALYSIS

Per serving with coulis: Calories 729, Protein 21g, Total fat 26g, Sat fat 7g, Trans fat 0g, Cholesterol 178mg, Carbohydrate 105g, Dietary fiber 13g, Sodium 170mg

Blackberry Coulis

MAKES ABOUT 1 CUP

---

3 cups fresh blackberries (about 18 ounces)
½ cup water
¼ cup sugar
3 tablespoons freshly squeezed lemon juice
2 tablespoons crème de cassis

Puree the blackberries in a food processor with the plastic blade (the metal blade tends to destroy the seeds and adds some bitterness). Press the blackberry puree through a fine sieve, pressing out all the juice (there should be about 1 cup of fresh blackberry juice).

Heat the water to a low simmer. Add the sugar and stir until the sugar is dissolved. Add the blackberry juice and simmer until the mixture is reduced to about 1 cup, about 25 minutes. Let the juice cool to room temperature. Stir in the lemon juice and crème de cassis and refrigerate until chilled.

BONUS YEARS DAILY PERCENTAGES
Per serving: Fruits and vegetables 5%

NUTRITIONAL ANALYSIS
Per ¼-cup serving: Calories 130, Protein 1g, Total fat 0g, Sat fat 0g, Trans fat 0g, Cholesterol 0mg, Carbohydrate 31g, Dietary fiber 3g, Sodium 0mg

Variation

Raspberry Coulis: Substitute raspberries for the blackberries and Chambord (black raspberry liqueur) or framboise (raspberry eau de vie) for the crème de cassis.

Turkey Breast
with Cranberry-Apple Relish

Bone-in turkey breast is one of my favorite ways to serve poultry. By keeping the bone and skin during roasting, you can add lots of flavor and ensure juicy, moist meat without adding much fat. The brining makes the turkey breast meltingly tender and moist.

Match the tang of the cranberries in the relish with a Zinfandel.

1 (about 2½-pound) turkey breast half with bone, preferably
    brined (see page 376) about 4 hours
2½ teaspoons poultry seasoning
freshly squeezed juice of 1 lemon
Cranberry-Apple Relish (optional; recipe follows)

Rinse the turkey breast in cold water, and pat dry with paper towels. Preheat the oven to 375 degrees. Using your fingers, carefully separate the turkey skin from the breast meat. Place 1¼ teaspoons of the poultry seasoning under the skin, and cover the turkey breast with the skin. Spread the remaining 1¼ teaspoons of the poultry seasoning over the skin and the underside of the turkey breast. Lightly spray the skin with olive oil cooking spray and then drizzle with the lemon juice.

Place the turkey breast on a cooking rack in a roasting pan. Roast for about 1½ hours, or until an instant-read thermometer registers 145 to 150 degrees; don't overcook.

Place an aluminum foil tent over the turkey breast and let rest for 15 minutes. Remove the skin and cut the meat across the diagonal into thin slices. (Refrigerate about 6 ounces of cooked turkey for lunch the next day.)

Serve with the relish, if using.

NUTRITIONAL ANALYSIS

Per serving (turkey only): Calories 263, Protein 39g, Total fat 10g, Sat fat 3g, Trans fat 0g, Cholesterol 101mg, Carbohydrate 1g, Dietary fiber 0g, Sodium 87mg

Cranberry-Apple Relish

MAKES 6 (½-CUP) SERVINGS

The relish can be prepared up to three days ahead and refrigerated.

1 cup freshly squeezed orange juice (2 medium oranges)
1 cup water
¾ cup packed light brown sugar
1 (12-ounce) package fresh or frozen cranberries
1 tablespoon grated orange zest
1 cup peeled, chopped tart apples
¼ cup apple cider vinegar
½ cup raisins
¾ cup chopped walnuts, toasted (see page 159)
½ teaspoon kosher salt
¼ teaspoon ground cinnamon
2 pinches red pepper flakes
2 tablespoons freshly squeezed lemon juice

Heat the orange juice and water in a heavy, 3-quart saucepan. Add the sugar and stir until dissolved. Add the remaining ingredients, except the lemon juice. Simmer for about 20 minutes. Cool for 10 minutes. Stir in the lemon juice and refrigerate until chilled, covered, for up to 4 days.

BONUS YEARS DAILY PERCENTAGES
Per serving: Fruits and vegetables 40%; Nuts 25%

NUTRITIONAL ANALYSIS
Per serving: Calories 306, Protein 3g, Total fat 10g, Sat fat 1g, Cholesterol 0mg, Carbohydrate 56g, Dietary fiber 5g, Sodium 171mg

Roasted Root-Vegetable Puree with Horseradish

MAKES 4 SERVINGS

⅔ pound parsnips, peeled and cut into ½-inch pieces
⅔ pound turnips, peeled and cut into ½-inch pieces
⅔ pound orange sweet potatoes (sometimes called yams),
  peeled and cut into ½-inch pieces
½ cup low-fat sour cream
1 tablespoon horseradish mustard or your favorite spicy
  mustard
kosher salt and freshly ground black pepper, to taste

Preheat the oven to 400 degrees. Place the parsnips, turnips, and sweet potatoes in a large ovenproof pan, and coat with cooking spray. Roast for 45 to 50 minutes, or until vegetables are soft, turning occasionally. Force the roasted vegetables through a ricer or food mill into a bowl. Stir in the sour cream and mustard and season with salt and pepper.

BONUS YEARS DAILY PERCENTAGES
Per serving: Fruits and vegetables 20%
NUTRITIONAL ANALYSIS
Per serving: Calories 150, Protein 4g, Total fat 1g, Sat fat 0g, Trans fat 0g,
Cholesterol 5mg, Carbohydrate 32g, Dietary fiber 7g, Sodium 138mg

Dr. Chef's Note

It is important that you use a ricer or food mill to puree the vegetables and not a food processor or blender, both of which will overwork the starch in the vegetables.

STEAMED BROCCOLI

BONUS YEARS DAILY PERCENTAGES

Per ½-cup serving: Fruits and vegetables 20%

NUTRITIONAL ANALYSIS

Per ½-cup serving: Calories 22, Protein 2g, Total fat 0g, Sat fat 0g, Cholesterol 0mg, Trans fat 0g, Carbohydrate 4g, Dietary fiber 2g, Sodium 21mg

Roasted Peppers, Fennel, and Artichokes with Baked Polenta

MAKES 4 SERVINGS

This is one of my favorite recipes. It's a complete meal by itself, but add a tossed green salad if you want something crunchy. Don't leave out the feta cheese; it makes the meal. Remember, feta cheese is salty, so taste before adding the salt.

1 tablespoon extra-virgin olive oil

1 medium onion (about 6 ounces), thinly sliced

1 (about 7-ounce) fennel bulb, thinly sliced (about 2 cups)

2 medium red bell peppers, roasted (see page 378), peeled, and chopped, or 1 (about 12-ounce) jar roasted red bell peppers, drained

1 (about 14-ounce) can artichoke hearts in water, drained and coarsely chopped

4 cloves garlic, thinly sliced

½ cup crumbled low-fat feta cheese (2 ounces)

¼ cup dry-packed, sun-dried tomatoes, rehydrated in ¾ cup hot water, coarsely chopped, and water reserved

2 tablespoons balsamic vinegar

½ teaspoon red pepper flakes

kosher salt, to taste

Baked Polenta (recipe follows)

Heat the olive oil in a 12-inch skillet over medium heat. Add the onion and fennel and sauté for 5 minutes. Add the bell peppers and artichoke hearts and simmer for 3 minutes. Add the garlic and sauté for 1 to 2 minutes.

Add the feta cheese, tomatoes, the tomato water, vinegar, and pepper flakes. Simmer for 2 minutes. Taste for seasoning and add salt if needed. Serve over the polenta.

BONUS YEARS DAILY PERCENTAGES

Per serving (without polenta): Fruits and vegetables 65%; Garlic 100%

NUTRITIONAL ANALYSIS

Per serving (without polenta): Calories 156, Protein 8g, Total fat 5g, Sat fat 1g, Trans fat 0g, Cholesterol 5mg, Carbohydrate 21g, Dietary fiber 4g, Sodium 466mg

Baked Polenta

This easy-to-prepare polenta doesn't require a lot of stirring and was adapted from Paula Wolfert's recipe in Mediterranean Grains and Greens *(HarperCollins, 1998).*

1 tablespoon extra-virgin olive oil
½ cup chopped onion (about 4 ounces)
3 cloves garlic, minced
1 cup coarse cornmeal or polenta
4 cups low-sodium chicken broth
½ teaspoon kosher salt
¼ cup freshly grated Parmesan cheese, or more to taste

Preheat the oven to 350 degrees. Heat the oil in an 8-inch nonstick ovenproof skillet over medium heat. Add the onion and sauté for about 3 minutes. Add the garlic and sauté for 2 minutes. Stir the cornmeal, broth, and salt into the onion and garlic in the skillet.

Transfer to the oven and bake for 45 minutes. Thoroughly stir in the Parmesan cheese and bake for 5 to 10 minutes, or until the polenta is of the desired consistency. Remove the skillet from the oven and transfer the polenta to a warm bowl. Divide among six deep plates.

BONUS YEARS DAILY PERCENTAGES
Per serving: Garlic 50%
NUTRITIONAL ANALYSIS
Per serving: Calories 256, Protein 9g, Total fat 7g, Sat fat 2g, Trans fat 0g, Cholesterol 8mg, Carbohydrate 40g, Dietary fiber 4g, Sodium 436mg

RED WINE

NUTRITIONAL ANALYSIS

Per 5 ounces: Calories 106, Protein 0g, Total fat 0g, Sat fat 0g, Trans fat 0g,
Cholesterol 0mg, Carbohydrate 2g, Dietary fiber 0g, Sodium 7mg

DARK CHOCOLATE

NUTRITIONAL ANALYSIS

Per 2 ounces: Calories 302, Protein 3g, Total fat 16g, Sat fat 10g, Trans fat 0g,
Cholesterol 0mg, Carbohydrate 36g, Dietary fiber 2g, Sodium 9mg

NUTS

NUTRITIONAL ANALYSIS

Per 1 ounce: Calories 168, Protein 5g, Total fat 14g, Sat fat 2g, Trans fat 0g,
Cholesterol 0mg, Carbohydrate 7g, Dietary fiber 2g, Sodium 3mg

DAY 9: MONDAY

Breakfast

½ cup raspberries
Scrambled Eggs with Herbs
1 slice whole wheat bread, toasted
BONUS YEARS POINTS: FRUITS AND VEGETABLES 20%
CALORIES: 225

Lunch

Turkey Gyros
BONUS YEARS POINTS: FRUITS AND VEGETABLES 20%;
GARLIC 100%
CALORIES: 358

Dinner

Farfalle with Monkfish,
Mushrooms, and Fennel
Mixed Baby Greens with Roasted
Garlic Vinaigrette (page 113)
BONUS YEARS POINTS: FRUITS AND VEGETABLES 100%;
FISH 100%; GARLIC 100%
CALORIES: 718

5 ounces wine
BONUS YEARS POINTS: WINE 100%
CALORIES: 106

Snacks

2 ounces dark chocolate
BONUS YEARS POINTS: CHOCOLATE 100%
CALORIES: 302

2 ounces unsalted dry-roasted
or natural nuts
BONUS YEARS POINTS: NUTS 100%
CALORIES: 337

DAY'S TOTAL BONUS YEARS POINTS: WINE 100%; CHOCOLATE 100%;
FRUITS AND VEGETABLES 140%; FISH 100%; GARLIC 100%; NUTS 100%
TOTAL CALORIES: 2,046

Scrambled Eggs with Herbs

―――

Scrambled eggs as a quick workday breakfast? Yes. Scrambled eggs take less than 3 minutes to cook and can be rolled in a whole-grain tortilla for an on-the-go breakfast if a sit-down breakfast isn't an option.

1½ cups egg substitute, or 6 eggs, lightly beaten
2 tablespoons fat-free milk
¼ cup minced flat-leaf parsley
2 tablespoons minced chives, or green onion tops
1 teaspoon minced basil
dash red pepper flakes, to taste
2 to 4 tablespoons freshly grated Parmesan cheese
kosher salt and freshly ground black pepper, to taste
1 tablespoon canola oil or no-trans fat margarine

Combine the egg substitute, milk, parsley, chives, basil, pepper flakes, and cheese in a medium bowl. Season with salt and black pepper.

Heat the oil in a 10-inch nonstick skillet over medium heat. Add the egg mixture and cook, stirring gently, until set.

NUTRITIONAL ANALYSIS

Per serving: Calories 126, Protein 13g, Total fat 7g, Sat fat 1g, Trans fat 0g, Cholesterol 3mg, Carbohydrate 1g, Dietary fiber 0g, Sodium 219mg

RASPBERRIES

BONUS YEARS DAILY PERCENTAGES

Per serving: Fruits and vegetables 20%

NUTRITIONAL ANALYSIS

Per ½-cup serving: Calories 30, Protein 0g, Total fat 0g, Sat fat 0g, Trans fat 0g, Cholesterol 0mg, Carbohydrate 7g, Dietary fiber 3g, Sodium 0mg

WHOLE WHEAT BREAD

NUTRITIONAL ANALYSIS

Per slice: Calories 69, Protein 3g, Total fat 1g, Sat fat 0g, Trans fat 0g, Cholesterol 0mg, Carbohydrate 13g, Dietary fiber 2g, Sodium 147mg

Turkey Gyros

MAKES 2 SERVINGS

6 ounces baked turkey breast (from yesterday's lunch,
   page 172), or from a deli, cut into ¼-inch dice
2 Roma tomatoes (6 ounces total), cored, seeded, and diced
½ cup plain low-fat yogurt
2 large cloves garlic, minced
2 tablespoons minced onion
2 tablespoons freshly squeezed lemon juice
1 tablespoon minced dill
kosher salt and freshly ground black pepper, to taste
2 large pita breads (3 ounces each)

Thoroughly mix all the ingredients, except the pitas, in a medium
bowl. Use half of the turkey mixture to fill each of the pitas.

To Make Ahead: Combine the filling ingredients, cover, and refrigerate. Fill the pitas just before eating.

BONUS YEARS DAILY PERCENTAGES

Per serving: Fruits and vegetables 20%; Garlic 100%

NUTRITIONAL ANALYSIS

Per serving: Calories 358, Protein 34g, Total fat 5g, Sat fat 1g, Trans fat 0g,
Cholesterol 80mg, Carbohydrate 44g, Dietary fiber 2g, Sodium 317mg

Farfalle with Monkfish, Mushrooms, and Fennel

Cuts of monkfish comes from the tail; the fish is sometimes called "poor man's lobster" because of its sweet taste. It is a hearty, meaty fish, which requires significant time to cook through. If you substitute another firm fish such as swordfish or shark, reduce the cooking time.

Drink Cabernet Sauvignon with the dish, just as you use in the cooking.

1½ tablespoons extra-virgin olive oil

1 medium onion (about 6 ounces), chopped

1 cup coarsely chopped fennel bulb (about 8 ounces)

10 ounces cremini or button mushrooms, stems removed and caps quartered

2 teaspoons fennel seed

4 cloves garlic, thinly sliced

¼ teaspoon red pepper flakes

1½ cups Cabernet Sauvignon wine

1 (28-ounce) can chopped Italian plum tomatoes in juice

3 tablespoons red wine vinegar

1½ pounds boneless monkfish, skin removed and cut into
 ¾-inch dice
kosher salt and freshly ground black pepper, to taste
12 ounces farfalle (butterfly pasta), preferably good-quality
 whole wheat pasta, cooked until al dente (tender but firm to
 the bite)

Heat the olive oil in a 12-inch skillet over medium-high heat. Add the onion and fennel and sauté for 3 minutes. Add the mushrooms and sauté until the mushrooms release their liquid and are slightly browned. Add the fennel seed, garlic, and pepper flakes and sauté for 1 minute.

Add the wine and simmer until reduced by half. Add the tomatoes and simmer, covered, for about 35 minutes. Add the vinegar and monkfish and simmer until the monkfish is tender and cooked through, about 15 minutes. Season the sauce with salt and pepper. Add the pasta to the sauce, thoroughly mix, heat until hot, and divide among four plates.

BONUS YEARS DAILY PERCENTAGES

Per serving: Fruits and vegetables 65%; Fish 100%; Garlic 100%

NUTRITIONAL ANALYSIS

Per serving: Calories 604, Protein 41g, Total fat 9g, Sat fat 1g, Trans fat 0g, Cholesterol 42mg, Carbohydrate 82g, Dietary fiber 11g, Sodium 544mg

Dr. Chef's Notes

Fennel seed and fennel bulbs come from two different plants. When cooked, the bulbs have a delicate anise flavor.

If you want to reduce the amount of sodium in this dish, use no-salt-added tomatoes.

RED WINE

NUTRITIONAL ANALYSIS

Per 5 ounces: Calories 106, Protein 0g, Total fat 0g, Sat fat 0g, Trans fat 0g, Cholesterol 0mg, Carbohydrate 2g, Dietary fiber 0g, Sodium 7mg

DARK CHOCOLATE

NUTRITIONAL ANALYSIS

Per 2 ounces: Calories 302, Protein 3g, Total fat 16g, Sat fat 10g, Trans fat 0g, Cholesterol 0mg, Carbohydrate 36g, Dietary fiber 2g, Sodium 9mg

NUTS

NUTRITIONAL ANALYSIS

Per 2 ounce: Calories 337, Protein 10g, Total fat 29g, Sat fat 4g, Trans fat 0g, Cholesterol 0mg, Carbohydrate 14g, Dietary fiber 5g, Sodium 7mg

DAY 10: TUESDAY

Breakfast

Applesauce-Oat Muffin

BONUS YEARS POINTS: FRUITS AND VEGETABLES 25%

CALORIES: 207

Lunch

Smoked Turkey Sandwich with
Corn-and-Tomato Salsa

BONUS YEARS POINTS: FRUITS AND VEGETABLES 45%

CALORIES: 373

Dinner

Velvet Chicken
½ cup steamed brown rice
Asian Fruit Salad

BONUS YEARS POINTS: FRUITS AND VEGETABLES 65%;
GARLIC 100%; NUTS 85%

CALORIES: 837

5 ounces wine

BONUS YEARS POINTS: WINE 100%

CALORIES: 106

Snacks

2 ounces dark chocolate

BONUS YEARS POINTS: CHOCOLATE 100%

CALORIES: 302

1½ tablespoons unsalted dry-
roasted or natural nuts (about
⅓ ounce)

BONUS YEARS POINTS: NUTS 15%

CALORIES: 55

DAY'S TOTAL BONUS YEARS POINTS: WINE 100%; CHOCOLATE 100%;
FRUITS AND VEGETABLES 135%; GARLIC 100%; NUTS 100%
TOTAL CALORIES: 1,880

Applesauce-Oat Muffins

The applesauce adds moistness and flavor; the oats contribute soluble fiber, which helps in reducing blood cholesterol levels.

1 cup old-fashioned rolled oats
1 cup unsweetened applesauce
1 cup unbleached all-purpose flour
1 cup white whole wheat or regular whole wheat flour
2 teaspoons baking powder
pinch kosher salt
¼ cup honey
¼ cup egg substitute, or 1 egg, lightly beaten
¼ cup canola oil
1 teaspoon vanilla extract
1 cup dried cranberries

Preheat the oven to 400 degrees. Spray 12 (2½- to 3-inch) nonstick muffin cups with cooking spray. Or line the muffin cups with paper cup liners.

Combine the oats and applesauce in a large bowl; let stand, stirring occasionally, about 15 minutes. Combine the flours, baking powder, and salt in a medium bowl. Add the honey, egg substitute, oil, and vanilla to the oat mixture. Add the oat mixture to the dry ingredients and stir just until the dry ingredients are moistened (batter will be lumpy). Stir in the cranberries.

Spoon the batter into the prepared muffin cups. Bake for about 20 minutes, or until tops spring back when pressed. Remove from the pan and place on a wire cooling rack. Serve warm or at room temperature. (Muffins will keep, covered, at room temperature for 2 days. They can be frozen for up to 3 months. Thaw in the microwave on low.)

BONUS YEARS DAILY PERCENTAGES

Per serving: Fruits and vegetables 25%

NUTRITIONAL ANALYSIS

Per muffin: Calories 207, Protein 4g, Total fat 5g, Sat fat 0g, Trans fat 0g, Cholesterol 0mg, Carbohydrate 37g, Dietary fiber 4g, Sodium 91mg

Smoked Turkey Sandwich
with Corn-and-Tomato Salsa

MAKES 4 SERVINGS

---

8 slices hearty whole wheat bread

mustard or low-fat sandwich spread of your choice, to taste

1 small red bell pepper (4 ounces), roasted (see page 378), peeled, and sliced, or 8 slices jarred roasted red bell peppers, drained

12 ounces sliced low-sodium turkey from the deli

arugula, watercress, or plain lettuce

Corn-and-Tomato Salsa (recipe follows)

Spread one side of each slice of the bread with the mustard. Top the bottom slice of each sandwich with 1 slice of the bell pepper, one-fourth of the smoked turkey, another bell pepper slice, and finally the arugula. Place the remaining bread slices, mustard sides down, over the arugula. Serve with the salsa.

BONUS YEARS DAILY PERCENTAGES

Per serving (without salsa): Fruits and vegetables 15%

NUTRITIONAL ANALYSIS

Per serving without salsa: Calories 331, Protein 23g, Total fat 5g, Sat fat 1g, Trans fat 0g, Cholesterol 37mg, Carbohydrate 49g, Dietary fiber 6g, Sodium 843mg

Corn-and-Tomato Salsa

MAKES 4 (½-CUP) SERVINGS

———

3 Roma tomatoes (about 12 ounces), seeds removed, and
   diced (2 cups)
½ cup cooked fresh or frozen corn kernels
½ cup diced green bell pepper (2 ounces)
⅓ cup diced red onion (1½ ounces)
1 tablespoon freshly squeezed lime juice
½ to 1 jalapeño pepper, seeds removed and finely diced
2 tablespoons finely chopped fresh cilantro
kosher salt and freshly ground black pepper, to taste

Thoroughly mix all the ingredients in a small bowl. Cover and refrigerate for at least 30 minutes for the flavors to blend.

To Make Ahead: Combine all the ingredients, cover, and refrigerate for up to 2 days.

BONUS YEARS DAILY PERCENTAGES
Per serving: Fruits and vegetables 30%
NUTRITIONAL ANALYSIS
Per serving: Calories 42, Protein 1g, Total fat 0g, Sat fat 0g, Trans fat 0g,
Cholesterol 0mg, Carbohydrate 10g, Dietary fiber 2g, Sodium 5mg

Variation

The salsa has a more robust flavor if the corn is roasted on the ear,
then cut off and combined with the other ingredients. See page 373
for directions on roasting vegetables.

Velvet Chicken

MAKES 4 SERVINGS

_____

Water blanching is adding ingredients to boiling water for a short time and then immediately cooling in iced water. Water blanching the marinated chicken gives it that velvety texture found in Chinese restaurants. This cooking method gives the broccoli and cauliflower a vibrant color, a crisp texture, and assures that they will be not be under- or overcooked, because their cooking times are different from the carrot and celery.

12 ounces boneless, skinless chicken breasts

1 tablespoon cornstarch

1½ tablespoons white wine

generous pinch ground white pepper

2½ cups broccoli florets (about 5 ounces), cut into bite-size pieces

2½ cups cauliflower florets (about 5 ounces), cut into bite-size pieces

1 tablespoon canola oil

1 celery stalk (about 2 ounces), cut in half lengthwise and then crosswise into ¼-inch slices

1 large carrot (about 6 ounces), peeled and cut on the diagonal into ¼-inch slices

1 tablespoon minced fresh ginger

4 cloves garlic, minced

1 cup coarsely chopped walnuts (about 4 ounces)

¾ cup low-sodium chicken broth

4½ tablespoons plum sauce

3 tablespoons low-sodium soy sauce

1 tablespoon sherry

1½ tablespoons cornstarch dissolved in 3 tablespoons water

C ut the chicken across the grain into 1½-inch matchstick-size strips. Combine the 1 tablespoon cornstarch, wine, and pepper in a medium bowl. Add the chicken and stir to coat with the cornstarch mixture; let stand for 15 minutes.

Bring a pot of water to a boil. Prepare a bowl of ice and water. Add the chicken to the boiling water. Remove with a slotted spoon after 1½ minutes and immediately place the chicken in the ice water for about 1 minute. Drain and reserve the chicken.

Add the broccoli and cauliflower florets to the boiling water. Drain after 1 minute and immediately cool in the ice water. Drain and reserve the vegetables.

Heat the oil in a nonstick skillet or wok over medium heat. Add the celery and carrot and stir-fry for about 1½ minutes. Add the ginger, garlic, and nuts and stir-fry about 1 minute; do not burn the garlic. Add the broth, plum sauce, soy sauce, and sherry, and bring to a low simmer. Add the reserved chicken and vegetables and heat until hot.

Stir in the cornstarch mixture and bring the sauce back to a simmer, stirring to thicken the sauce.

BONUS YEARS DAILY PERCENTAGES

Per serving: Fruits and vegetables 30%; Garlic 100%; Nuts 50%

NUTRITIONAL ANALYSIS

Per serving: Calories 433, Protein 28g, Total fat 25g, Sat fat 2g, Cholesterol 50mg, Carbohydrate 27g, Dietary fiber 5g, Sodium 682mg

STEAMED BROWN RICE

NUTRITIONAL ANALYSIS

Per ½-cup serving: Calories 108, Protein 2g, Total fat 0g, Sat fat 0g, Trans fat 0g, Cholesterol 0mg, Carbohydrate 22g, Dietary fiber 2g, Sodium 5mg

Asian Fruit Salad

MAKES 6 SERVINGS

---

1 (11-ounce) can Mandarin oranges, drained

1 (15-ounce) can lychees, drained

2 Asian pears, cut into 1-inch cubes or use a melon baller

2 kiwifruit, peeled and cut into wedges

2 tablespoons freshly squeezed orange juice

2 tablespoons orange liqueur, such as triple sec or Grand Marnier

2 tablespoons sugar

1 tablespoon freshly squeezed lime juice

1 cup chopped roasted almonds

mint sprigs, for garnish

Mix all of the fruit in a large bowl; cover and refrigerate for at least 1 hour.

In a small bowl, mix the orange juice, liqueur, sugar, and lime juice; cover and refrigerate.

Before serving, pour the juice mixture over the fruit and gently mix. Divide among four plates, top with the almonds and mint.

BONUS YEARS DAILY PERCENTAGES

Per serving: Fruits and vegetables 35%; Nuts 35%

NUTRITIONAL ANALYSIS

Per serving: Calories 296, Protein 6g, Total fat 12g, Sat fat 1g, Trans fat 0g, Cholesterol 0mg, Carbohydrate 42g, Dietary fiber 6g, Sodium 4mg

Dr. Chef's Note

Lychees are sometimes found in the Asian section of the supermarket rather than with the canned fruit.

RED WINE

NUTRITIONAL ANALYSIS

Per 5 ounces: Calories 106, Protein 0g, Total fat 0g, Sat fat 0g, Trans fat 0g, Cholesterol 0mg, Carbohydrate 2g, Dietary fiber 0g, Sodium 7mg

DARK CHOCOLATE

NUTRITIONAL ANALYSIS

Per 2 ounces: Calories 302, Protein 3g, Total fat 16g, Sat fat 10g, Trans fat 0g, Cholesterol 0mg, Carbohydrate 36g, Dietary fiber 2g, Sodium 9mg

NUTS

NUTRITIONAL ANALYSIS

Per ⅓ ounce: Calories 55, Protein 1g, Total fat 5g, Sat fat 1g, Trans fat 0g, Cholesterol 0mg, Carbohydrate 2g, Dietary fiber 1g, Sodium 2mg

DAY 11: WEDNESDAY

Breakfast

Quick Berry-Yogurt Smoothie
BONUS YEARS POINTS: FRUITS AND VEGETABLES 30%
CALORIES: 159

Lunch

Asian-Style Chicken Salad with
Peanut Sauce
BONUS YEARS POINTS: FRUITS AND VEGETABLES 45%;
NUTS 25%
CALORIES: 397

Dinner

Steamed Salmon Steaks
Roasted Mushrooms and
Asparagus
Roasted new potatoes
BONUS YEARS POINTS: FRUITS AND VEGETABLES 25%;
FISH 100%; GARLIC 100%
CALORIES: 503

5 ounces wine
BONUS YEARS POINTS: WINE 100%
CALORIES: 106

Snacks

2 ounces dark chocolate
BONUS YEARS POINTS: CHOCOLATE 100%
CALORIES: 302

1½ ounces unsalted dry-roasted
or natural nuts
BONUS YEARS POINTS: NUTS 75%
CALORIES: 253

DAY'S TOTAL BONUS YEARS POINTS: WINE 100%; CHOCOLATE 100%;
FRUITS AND VEGETABLES 100%; FISH 100%; GARLIC 100%; NUTS 100%
TOTAL CALORIES: 1,720

Quick Berry-Yogurt Smoothie

MAKES 2 SERVINGS

1 cup frozen strawberries (about 8 ounces), halved if large, or
raspberries
1 (6-ounce) container strawberry or raspberry yogurt
1 cup freshly squeezed orange juice

Combine the berries, yogurt, and ½ cup of the orange juice in a blender. Blend until smooth. Add the remaining orange juice and blend until combined. Pour into two glasses and serve.

BONUS YEARS DAILY PERCENTAGES
Per serving: Fruits and vegetables 30%

NUTRITIONAL ANALYSIS
Per serving: Calories 159, Protein 5g, Total fat 1g, Sat fat 0g, Trans fat 0g, Cholesterol 0mg, Carbohydrate 34g, Dietary Fiber 2g, Sodium 54mg

Asian-Style Chicken Salad with Peanut Sauce

MAKES 4 SERVINGS

Peanut Sauce

½ cup low-sodium chicken broth
¼ cup reduced-fat peanut butter
¼ cup low-sodium soy sauce
2 tablespoons sugar
¼ cup unseasoned rice vinegar
1 teaspoon Asian chili paste
1 teaspoon Asian sesame oil
1 tablespoon dry mustard
1 teaspoon arrowroot, dissolved in 2 tablespoons cold water

12 ounces cooked boneless, skinless chicken breast, cut into bite-size pieces
1 medium red bell pepper (6 ounces), cut into matchstick-size lengths
1 large carrot (6 ounces), peeled and cut into matchstick-size lengths
1 cup sugar snap peas (4 ounces), trimmed and cut in half on the diagonal
½ cup minced green onion tops
2 tablespoons chopped cilantro
8 cups mixed greens (about 12 ounces)
1 (11-ounce) can Mandarin oranges, drained (about 6 ounces after draining)
¾ cup chow mein noodles (optional)

Make the peanut sauce: Heat the broth in a small saucepan over medium heat. Add the peanut butter and stir until melted. Stir in the remaining sauce ingredients except the arrowroot mixture. Whisk in the arrowroot mixture and simmer, stirring, until the sauce thickens. Transfer to a bowl, cover, and refrigerate until chilled.

Combine the chicken, bell pepper, carrot, peas, green onion, and cilantro in a medium bowl.

Divide the mixed greens among four plates. Top each serving with one-fourth of the chicken-vegetable mixture. Top each salad with equal portions of the oranges and noodles (if using). Drizzle the sauce over the salads.

To Make Ahead: Prepare the sauce and refrigerate. Combine the chicken and vegetables in a bowl, cover, and refrigerate. Add the greens, oranges, and noodles (if using) as directed just before serving and drizzle with the sauce.

BONUS YEARS DAILY PERCENTAGES

Per serving: Fruits and vegetables 45%; Nuts 25%

NUTRITIONAL ANALYSIS

Per serving: Calories 397, Protein 34g, Total fat 11g, Sat fat 2g, Trans fat 0g, Cholesterol 66mg, Carbohydrate 42g, Dietary fiber 7g, Sodium 896mg

Steamed Salmon Steaks

MAKES 4 SERVINGS

A fast weeknight recipe, it demonstrates how easy it is to prepare your Bonus Years seafood.

4 (6-ounce) salmon steaks
kosher salt and freshly ground black pepper, to taste
½ medium onion (about 3 ounces), thinly sliced
1½ tablespoons chopped dill
3 tablespoons chopped flat-leaf parsley
3 tablespoons dry white wine
3 tablespoons freshly squeezed lemon juice
1 teaspoon arrowroot dissolved in 2 teaspoons cold milk

Season the salmon with salt and pepper. Place the salmon on a platter that will fit in your steamer, cover with the onion, then the dill and parsley. Pour the wine and lemon juice over the salmon.

Place the platter in a steamer over boiling water. Cover and steam for 10 to 12 minutes, or until the salmon is opaque. Remove the salmon and onion to a serving dish, cover, and keep warm. Pour the liquid that remains on the platter into a small saucepan; whisk in the arrowroot mixture. Cook, whisking, over low heat until thickened. Season with salt and pepper and serve over the salmon.

BONUS YEARS DAILY PERCENTAGES
Per serving: Fruit and vegetables 5%; Fish 100%

NUTRITIONAL ANALYSIS
Per serving: Calories 325, Protein 34g, Total fat 18g, Sat fat 4g, Trans fat 0g, Cholesterol 112mg, Carbohydrate 3g, Dietary fiber 0g, Sodium 83mg

Roasted Mushrooms and Asparagus

MAKES 4 SERVINGS

1 pound medium-thickness asparagus
4 cloves garlic, unpeeled
kosher salt and freshly ground black pepper, to taste
3 medium portobello mushrooms (about 8 ounces)
3 tablespoons low-sodium or mushroom-flavored soy sauce
½ tablespoon extra-virgin olive oil
1 tablespoon freshly squeezed lemon juice

Preheat the oven to 400 degrees. Snap off the tough ends of the asparagus and peel the stalks. Place the asparagus and garlic in a large baking dish. Lightly coat with cooking spray. Season the asparagus with salt and pepper. Roast for 10 minutes.

Meanwhile, cut off the stems of the mushrooms. Thoroughly rinse the caps under cold water and pat dry. Score the caps by making 3 very shallow cuts in each cap and then rotating a quarter of a turn and making another 3 cuts in that direction (making a checkerboard appearance). Lightly coat the caps and gills of the mushrooms with cooking spray. Brush the gills of the mushrooms with the soy sauce.

Add the mushrooms to the asparagus and roast for 10 minutes, or until the asparagus is crisp-tender.

Remove from the oven. Coarsely chop the mushrooms and cut the asparagus into 1½-inch-long pieces. Peel the garlic and mash. Transfer the asparagus to a bowl and drizzle with the olive oil and lemon juice. Add the garlic and mushrooms and mix to combine.

BONUS YEARS DAILY PERCENTAGES

Per serving: Fruits and vegetables 20%; Garlic 100%

NUTRITIONAL ANALYSIS

Per serving: Calories 68, Protein 5g, Total fat 2g, Sat fat 0g, Trans fat 0g,
Cholesterol 0mg, Carbohydrate 9g, Dietary fiber 3g, Sodium 455mg

ROASTED NEW POTATOES

NUTRITIONAL ANALYSIS

Per serving: Calories 110, Protein 3g, Total fat 3g, Sat fat .5g, Trans fat 0g,
Cholesterol 0mg, Carbohydrate 20g, Dietary fiber 2g, Sodium 30mg

RED WINE

NUTRITIONAL ANALYSIS

Per 5 ounces: Calories 106, Protein 0g, Total fat 0g, Sat fat 0g, Trans fat 0g,
Cholesterol 0mg, Carbohydrate 2g, Dietary fiber 0g, Sodium 7mg

DARK CHOCOLATE

NUTRITIONAL ANALYSIS

Per 2 ounces: Calories 302, Protein 3g, Total fat 16g, Sat fat 10g, Trans fat 0g,
Cholesterol 0mg, Carbohydrate 36g, Dietary fiber 2g, Sodium 9mg

NUTS

NUTRITIONAL ANALYSIS

Per 1½ ounces: Calories 253, Protein 7g, Total fat 22g, Sat fat 3g, Trans fat 0g,
Cholesterol 0mg, Carbohydrate 11g, Dietary fiber 4g, Sodium 5mg

DAY 12: THURSDAY

Breakfast

Spiced Steel-Cut Oatmeal

BONUS YEARS POINTS: FRUITS AND VEGETABLES 35%;
NUTS 50%

CALORIES: 532

Lunch

Middle Eastern Pita Salad

BONUS YEARS POINTS: FRUITS AND VEGETABLES 45%

CALORIES: 289

Dinner

Three-Pepper and Beef Stir-fry
½ cup cooked soba noodles

BONUS YEARS POINTS: FRUITS AND VEGETABLES 30%;
GARLIC 100%

CALORIES: 364

5 ounces wine

BONUS YEARS POINTS: WINE 100%

CALORIES: 106

Snacks

2 ounces dark chocolate

BONUS YEARS POINTS: CHOCOLATE 100%

CALORIES: 302

1 ounce unsalted dry-roasted
or natural nuts

BONUS YEARS POINTS: NUTS 50%

CALORIES: 160

DAY'S TOTAL BONUS YEARS POINTS: WINE 100%; CHOCOLATE 100%;
FRUITS AND VEGETABLES 110%; GARLIC 100%; NUTS 100%
TOTAL CALORIES: 1,761

Spiced Steel-Cut Oatmeal

---

2 teaspoons canola oil

1 cup steel-cut oats

3 cups apple juice, heated to a simmer

¼ teaspoon ground cinnamon

1 teaspoon ground nutmeg

1 tablespoon light brown sugar

1 cup fat-free milk

3 cups mixed berries of your choice

4 ounces chopped nuts (1 cup)

Heat the oil in a heavy 3- to 4-quart saucepan over medium heat. Add the oats and sauté for about 3 minutes, stirring often. Add the apple juice, cinnamon, nutmeg, and brown sugar. Cover and simmer until all the liquid has evaporated, about 20 minutes. Stir and divide among four breakfast bowls. Top each serving with ¼ cup of the milk, ¾ cup of the berries, and ¼ cup of the nuts.

BONUS YEARS DAILY PERCENTAGES

Per serving: Fruit and vegetables 35%; Nuts 50%

NUTRITIONAL ANALYSIS

Per serving: Calories 532, Protein 15g, Total fat 20g, Sat fat 2g, Trans fat 0g, Cholesterol 1mg, Carbohydrate 74g, Dietary fiber 15g, Sodium 39mg

Middle Eastern Pita Salad

MAKES 4 SANDWICHES

2 Roma tomatoes (6 ounces), chopped into small dice
½ hothouse or English cucumber (7 ounces), peeled and
   chopped into small dice
1 small red bell pepper (4 ounces), chopped into small dice
1 small green bell pepper (4 ounces), chopped into small dice
⅔ bunch radishes (3 ounces), chopped into small dice
3 to 4 green onions (green parts only), chopped into
   small dice
½ cup coarsely chopped pitted green olives (2 ounces)
3 tablespoons finely chopped dill
2 tablespoons extra-virgin olive oil
2 tablespoons freshly squeezed lemon juice
kosher salt and freshly ground black pepper, to taste
4 large (about 7-inch) pita breads (3 ounces each), cut in half
   crosswise and pockets opened

Mix all the vegetables, olives, and dill together in a medium bowl. Add the olive oil, lemon juice, salt, and pepper and toss to combine. Fill the pitas with the vegetable mixture.

To Make Ahead: Combine the vegetables, olives, and dill in a bowl, cover, and refrigerate. Toss with the olive oil and lemon juice and stuff into the pita pockets just before serving.

BONUS YEARS DAILY PERCENTAGES

Per serving: Fruits and vegetables 45%

NUTRITIONAL ANALYSIS

Per serving: Calories 289, Protein 7g, Total fat 10g, Sat fat 1g, Trans fat 0g, Cholesterol mg, Carbohydrate 43g, Dietary fiber 3g, Sodium 573mg

Three-Pepper and Beef Stir-fry

A simple stir-fry is made special by marinating the beef in the cornstarch and wine, a wonderful way to prepare tender and succulent meats and poultry.

Serve a simple, soft red wine, such as an easy drinking Cabernet Sauvignon or Syrah.

1 (1-pound) beef flank steak

1 tablespoon dry sherry or Chinese rice wine

1 egg white

2 tablespoons low-sodium soy sauce

⅛ teaspoon freshly ground black pepper

1 tablespoon cornstarch

1 tablespoon canola or grapeseed oil

2 cups sliced onions in matchstick-size lengths (about 8 ounces)

1 small green bell pepper (4 ounces), cut into matchstick pieces

1 small red bell pepper (4 ounces), cut into matchstick pieces

1 tablespoon minced garlic

1 tablespoon minced fresh ginger

½ teaspoon red pepper flakes

¼ to ½ teaspoon kosher salt

½ teaspoon sugar

1 teaspoon Asian sesame oil

Place the flank steak in the freezer for about 30 minutes to make it easier to slice. Remove the meat from the freezer, and cut crosswise against the grain into ¼-inch strips, then cut these strips lengthwise in half and then into 2- to 3-inch-long slices. Mix the sherry, egg white, 1 tablespoon of the soy sauce, the black pepper and cornstarch in a medium bowl to form a paste. Add the steak and stir to coat with the cornstarch mixture. Let stand for 30 minutes to 1 hour.

Meanwhile, bring a small saucepan of water to a boil. Prepare a bowl of ice and water. Drain off the excess marinade from the beef. Add the beef to the boiling water and drain after 1 minute. Immediately transfer the beef to the ice water to stop the cooking. Drain the beef, pat dry, and reserve.

Heat the oil in a nonstick 12-inch skillet over medium heat. Add the onions and stir-fry for 3 minutes. Add the bell peppers and stir-fry for 2 to 3 minutes. Add the reserved beef, mix thoroughly, and cook for 2 to 3 minutes. Add the garlic and ginger and stir-fry for about 2 minutes. Stir in the remaining 1 tablespoon of soy sauce, the pepper flakes, salt, sugar, and sesame oil, combining the seasonings with the meat and the vegetables.

BONUS YEARS DAILY PERCENTAGES

Per serving: Fruits and vegetables 30%; Garlic 100%

NUTRITIONAL ANALYSIS

Per serving: Calories 308, Protein 25g, Total fat 17g, Sat fat 6g, Trans fat 0g, Cholesterol 59mg, Carbohydrate 13g, Sodium 515mg

COOKED SOBA NOODLES

NUTRITIONAL ANALYSIS

Per ½-cup serving: Calories 56, Protein 3g, Total fat 0g, Sat fat 0g, Trans fat 0g, Cholesterol 0mg, Carbohydrate 12g, Dietary fiber 0g, Sodium 34mg

RED WINE

NUTRITIONAL ANALYSIS

Per 5 ounces: Calories 106, Protein 0g, Total fat 0g, Sat fat 0g, Trans fat 0g, Cholesterol 0mg, Carbohydrate 2g, Dietary fiber 0g, Sodium 7mg

DARK CHOCOLATE

NUTRITIONAL ANALYSIS

Per 2 ounces: Calories 302, Protein 3g, Total fat 16g, Sat fat 10g, Trans fat 0g, Cholesterol 0mg, Carbohydrate 36g, Dietary fiber 2g, Sodium 9mg

NUTS

NUTRITIONAL ANALYSIS

Per 1 ounce: Calories 168, Protein 5g, Total fat 14g, Sat fat 2g, Trans fat 0g, Cholesterol 0mg, Carbohydrate 7g, Dietary fiber 2g, Sodium 3mg

DAY 13: FRIDAY

Breakfast

Muesli and Berry Breakfast
BONUS YEARS POINTS: FRUITS AND VEGETABLES 20%;
NUTS 25%
CALORIES: 397

Lunch

Chicken Spinach Salad with Plum Sauce Vinaigrette
BONUS YEARS POINTS: FRUITS AND VEGETABLES 25%
CALORIES: 278

Dinner

Shrimp Creole with Rice Mixed Fruit Compote
BONUS YEARS POINTS: FRUITS AND VEGETABLES 75%;
FISH 80%; GARLIC 100%; NUTS 25%
CALORIES: 700

5 ounces wine
BONUS YEARS POINTS: WINE 100%
CALORIES: 106

Snacks

2 ounces dark chocolate
BONUS YEARS POINTS: CHOCOLATE 100%
CALORIES: 302

1 ounce unsalted dry-roasted or natural nuts
BONUS YEARS POINTS: NUTS 50%
CALORIES: 168

DAY'S TOTAL BONUS YEARS POINTS: WINE **100%**; CHOCOLATE **100%**;
FRUITS AND VEGETABLES **120%**; FISH **80%**; GARLIC **100%**; NUTS **100%**
TOTAL CALORIES: **1,951**

Muesli and Berry Breakfast

MAKES 1 SERVING

¾ cup low-fat muesli or other low-fat, high-fiber cereal
½ cup fat-free milk
½ cup fresh berries
2 tablespoons chopped nuts (½ ounce)

Mix the muesli and milk in a serving bowl and top with the berries and nuts.

BONUS YEARS DAILY PERCENTAGES

Per serving: Fruits and vegetables 20%; Nuts 25%

NUTRITIONAL ANALYSIS

Per serving: Calories 397, Protein 14g, Total fat 13g, Sat fat 1g, Trans fat 0g, Cholesterol 2mg, Carbohydrate 64g, Dietary fiber 10g, Sodium 150mg

Chicken Spinach Salad
with Plum Sauce Vinaigrette

MAKES 4 SERVINGS; 10 TABLESPOONS VINAIGRETTE

This combination of Japanese and Chinese condiments makes a light, tangy vinaigrette that is one of my favorites.

PLUM SAUCE VINAIGRETTE

3 tablespoons mirin (rice wine)
2 tablespoons white (mild) shiro miso
1½ tablespoons plum sauce
2 teaspoons Asian sesame oil
1 tablespoon unseasoned rice vinegar
1 tablespoon low-sodium soy sauce
1 tablespoon water
1½ teaspoons Dijon mustard
¼ teaspoon Asian chili paste

1 cup thinly sliced red onion (4 ounces)
8 cups loosely packed fresh spinach (about 6 ounces), large
    stems removed, washed, and spun dry
1½ cups thinly sliced button mushrooms
1 cup julienned carrots (3 ounces)
12 ounces cubed, cooked chicken
2 tablespoons freshly squeezed lime juice

To make the vinaigrette, thoroughly whisk all the ingredients together in a small bowl.

To make the salad, place the onion in a bowl of cold water for about 20 minutes, remove, and spin the onion dry.

Thoroughly toss all the ingredients, except the vinaigrette and lime juice, in a large bowl. Add the vinaigrette and lime juice; mix until evenly coated.

To Make Ahead: Make the vinaigrette, cover, and refrigerate. Combine all the remaining ingredients, except the lime juice, in a bowl, cover, and refrigerate. Bring the vinaigrette to room temperature and whisk again before tossing with the salad and lime juice.

BONUS YEARS DAILY PERCENTAGES

Per serving: Fruits and vegetables 25%

NUTRITIONAL ANALYSIS

Per serving: Calories 278, Protein 31g, Total fat 7g, Sat fat 1g, Trans fat 0g, Cholesterol 72mg, Carbohydrate 20g, Dietary fiber 5g, Sodium 706mg

Shrimp Creole with Rice

MAKES 4 SERVINGS

This dish is seasoned with onion, celery, and bell peppers, sometimes called the Holy Trinity in Creole cooking in New Orleans.

1 tablespoon canola or grapeseed oil

1 large onion (8 ounces), diced (1¼ cups)

2 celery stalks (4 ounces), cut into ½-inch dice (1 cup)

1 small green bell pepper (4 ounces), cut into ¼-inch dice
  (1 cup)

1½ teaspoons Creole or Cajun seasoning

4 cloves garlic, thinly sliced

1 tablespoon tomato paste

1 (14.5-ounce) can diced tomatoes, drained

1¼ cups low-sodium chicken broth

1¼ pounds shrimp (21 to 25 per pound), peeled and deveined

kosher salt and freshly ground black pepper, to taste

2 cups cooked white rice

¼ cup chopped flat-leaf parsley, for garnish

Heat the oil in a 12-inch skillet over medium heat. Add the onion, celery, and bell pepper and sauté for 5 minutes. Add the Creole seasoning and garlic and sauté for 1 minute. Stir in the tomato paste and cook for 1 minute. Add the tomatoes and broth. Reduce the heat to low and simmer for about 7 minutes. Add the shrimp and simmer until the shrimp are just cooked through, 3 to 5 minutes. Season with salt and pepper.

Divide the rice among four plates, top each serving with one-fourth of the shrimp and tomato sauce, and garnish with the parsley.

BONUS YEARS DAILY PERCENTAGES

Per serving: Fruits and vegetables 50%; Fish 80%; Garlic 100%

NUTRITIONAL ANALYSIS

Per serving: Calories 374, Protein 34g, Total fat 7g, Sat fat 1g, Trans fat 0g, Cholesterol 217mg, Carbohydrate 43g, Dietary fiber 3g, Sodium 421mg

Mixed Fruit Compote

1 (8-ounce) package mixed dried fruit
grated fresh zest and juice of 2 medium oranges (about
    1 cup juice)
grated fresh zest and juice of 1 lemon
¼ cup packed light brown sugar
1 cinnamon stick
¼ cup orange liqueur, such as triple sec or Grand Marnier
    (optional, but strongly recommended)
½ cup coarsely chopped almonds (2 ounces)

Coarsely chop the dried fruit. Place the dried fruit in a heavy, 2- or 3-quart saucepan. Add the orange zest and juice. Add the lemon zest and juice, reserving 1 tablespoon lemon juice. Add the sugar and cinnamon stick. Simmer over low heat until the fruit is tender and the juices nicely thickened, about 15 minutes. Take the saucepan off the heat and let cool for about 5 minutes. Stir in the liqueur (if using) and the reserved 1 tablespoon lemon juice. Transfer to a bowl, cover, and refrigerate until chilled. Discard the cinnamon stick. To serve, divide among four small bowls and top with the almonds.

BONUS YEARS DAILY PERCENTAGES
Per serving: Fruits and vegetables 25%; Nuts 25%

NUTRITIONAL ANALYSIS
Per serving: Calories 326, Protein 5g, Total fat 9g, Sat fat 1g, Trans fat 0g,
Cholesterol 0mg, Carbohydrate 60g, Dietary fiber 7g, Sodium 16mg

RED WINE
NUTRITIONAL ANALYSIS
Per 5 ounces: Calories 106, Protein 0g, Total fat 0g, Sat fat 0g, Trans fat 0g, Cholesterol 0mg, Carbohydrate 2g, Dietary fiber 0g, Sodium 7mg

DARK CHOCOLATE
NUTRITIONAL ANALYSIS
Per 5 ounces: Calories 106, Protein 0g, Total fat 0g, Sat fat 0g, Trans fat 0g, Cholesterol 0mg, Carbohydrate 2g, Dietary fiber 0g, Sodium 7mg

NUTS
NUTRITIONAL ANALYSIS
Per 1 ounce: Calories 168, Protein 5g, Total fat 14g, Sat fat 2g, Trans fat 0g, Cholesterol 0mg, Carbohydrate 7g, Dietary fiber 2g, Sodium 3mg

DAY 14: SATURDAY

Breakfast

Garden Frittata
with Sun-Dried Tomatoes
BONUS YEARS POINTS: FRUITS AND VEGETABLES 30%;
GARLIC 100%
CALORIES: 227

Lunch

Greek Salad
½ piece whole wheat pita bread
BONUS YEARS POINTS: FRUITS AND VEGETABLES 55%
CALORIES: 300

Dinner

Broiled Tuscan-Style Flank Steak
Ice cream with Raspberry Coulis
(page 171)
BONUS YEARS POINTS: FRUITS AND VEGETABLES 35%;
GARLIC 100%
CALORIES: 833

5 ounces wine
BONUS YEARS POINTS: WINE 100%
CALORIES: 106

Snacks

2 ounces dark chocolate
BONUS YEARS POINTS: CHOCOLATE 100%
CALORIES: 302

2 ounces unsalted dry-roasted
or natural nuts
BONUS YEARS POINTS: NUTS 100%
CALORIES: 337

DAY'S TOTAL BONUS YEARS POINTS: WINE **100%**; CHOCOLATE **100%**;
FRUITS AND VEGETABLES **120%**; GARLIC **200%**; NUTS **100%**
TOTAL CALORIES: **2,105**

Garden Frittata
with Sun-Dried Tomatoes

MAKES 4 SERVINGS

1¼ cups egg substitute, or 5 eggs, at room temperature
kosher salt and freshly ground black pepper, to taste
⅔ cup freshly grated Parmesan cheese
2 teaspoons extra-virgin olive oil
1 green onion (white and green parts), thinly sliced on the
   diagonal
1 zucchini (6 to 7 ounces), cut into ¼-inch dice (about 1 cup)
1 small red bell pepper (about 4 ounces), cut into ¼-inch dice
   (about 1 cup)
4 cloves garlic, thinly sliced
1 cup frozen green peas, thawed
½ cup dry-packed sun-dried tomatoes, rehydrated in ¾ cup
   hot water, drained, and thinly sliced
2 tablespoons sweet paprika

Season the egg substitute with salt and pepper; stir briefly with a
fork. Add ¼ cup of the cheese and set aside.

Heat a 12-inch ovenproof nonstick skillet over medium-high heat.
Add the oil, and heat until it begins to shimmer. Add the green onion
and sauté for about 30 seconds. Add the zucchini and bell pepper and
sauté for about 2 minutes. Add the garlic and peas and cook until the
vegetables are crisp-tender, 2 or 3 minutes.

Preheat the broiler. Pour the egg mixture into the skillet and reduce the heat to low. Stir until curds begin to form, and then cook until the eggs are just slightly creamy on top, about 4 minutes. Top with
the remaining cheese, tomatoes, and paprika. Place under the broiler
for 2 to 4 minutes, or until the frittata begins to brown; watch it

closely to keep it from burning. Remove the frittata from the oven, slide it onto a plate, and divide into four servings.

BONUS YEARS DAILY PERCENTAGES

Per serving: Fruits and vegetables 30%; Garlic 100%

NUTRITIONAL ANALYSIS

Per serving: Calories 227, Protein 19g, Total fat 10g, Sat fat 3g, Trans fat 0g, Cholesterol 11mg, Carbohydrate 17g, Dietary fiber 5g, Sodium 531mg

Greek Salad

4 tablespoons thickened chicken broth (see page 377)

2 tablespoons extra-virgin olive oil

3 tablespoons freshly squeezed lemon juice

½ teaspoon dried oregano

12 black olives (2 ounces), such as kalamatas, pitted and
coarsely sliced

1½ cups thinly sliced red onion (3 ounces)

1 small red bell pepper (4 ounces), cut into rings

1 large tomato (10 ounces), cut into 16 wedges

½ hothouse or English cucumber (7 ounces), unpeeled, cut
into thin rings

6 cups loosely packed mixed salad greens (about 5 ounces)

kosher salt and freshly ground black pepper, to taste

1 cup chopped low-fat feta cheese

Whisk together the thickened broth, olive oil, and lemon juice.
Add the oregano.

In a large salad bowl, mix the olives, onion, bell pepper, tomato,
and cucumber. Add the olive oil mixture and let stand for about
30 minutes, or up to 4 hours in the refrigerator. Add the salad greens
and toss to combine. Season with salt and pepper, remembering that
the feta is salty. Divide among four plates and garnish each plate with
one-fourth of the feta cheese.

Per 1½-cup serving: Fruits and vegetables 55%

NUTRITIONAL ANALYSIS

Per 1½-cup serving: Calories 215, Protein 9g, Total fat 14g, Sat fat 3g, Trans fat 0g, Cholesterol 10mg, Carbohydrate 17g, Dietary fiber 5g, Sodium 591mg

WHOLE WHEAT PITA BREAD

NUTRITIONAL ANALYSIS

Per ½ piece: Calories 85, Protein 3g, Total fat 1g, Sat fat 0g, Trans fat 0g, Cholesterol 0mg, Carbohydrate 18g, Dietary fiber 2g, Sodium 170mg

Broiled Tuscan-Style Flank Steak

MAKES 4 SERVINGS

Seared steak and cannellini beans are staples of Tuscan cuisine, so why not combine them! Heating the olive oil with the garlic and seasonings adds flavor to the oil.

Serve a Chianti Classico wine with the steak.

⅓ cup extra-virgin olive oil
1 tablespoon Italian seasoning
4 large cloves garlic, thinly sliced
⅓ cup thickened chicken broth (see page 377)
⅓ cup freshly squeezed lemon juice
kosher salt and freshly ground black pepper, to taste
1 (1¾-pound) beef flank steak
2 cups cooked cannellini or great northern beans, drained
  (see Dr. Chef's Note, page 111)
2 medium Roma tomatoes (about 6 ounces), cored, seeds
  removed, and finely diced
¼ cup chopped flat-leaf parsley

Heat the olive oil in a small saucepan over low heat. Add the Italian seasoning and garlic, and cook for about 3 minutes, stirring often.

Remove the pan from the heat, add the broth, lemon juice, salt, and pepper, and mix thoroughly. Pour into a glass bowl and let cool in the refrigerator for about 5 minutes. Add the steak to the lemon juice mixture and let marinate for 45 minutes at room temperature or up to 2 hours in the refrigerator.

Meanwhile, thoroughly mix the beans, tomatoes, and parsley in a small bowl.

Preheat the broiler. Drain the steak, reserving the marinade. Broil the steak for 4½ minutes on each side. Remove the steak, cover, and let stand for about 10 minutes.

Bring the reserved marinade to a low boil. Pour ¼ cup of the marinade over the bean mixture. Season the beans with salt and pepper. Slice the steak across the grain into ⅛-inch-thick slices. Reserve one-fourth of the sliced steak for lunch the next day. Divide the remaining sliced steak and the bean mixture among four plates.

BONUS YEARS DAILY PERCENTAGES

Per serving: Fruits and vegetables 30%; Garlic 100%

NUTRITIONAL ANALYSIS

Per serving: Calories 593, Protein 44, Total fat 40g, Sat fat 11g, Trans fat 0g, Cholesterol 103mg, Carbohydrate 14g, Dietary fiber 4g, Sodium 157mg

½ CUP LIGHT ICE CREAM WITH ¼ CUP RASPBERRY COULIS
(page 171)

BONUS YEARS DAILY PERCENTAGES

Per serving: Fruits and vegetables 5%

NUTRITIONAL ANALYSIS

Per serving: Calories 240, Protein 4g, Total fat 2g, Sat fat 1g, Trans fat 0g, Cholesterol 5mg, Carbohydrate 50g, Dietary fiber 4g, Sodium 45mg

RED WINE

NUTRITIONAL ANALYSIS

Per 5 ounces: Calories 106, Protein 0g, Total fat 0g, Sat fat 0g, Trans fat 0g, Cholesterol 0mg, Carbohydrate 2g, Dietary fiber 0g, Sodium 7mg

DARK CHOCOLATE

NUTRITIONAL ANALYSIS

Per 2 ounces: Calories 302, Protein 3g, Total fat 16g, Sat fat 10g, Trans fat 0g, Cholesterol 0mg, Carbohydrate 36g, Dietary fiber 2g, Sodium 9mg

NUTS

NUTRITIONAL ANALYSIS

Per 2 ounces: Calories 337, Protein 10g, Total fat 29g, Sat fat 4g, Trans fat 0g, Cholesterol 0mg, Carbohydrate 14g, Dietary fiber 5g, Sodium 7mg

DAY 15: SUNDAY

Breakfast

Chocolate Waffles
with Orange-Raspberry Syrup
BONUS YEARS POINTS: CHOCOLATE 25%;
FRUITS AND VEGETABLES 10%

CALORIES: 217

Lunch

Oven-Roasted Pork Chops with
Sun-Dried Cherry Wine Sauce
Roasted Root-Vegetable Puree with
Horseradish (page 175)
½ cup steamed kale or other greens
BONUS YEARS POINTS: FRUITS AND VEGETABLES 50%

CALORIES: 451

Dinner

Bulgur Pilaf
Tossed green salad with
low-fat dressing
Ice Cream with
Chocolate–Peanut Butter Sauce
BONUS YEARS POINTS: CHOCOLATE 50%; FRUITS AND
VEGETABLES 80%; GARLIC 100%; NUTS 100%

CALORIES: 1,020

5 ounces wine
BONUS YEARS POINTS: WINE 100%

CALORIES: 106

Snacks

½ ounce dark chocolate
BONUS YEARS POINTS: CHOCOLATE 25%

CALORIES: 75

DAY'S TOTAL BONUS YEARS POINTS: WINE 100%; CHOCOLATE 100%;
FRUITS AND VEGETABLES 140%; GARLIC 100%; NUTS 100%

TOTAL CALORIES: 1,869

Chocolate Waffles
with Orange-Raspberry Syrup

MAKES ABOUT 4 WAFFLES; 8 SERVINGS

¾ cup unbleached all-purpose flour
¾ cup white whole wheat or regular whole wheat flour
⅓ cup unsweetened cocoa powder (not Dutch processed)
1½ tablespoons sugar
2 teaspoons baking powder
¼ teaspoon baking soda
pinch kosher salt
1½ cups low-fat buttermilk
½ cup egg substitute, or 2 eggs, lightly beaten
2 tablespoons canola oil
1 teaspoon vanilla extract
Orange-Raspberry Syrup (recipe follows)
8 tablespoons chopped pecans (optional)

Preheat a nonstick waffle iron. Combine the flours, cocoa powder, sugar, baking powder, baking soda, and salt in a medium bowl. Combine the buttermilk, egg substitute, oil, and vanilla in another bowl. Add the buttermilk mixture to the dry ingredients and stir just until combined.

Spoon the batter into the hot waffle iron and cook according to manufacturer's directions. (Waffles can be cooled and wrapped individually in plastic wrap and placed in a plastic freezer bag or container and frozen up to 1 month. Heat in a toaster or 350-degree oven.) Serve with syrup and sprinkle each serving with 1 tablespoon of the pecans, if using.

BONUS YEARS DAILY PERCENTAGES

Per serving: Chocolate 25%

NUTRITIONAL ANALYSIS

Per serving (without syrup): Calories 174, Protein 6g, Total fat 6g, Sat fat 0g, Trans fat 0g, Cholesterol 2mg, Carbohydrate 24g, Dietary fiber 3g, Sodium 237mg

Orange-Raspberry Syrup

1 cup freshly squeezed orange juice
2 teaspoons cornstarch
2 tablespoons mild honey, or to taste
1½ cups fresh raspberries or frozen unsweetened raspberries
1 tablespoon grated fresh orange zest

Combine a little of the orange juice with the cornstarch in a medium saucepan. Whisk in the remaining orange juice and honey. Cook, stirring constantly, over medium heat until the mixture is bubbly and slightly thickened. Stir in the raspberries and orange zest. Serve warm.

BONUS YEARS DAILY PERCENTAGES
Per serving: Fruits and vegetables 10%

NUTRITIONAL ANALYSIS
Per serving: Calories 43, Protein 0g, Total fat 0g, Sat fat 0g, Trans fat 0g, Cholesterol 0mg, Carbohydrate 11g, Dietary fiber 2g, Sodium 1mg

Oven-Roasted Pork Chops
with Sun-Dried Cherry Wine Sauce

MAKES 4 SERVINGS

The rich, tangy sauce will go well with a Valpolicella or Beaujolais wine.

4 (1- to 1¼-inch) bone-in loin or rib pork chops (about
   2 pounds total), preferably brined (see page 376) for 2 hours
¾ cup freshly squeezed orange juice
1 tablespoon red wine vinegar
¾ cup sun-dried cherries
2 tablespoons extra-virgin olive oil
2 tablespoons chopped shallot
½ teaspoon dried thyme
¼ cup dry red wine
1½ cups low-sodium chicken broth, preferably dark broth
¾ teaspoon light brown sugar
kosher salt and freshly ground black pepper, to taste
½ teaspoon arrowroot dissolved in ½ teaspoon water

Rinse the pork under cold water and pat dry.
Bring the orange juice and vinegar to a low simmer in a small saucepan. Remove from the heat and add the cherries to the liquid to reconstitute.

Preheat the oven to 350 degrees. Heat 1½ tablespoons of the olive oil in a large skillet over medium heat. Reduce the heat to low and add the pork chops and cook until they are nicely browned on both sides, about 6 minutes total cooking time.

Transfer the chops to a baking pan; reserve the drippings in the skillet. Bake for 7 to 9 minutes, or until the pork chops are still a bit pink in the center (about 140 degrees on an instant-read thermometer). Remove the pork chops from the oven, cover, and keep warm.

Add the remaining ½ tablespoon olive oil to the drippings in the skillet and heat over medium heat. Add the shallot and sauté for 1 to 2 minutes. Add the thyme and sauté for 1 minute. Add the wine and broth and simmer until reduced to 1 cup. Add the cherries and their soaking liquid and simmer until the liquid is reduced to about ¾ cup. Stir in the brown sugar, and season with salt and pepper. Stir in the arrowroot mixture and cook, stirring, until thickened.

To serve, place a pork chop on each of four plates and top with one-fourth of the cherry wine sauce.

BONUS YEARS DAILY PERCENTAGES
Per serving: Fruits and vegetables 10%

NUTRITIONAL ANALYSIS
Per serving: Calories 433, Protein 32g, Total fat 17g, Sat fat 4g, Trans fat 0g, Cholesterol 89mg, Carbohydrate 28g, Dietary fiber 1g, Sodium 102mg

Dr. Chef's Note

Brining pork chops (page 376) assures moist and flavorful meat. Don't overcook; remove the pork from the oven when the meat reaches an internal temperature of 140 degrees.

KALE

BONUS YEARS DAILY PERCENTAGES
Per ½-cup serving, cooked: Fruits and vegetables 20%

NUTRITIONAL ANALYSIS
Per ½-cup serving, cooked: Calories 18, Protein 1g, Total fat 0g, Sat fat 0g, Trans fat 0g, Cholesterol 0mg, Carbohydrate 3g, Dietary fiber 1g, Sodium 15mg

Bulgur Pilaf

This is a hearty dish that can serve as a vegetarian entrée. Sautéing the barley in oil, the traditional method for making pilaf, adds a nuttiness to the flavor and ensures the individual grains will be separate and fluffy.

1½ tablespoons canola oil

1½ teaspoons ground, toasted cumin seed (see page 378)

1 large red onion (about 8 ounces), coarsely diced (2 cups)

6 large cloves garlic, minced

1½ cups coarse-grain bulgur wheat

2¼ cups low-sodium vegetable or chicken broth, brought to a simmer

1 (14.5-ounce) can diced tomatoes

3 medium carrots (about 10 ounces), cut into ¾-inch dice (about 2½ cups)

1¼ pounds new red potatoes, cut into ¾-inch dice, or baby red potatoes, cut into eighths

1 teaspoon salt

½ teaspoon freshly ground black pepper

¾ cup minced flat-leaf parsley

Heat the oil in a heavy, 4-quart saucepan over medium heat. Add the cumin and sauté for about 30 seconds. Add the onion and sauté until it begins to soften, for about 3 minutes. Add the garlic and sauté for 2 minutes. Add the bulgur to the saucepan and sauté for 4 to 5 minutes, stirring constantly.

Add the stock, tomatoes with their juices, carrots, potatoes, salt, and pepper. Bring to a low boil; reduce the heat, cover, and simmer for about 20 minutes. Remove from the heat, and let sit for 10 minutes. Stir in the parsley. Reserve 2 cups for lunch. Divide the remaining bulgur among four plates.

BONUS YEARS DAILY PERCENTAGES

Per 1½-cup serving: Fruits and vegetables 60%; Garlic 100%

Per 1-cup serving: Fruits and vegetables 45%; Garlic 50%

NUTRITIONAL ANALYSIS

Per 1½-cup serving: Calories 321, Protein 10g, Total fat 6g, Sat fat 1g, Trans fat 0g, Cholesterol 0mg, Carbohydrate 61g, Dietary fiber 12g, Sodium 549mg

Per 1-cup serving: Calories 214, Protein 7g, Total fat 4g, Sat fat 0g, Trans fat 0g, Cholesterol 0mg, Carbohydrate 41g, Dietary fiber 8g, Sodium 366mg

TOSSED GREEN SALAD WITH LOW-FAT DRESSING

BONUS YEARS DAILY PERCENTAGES

Per ½-cup serving: Fruits and vegetables 20%

NUTRITIONAL ANALYSIS

Per ½-cup serving: Calories, Protein 1g, Total fat 3g, Sat fat 0g, Trans fat 0g, Cholesterol 0mg, Carbohydrate 4g, Dietary fiber 2g, Sodium 257mg

Ice Cream with
Chocolate–Peanut Butter Sauce

MAKES 4 SERVINGS

———

The sauce can be made ahead and warmed in the microwave before serving.

4 ounces semisweet or bittersweet chocolate, coarsely
   chopped
1 cup crunchy natural peanut butter
2 cups reduced-fat vanilla ice cream

Place the chocolate in a microwave-safe bowl. Microwave on medium until melted, stirring after every minute (time will vary depending on the power of the microwave). Cool slightly and stir in peanut butter.

Divide ice cream among four dessert dishes. Top with warm sauce.

BONUS YEARS DAILY PERCENTAGES
Per serving: Chocolate 50%; Nuts 100%

NUTRITIONAL ANALYSIS
Per serving: Calories 654, Protein 19g, Total fat 45g, Sat fat 11g, Trans fat 0g, Cholesterol 5mg, Carbohydrate 46g, Dietary fiber 6g, Sodium 285mg

RED WINE

NUTRITIONAL ANALYSIS

Per 5 ounces: Calories 106, Protein 0g, Total fat 0g, Sat fat 0g, Trans fat 0g, Cholesterol 0mg, Carbohydrate 2g, Dietary fiber 0g, Sodium 7mg

DARK CHOCOLATE

NUTRITIONAL ANALYSIS

Per ½ ounce: Calories 75, Protein 1g, Total fat 4g, Sat fat 2g, Trans fat 0g, Cholesterol 0mg, Carbohydrate 9g, Dietary fiber 1g, Sodium 2mg

DAY 16: MONDAY

Breakfast

Creamy Old-fashioned Oatmeal
with Dried Cranberries and
Slivered Almonds
BONUS YEARS POINTS: FRUITS AND VEGETABLES 20%;
NUTS 50%
CALORIES: 459

Lunch

Ramen Noodle Salad with
Balsamic Cilantro Vinaigrette
BONUS YEARS POINTS: FRUITS AND VEGETABLES 20%;
GARLIC 100%
CALORIES: 224

Dinner

Oven-Fried Cajun Catfish
Cajun Okra-Tomato Braise
½ cup steamed brown rice
BONUS YEARS POINTS: FRUITS AND VEGETABLES 35%;
FISH 100%
CALORIES: 528

5 ounces wine
BONUS YEARS POINTS: WINE 100%
CALORIES: 106

Snacks

2 ounces dark chocolate
BONUS YEARS POINTS: CHOCOLATE 100%
CALORIES: 302

1 ounce unsalted dry-roasted
or natural nuts
BONUS YEARS POINTS: NUTS 50%
CALORIES: 168

25 grapes
BONUS YEARS POINTS: FRUITS AND VEGETABLES 25%
CALORIES: 89

DAY'S TOTAL BONUS YEARS POINTS: WINE 100%; CHOCOLATE 100%;
FRUITS AND VEGETABLES 100%; FISH 100%; GARLIC 100%; NUTS 100%

TOTAL CALORIES: 1,876

Creamy Old-fashioned Oatmeal with Dried Cranberries and Slivered Almonds

MAKES 4 SERVINGS

1½ cups old-fashioned rolled oats
about 4 cups fat-free milk
1 cup water
½ cup dried cranberries
dash kosher salt
1 cup slivered almonds (4 ounces)

Combine the oats, 2 cups of the milk, water, cranberries, and salt in a medium saucepan over medium heat. Bring to a boil, stirring occasionally. Reduce the heat and simmer for 5 minutes. Cover and let stand 5 minutes.

Spoon the oatmeal into four bowls. Top each serving with about ½ cup of the remaining milk and ¼ cup of the almonds.

BONUS YEARS DAILY PERCENTAGES
Per serving: Fruits and vegetables 20%; Nuts 50%

NUTRITIONAL ANALYSIS
Per serving: Calories 459, Protein 20g, Total fat 20g, Sat fat 2g, Trans fat 0g, Cholesterol 5mg, Carbohydrate 53g, Dietary fiber 8g, Sodium 131mg

Ramen Noodle Salad
with Balsamic Cilantro Vinaigrette

MAKES 4 (1½-CUP) SERVINGS

Ramen noodles are great for a light Asian salad. The combination of the balsamic vinegar and the mirin give the vinaigrette a smooth and mellow flavor.

BALSAMIC CILANTRO VINAIGRETTE

¼ cup low-sodium soy sauce
2 tablespoons balsamic vinegar
2 tablespoons unseasoned rice wine vinegar
1 tablespoon mirin or sweet sherry
1 tablespoon sugar
1 tablespoon Asian sesame oil
2 tablespoons minced cilantro
4 large cloves garlic, minced

10 dried shiitake mushrooms, or 8 ounces fresh shiitake or
  brown mushrooms (about 1½ cups sliced)
2 (3-ounce) packages low-fat ramen noodles (90% less fat
  than the traditional fried variety, available in health food
  stores)
2 teaspoons Asian sesame oil
4 ounces snow peas
1 medium carrot (about 3 ounces), cut into matchstick-size
  pieces
1 large red bell pepper (about 6 ounces), cut into matchstick-
  size pieces
3 green onions, cut diagonally into thin slices
¼ teaspoon Asian chili paste

Make the vinaigrette: Combine all the ingredients in a bowl and whisk to combine. Set aside.

Soak the dried mushrooms in hot water for 30 minutes. Rinse, discard the stems, and cut the caps into thin slivers. If using fresh mushrooms, cut them into thin slivers.

Prepare the noodles according to the package directions, discarding the packaged seasonings. Drain the noodles, toss with the oil, and chill in the refrigerator.

Bring a pot of water to a boil. Prepare a bowl of ice and water. Add the snow peas to the boiling water. Remove after 1 minute, and place in an ice water bath for a few minutes to stop the cooking. Snap off the ends, remove the strings, and cut lengthwise into thin slivers.

Thoroughly mix the mushrooms, noodles, snow peas, carrot, bell pepper, onions, chili paste, and vinaigrette. Divide among four plates.

To Make Ahead: Prepare the vinaigrette and refrigerate. Combine the remaining ingredients, cover, and refrigerate. Bring the vinaigrette to room temperature and whisk before tossing with the salad.

BONUS YEARS DAILY PERCENTAGES

Per serving: Fruits and vegetables 20%; Garlic 100%

NUTRITIONAL ANALYSIS

Per serving: Calories 224, Protein 6g, Total fat 6g, Sat fat 1g, Trans fat 0g, Cholesterol 0mg, Carbohydrate 37g, Dietary fiber 4g, Sodium 624mg

Oven-Fried
Cajun Catfish

MAKES 4 SERVINGS

Coating foods with buttermilk, egg white, and crumbs makes an easy-to-prepare and healthy coating for oven frying. The technique works equally well with chicken breasts, which should be pounded to about ½-inch thickness for quicker cooking.

1 (about 5-ounce) box plain melba toast
1½ tablespoons plus 1½ teaspoons Cajun seasoning
⅓ cup low-fat buttermilk
1 large egg white
4 (5- to 6-ounce) catfish fillets

In a food processor or with a mallet, grind the melba toast into a mixture of finely ground and coarsely ground crumbs (this gives a good crunchy texture to the coating). Mix the toast crumbs with the 1½ tablespoons Cajun seasoning in a shallow bowl.

Thoroughly mix the buttermilk, egg white, and the 1½ teaspoons Cajun seasoning in another shallow bowl. Dip each catfish fillet in the buttermilk mixture until it is evenly coated, letting the excess buttermilk drip off. Then dip each catfish fillet in the crumb mixture, being careful to coat each side evenly. Place the fish fillets in the refrigerator for 15 minutes to allow the coating to set.

Preheat the oven to 400 degrees. Mist both sides of the catfish fillets with cooking spray. Place them on a wire rack over a baking sheet. Bake for about 14 minutes, or until the coating is brown and crisp and the fillets are opaque in the center.

BONUS YEARS DAILY PERCENTAGES

Per serving: Fish 100%

NUTRITIONAL ANALYSIS

Per serving: Calories 342, Protein 28g, Total fat 12g, Sat fat 3g, Trans fat 0g, Cholesterol 67mg, Carbohydrate 28g, Dietary fiber 2g, Sodium 643mg

Cajun Okra-Tomato Braise

1 tablespoon extra-virgin olive oil

2 cups ¼-inch-dice onions

1 stalk celery, cut into ¼-inch dice

1 green bell pepper (6 ounces), cut into ¼-inch dice

⅓ pound smoked ham, diced

½ teaspoon dried thyme

12 ounces okra, ends removed and pods cut into ¼-inch-thick
slices

2 tablespoons cider vinegar

1 (14-ounce) can stewed tomatoes

½ cup low-sodium chicken broth

kosher salt, freshly ground black pepper, and Cajun
seasonings, to taste

Heat the oil in a nonstick skillet over medium heat. Add the onions, celery, bell pepper, and ham and sauté, stirring occasionally, until all the vegetables begin to soften, about 5 minutes. Add the thyme and sauté for 30 seconds. Add the okra and vinegar and sauté, stirring occasionally, until the stringiness of the okra begins to disappear, about 7 minutes.

Add the tomatoes with their juices and the broth. Bring to a simmer, cover, and cook until the okra has lost all its stringiness, about 20 minutes. Uncover, season with salt, pepper, and Cajun seasonings, and simmer, uncovered, until the pan juices are the desired thickness, about 5 minutes.

BONUS YEARS DAILY PERCENTAGES

Per serving: Fruits and vegetables 35%

NUTRITIONAL ANALYSIS

Per serving: Calories 78, Protein 4g, Total fat 2g, Sat fat 0g, Trans fat 0g, Cholesterol 5mg, Carbohydrate 11g, Dietary fiber 3g, Sodium 129mg

STEAMED BROWN RICE

NUTRITIONAL ANALYSIS

Per ½-cup serving: Calories 108, Protein 2g, Total fat 0g, Sat fat 0g, Trans fat 0g, Cholesterol 0mg, Carbohydrate 22g, Dietary fiber 2g, Sodium 5mg

RED WINE

NUTRITIONAL ANALYSIS

Per 5 ounces: Calories 106, Protein 0g, Total fat 0g, Sat fat 0g, Trans fat 0g, Cholesterol 0mg, Carbohydrate 2g, Dietary fiber 0g, Sodium 7mg

DARK CHOCOLATE

NUTRITIONAL ANALYSIS

Per 2 ounces: Calories 302, Protein 3g, Total fat 16g, Sat fat 10g, Trans fat 0g, Cholesterol 0mg, Carbohydrate 36g, Dietary fiber 2g, Sodium 9mg

NUTS

NUTRITIONAL ANALYSIS

Per 1 ounce: Calories 168, Protein 5g, Total fat 14g, Sat fat 2g, Trans fat 0g, Cholesterol 0mg, Carbohydrate 7g, Dietary fiber 2g, Sodium 3mg

GRAPES

NUTRITIONAL ANALYSIS

Per 25: Calories 89, Protein 1g, Total fat 1g, Sat fat 0g, Trans fat 0g, Cholesterol 0mg, Carbohydrate 22g, Dietary fiber 1g, Sodium 2mg

DAY 17: TUESDAY

Breakfast

Cereal and Fruit Breakfast
BONUS YEARS POINTS: FRUITS AND VEGETABLES 15%
CALORIES: 188

Lunch

Bulgur Pilaf (page 232)
BONUS YEARS POINTS: FRUITS AND VEGETABLES 45%;
GARLIC 50%
CALORIES: 214

Dinner

Steak and Chickpea Salad
Breadsticks
Mocha Soufflé Cake
BONUS YEARS POINTS: FRUITS AND VEGETABLES 55%;
GARLIC 50%; CHOCOLATE 25%
CALORIES: 674

5 ounces wine
BONUS YEARS POINTS: WINE 100%
CALORIES: 106

Snacks

1½ ounces dark chocolate
BONUS YEARS POINTS: CHOCOLATE 100%
CALORIES: 227

2 ounces unsalted dry-roasted
or natural nuts
BONUS YEARS POINTS: NUTS 100%
CALORIES: 337

DAY'S TOTAL BONUS YEARS POINTS: WINE 100%; CHOCOLATE 100%;
FRUITS AND VEGETABLES 115%; GARLIC 100%; NUTS 100%
TOTAL CALORIES: 1,640

Cereal and Fruit Breakfast

MAKES 1 SERVING

⅔ cup high-fiber cereal topped with ½ cup blueberries
½ cup fat-free milk

BONUS YEARS DAILY PERCENTAGES

Per serving: Fruits and vegetables 15%

NUTRITIONAL ANALYSIS

Per serving: Calories 188, Protein 8g, Total fat 1g, Sat fat 0g, Trans fat 0g, Cholesterol 2mg, Carbohydrate 42g, Dietary fiber 7g, Sodium 173mg

Steak and Chickpea Salad

MAKES 4 SERVINGS, WITH LEFTOVERS

Pan roasting with an initial sear on a stovetop grill pan marks the steaks and guarantees a beautiful presentation. Finishing cooking in the oven assures a juicy steak, which is not overdone or burned on the surface.

Serve a tangy, good red wine, such as a Pinot Noir, Beaujolais, or Washington State Syrah, to match the vinegar in the dressing.

1 (1¾- to 2-pound) beef boneless top sirloin steak (about
  1 inch thick)
1½ cups Roasted Garlic Vinaigrette (page 113) or other low-
  fat Italian vinaigrette
4 Roma tomatoes (about 12 ounces total), each cut into
  8 wedges
1 cup cooked dried chickpeas (see page 266), drained
1 large red onion (8 ounces), thinly sliced
6 cups torn romaine lettuce (about 8 ounces), washed
  and dried

Marinate the steak in 1 cup of the vinaigrette for at least 30 minutes at room temperature or for up to 2 hours in the refrigerator.

Marinate the tomato wedges and the chickpeas in the remaining ½ cup of the vinaigrette for 30 minutes.

Place the onion in ice-cold water for 20 minutes. Remove the onion and drain well.

Preheat the oven to 375 degrees. Remove the steak from the marinade, reserving the marinade, and pat dry. Preheat a ridged stovetop grill pan over medium-high heat. Cook the steak on the grill pan for

4 minutes on each side, rotating a quarter turn after 2 minutes on a side to give grill markings.

Transfer the steak to the oven and cook for about 13 minutes for medium rare; the internal temperature of the steak should be about 135 degrees on an instant-read thermometer when it leaves the oven. Cover the steak and let it rest for 10 minutes. Cut the steak into ⅛-inch-thick slices. Reserve one-fourth of the slices and refrigerate them for sandwiches for the next day.

Meanwhile, place the reserved meat marinade in a small saucepan over low heat and bring to a boil. Remove the tomatoes and the chickpeas from their marinade, and add the vegetable marinade to the simmered marinade.

Toss the lettuce with the chickpeas and tomatoes and the onion. Add ¾ to 1 cup of the marinade and toss to combine. Divide the salad among four plates and top each salad with one-fourth of the remaining steak slices.

BONUS YEARS DAILY PERCENTAGES
Per serving: Fruits and vegetables 55%; Garlic 50%

NUTRITIONAL ANALYSIS
Per serving: Calories 430, Protein 48g, Total fat 15g, Sat fat 5g, Trans fat 0g, Cholesterol 121mg, Carbohydrate 22g, Dietary fiber 6g, Sodium 388mg

BREADSTICKS

NUTRITIONAL ANALYSIS
Per 2 small: Calories 41, Protein 1g, Total fat 1g, Sat fat 0g, Trans fat 0g, Cholesterol 0mg, Carbohydrate 7g, Dietary fiber 0g, Sodium 66mg

Mocha Soufflé Cake

Festive enough for entertaining, this make-ahead dessert can be served with Raspberry Coulis, page 171, or simply sprinkled with powdered sugar.

½ cup plus 2 tablespoons sugar

2 tablespoons unsweetened cocoa powder (not Dutch processed)

1 tablespoon cornstarch

2 teaspoons instant espresso powder

1 cup fat-free milk

4 ounces (½ cup) light cream cheese, in pieces

2 to 3 ounces bittersweet chocolate, in pieces

1 teaspoon vanilla extract

4 egg whites

pinch cream of tartar

powdered sugar (optional)

chocolate-covered coffee beans (optional)

Preheat the oven to 350 degrees. Spray an 8-inch springform pan with cooking spray. Combine the ½ cup sugar, cocoa powder, cornstarch, and espresso powder in a small saucepan. Add a little of the milk and stir to make a thin paste. Whisk in the remaining milk. Add the cream cheese. Cook, stirring over medium heat until bubbly and the cream cheese is melted. Remove from the heat and stir in the chocolate and vanilla, stirring until the chocolate is melted.

In a stainless steel bowl, beat the egg whites and cream of tartar with an electric mixer until soft peaks form. Gradually add the 2 tablespoons sugar and beat until stiff peaks form. Stir a little of the egg whites into the chocolate mixture. Add the chocolate mixture to the egg whites and fold in until no white streaks remain. Transfer the mixture to the prepared pan. Bake for about 30 minutes, or until a knife inserted off-center comes out clean. Cool. Cover and refrigerate until chilled. Remove the pan rim, sprinkle with powdered sugar (if using), and cut into wedges. Garnish each serving with coffee beans (if using).

To Make Ahead: The dessert can be made up to 2 days ahead. It is best served chilled.

BONUS YEARS DAILY PERCENTAGES

Per serving: Chocolate 25%

NUTRITIONAL ANALYSIS

Per serving: Calories 203, Protein 6g, Total fat 6g, Sat fat 4g, Trans fat 0g, Cholesterol 10mg, Carbohydrate 33g, Dietary fiber 1g, Sodium 149mg

---

RED WINE

NUTRITIONAL ANALYSIS

Per 5 ounces: Calories 106, Protein 0g, Total fat 0g, Sat fat 0g, Trans fat 0g, Cholesterol 0mg, Carbohydrate 2g, Dietary fiber 0g, Sodium 7mg

DARK CHOCOLATE

NUTRITIONAL ANALYSIS

Per 1½ ounces: Calories 227, Protein 2g, Total fat 12, Sat fat 7, Trans fat 0g, Cholesterol 0mg, Carbohydrate 27, Dietary fiber 2g, Sodium 7mg

NUTS

NUTRITIONAL ANALYSIS

Per 2 ounces: Calories 337, Protein 10g, Total fat 29g, Sat fat 4g, Trans fat 0g, Cholesterol 0mg, Carbohydrate 14g, Dietary fiber 5g, Sodium 7mg

DAY 18: WEDNESDAY

Breakfast

Peanut Butter–Chocolate Smoothie
BONUS YEARS POINTS: CHOCOLATE 50%; FRUITS
AND VEGETABLES 10%; NUTS 50%
CALORIES: 422

Lunch

Steak and Red-Onion Sandwich
BONUS YEARS POINTS: FRUITS AND VEGETABLES 20%
CALORIES: 516

Dinner

Sear-Roasted Sea Bass with Olives,
Capers, and Tomatoes
½ cup cooked couscous with
1 tablespoon raisins
BONUS YEARS POINTS: FRUITS AND VEGETABLES 60%;
FISH 100%; GARLIC 100%
CALORIES: 431

5 ounces wine
BONUS YEARS POINTS: WINE 100%
CALORIES: 106

Snacks

1 ounce dark chocolate
BONUS YEARS POINTS: CHOCOLATE 50%
CALORIES: 151

1 ounce unsalted dry-roasted
or natural nuts
BONUS YEARS POINTS: NUTS 50%
CALORIES: 168

1 medium apple
BONUS YEARS POINTS: FRUITS AND VEGETABLES 20%
CALORIES: 80

DAY'S TOTAL BONUS YEARS POINTS: WINE 100%; CHOCOLATE 100%;
FRUITS AND VEGETABLES 110%; FISH 100%; GARLIC 200%; NUTS 100%
TOTAL CALORIES: 1,874

Peanut Butter–Chocolate Smoothie

MAKES 2 SERVINGS

¼ cup unsweetened cocoa powder (not Dutch processed)
¼ cup hot water
4 to 6 tablespoons natural peanut butter
1 frozen peeled medium banana, cut into chunks
1 (6-ounce) container vanilla fat-free yogurt
1 cup fat-free milk or soymilk

Add the cocoa powder and hot water to a blender. Blend until combined. Add the peanut butter, banana, yogurt, and ½ cup of the milk. Blend until smooth. Add the remaining milk and blend until combined. Pour into two glasses and serve.

BONUS YEARS DAILY PERCENTAGES
Per serving: Chocolate 50%; Fruits and vegetables 10%; Nuts 50%

NUTRITIONAL ANALYSIS
Per serving: Calories 422, Protein 21g, Total fat 18g, Sat fat 3g, Trans fat 0g, Cholesterol 4mg, Carbohydrate 54g, Dietary fiber 7g, Sodium 231mg

Steak and Red-Onion Sandwich

½ cup (2 ounces) sliced red onion

2 (3-ounce) demi baguettes, or 2 (3-ounce) pieces of a regular
baguette, cut into 4 slices

2 tablespoons prepared mustard or your favorite low-fat
spread

1½ cups torn lettuce or mixed salad leaves (about 2 ounces)

½ small red bell pepper, roasted (page 378), peeled, and
sliced, or 2 slices jarred roasted red bell pepper (about 2
ounces), drained

6 to 7 ounces grilled steak slices (page 246)

Place the onion in ice-cold water for about 15 minutes; drain well.
Slice the baguettes in half. Spread 1 tablespoon of the mustard
on the bottom slice of each baguette. Then top each with half of the
lettuce, onion, bell pepper, and steak. Cover each sandwich with a
baguette top. Wrap in plastic wrap and refrigerate until needed.

BONUS YEARS DAILY PERCENTAGES

Per serving: Fruits and vegetables 20%

NUTRITIONAL ANALYSIS

Per serving: Calories 516, Protein 31g, Total fat 13g, Sat fat 3g, Trans fat 0g,
Cholesterol 60mg, Carbohydrate 70g, Dietary fiber 7g, Sodium 735mg

Variation

Substitute lean roast beef from the deli for the steak.

Sear-Roasted Sea Bass
with Olives, Capers, and Tomatoes

MAKES 4 SERVINGS

This is a basic recipe with endless variations, which when mastered will expand your culinary repertoire. Artichokes, fennel, and sun-dried tomatoes are some of the easily substituted vegetables. Halibut or escalar would also do well in this dish.

4 (5- to 6-ounce) skinned sea bass fillets (about 1 inch thick)
kosher salt and freshly ground black pepper, to taste
2 tablespoons extra-virgin olive oil
1 medium onion (6 ounces), thinly sliced
4 cloves garlic, thinly sliced
¾ cup dry white wine, such as Sauvignon Blanc
1 pound fresh tomatoes, peeled, seeded, and coarsely chopped
1½ tablespoons capers, drained
¾ cup coarsely chopped pitted black olives (3 ounces), such as
   Niçoise
¼ cup low-sodium chicken broth
2 tablespoons freshly squeezed lemon juice
pinch red pepper flakes
3 tablespoons chopped flat-leaf parsley, for garnish

Preheat the oven to 375 degrees. Season the sea bass with salt and black pepper. Heat 1 tablespoon of the oil in a 12-inch nonstick skillet over medium heat until it is just below smoking. Add the sea bass and cook for 3 minutes. (Do not move the fillets before the 3 minutes are up or they will stick.) Remove the sea bass, cover, and keep warm.

Heat the remaining 1 tablespoon oil in the same skillet over medium heat. Add the onion and sauté, stirring occasionally, for about 5 minutes. Add the garlic and sauté for 1 minute. Add the wine, tomatoes, capers, and olives and simmer over medium-low heat until the wine mostly evaporates, about 10 minutes. Stir in the broth and lemon juice.

Add the sea bass back to the skillet, and cover with the sauce. Transfer to the oven and cook for 5 to 7 minutes, or until the sea bass is just opaque. Remove from the oven, and transfer the sea bass to four plates. Season the sauce with the red pepper flakes, salt, and black pepper and spoon over the sea bass. (If the sauce is a bit thin, you can heat it on the stovetop for a few minutes to reduce it to the desired consistency.) Garnish with the parsley.

BONUS YEARS DAILY PERCENTAGES

Per serving: Fruits and vegetables 40%; Fish 100%; Garlic 100%

NUTRITIONAL ANALYSIS

Per serving: Calories 343, Protein 36g, Total fat 14g, Sat fat 2g, Trans fat 0g, Cholesterol 75mg, Carbohydrate 12g, Dietary fiber 3g, Sodium 462mg

COOKED COUSCOUS WITH 1 TABLESPOON RAISINS

BONUS YEARS DAILY PERCENTAGE

Per serving: Fruits and vegetables 20%

NUTRITIONAL ANALYSIS

Per ½-cup serving: Calories 88, Protein 3g, Total fat 0g, Sat fat 0g, Trans fat 0g, Cholesterol 0mg, Carbohydrate 18g, Dietary fiber 1g, Sodium 4mg

RED WINE

NUTRITIONAL ANALYSIS

Per 5 ounces: Calories 106, Protein 0g, Total fat 0g, Sat fat 0g, Trans fat 0g, Cholesterol 0mg, Carbohydrate 2g, Dietary fiber 0g, Sodium 7mg

DARK CHOCOLATE

NUTRITIONAL ANALYSIS

Per 1 ounce: Calories 151, Protein 1g, Total fat 8g, Sat fat 5g, Trans fat 0g, Cholesterol 0mg, Carbohydrate 18g, Dietary fiber 1g, Sodium 5mg

NUTS

NUTRITIONAL ANALYSIS

Per 1 ounce: Calories 168, Protein 5g, Total fat 14g, Sat fat 2g, Trans fat 0g, Cholesterol 0mg, Carbohydrate 7g, Dietary fiber 2g, Sodium 3mg

APPLE

BONUS YEARS DAILY PERCENTAGES

Per apple: Fruits and vegetables 20%

NUTRITIONAL ANALYSIS

Per apple: Calories 80, Protein 0g, Total fat 0g, Sat fat 0g, Trans fat 0g, Cholesterol 0mg, Carbohydrate 22g, Dietary fiber 5g, Sodium 0mg

DAY 19: THURSDAY

Breakfast

½ whole wheat bagel, toasted
2 tablespoons nut butter
½ medium banana
BONUS YEARS POINTS: FRUITS AND VEGETABLES 10%;
NUTS 50%
CALORIES: 314

Lunch

Italian Pasta Vegetable Salad
BONUS YEARS POINTS: FRUITS AND VEGETABLES 30%;
GARLIC 100%
CALORIES: 275

Dinner

Sole Poached in Seafood Court
Bouillon
Almond Rice Pilaf
½ cup steamed broccoli
BONUS YEARS POINTS: FRUITS AND VEGETABLES 40%;
FISH 100%; NUTS 25%
CALORIES: 539

5 ounces wine
BONUS YEARS POINTS: WINE 100%
CALORIES: 106

Snacks

2 ounces dark chocolate
BONUS YEARS POINTS: CHOCOLATE 100%
CALORIES: 302

½ ounce unsalted dry-roasted
or natural nuts
BONUS YEARS POINTS: NUTS 25%
CALORIES: 84

1 pear
BONUS YEARS POINTS: FRUITS AND VEGETABLES 20%
CALORIES: 98

DAY'S TOTAL BONUS YEARS POINTS: WINE 100%; CHOCOLATE 100%;
FRUITS AND VEGETABLES 110%; FISH 20%; GARLIC 200%; NUTS 100%
TOTAL CALORIES: 2,158

WHOLE WHEAT BAGEL

NUTRITIONAL ANALYSIS

Per ½ bagel: Calories 72, Protein 3g, Total fat 1g, Sat fat 0g, Trans fat 0g, Cholesterol 0mg, Carbohydrate 15g, Dietary fiber 2g, Sodium 148mg

NUT BUTTER (SUCH AS ALMOND OR PEANUT)

BONUS YEARS DAILY PERCENTAGES

Per 2 tablespoons: Nuts 50%

NUTRITIONAL ANALYSIS

Per 2 tablespoons: Calories 188, Protein 8g, Total fat 16g, Sat fat 3g, Trans fat 0g, Cholesterol 0mg, Carbohydrate 6g, Dietary fiber 2g, Sodium 148mg

BANANA

BONUS YEARS DAILY PERCENTAGES

Per ½ banana: Fruits and vegetables 10%

NUTRITIONAL ANALYSIS

Per ½ banana: Calories 54, Protein 1g, Total fat 0g, Sat fat 0g, Trans fat 0g, Cholesterol 0mg, Carbohydrate 14g, Dietary fiber 1g, Sodium 0mg

Italian Pasta Vegetable Salad

MAKES 4 SERVINGS

6 ounces farfalle (butterfly) or conchiglie (shell) pasta
(about 3 cups)
1 (12-ounce) bag mixed vegetables, such as carrots, broccoli,
and snow peas (from the produce refrigerated section)
½ cup finely chopped red onion (2 ounces)
1 cup roughly chopped pitted black olives (4 ounces)
¾ cup Roasted Garlic Vinaigrette (page 113) or other low-fat
Italian vinaigrette
¼ cup freshly grated Parmesan cheese

Cook the pasta according to package directions until al dente. Drain and reserve.

Bring a large pot of water to a boil. Prepare a large bowl of ice and water. Add the vegetables to the boiling water and drain after 1 minute. Immediately transfer them to the ice water to stop the cooking. Drain the vegetables. Cut the large florets and snow peas in half.

Mix the pasta, vegetables, onion, olives, and vinaigrette together in a large bowl. Divide among four plates, and top each serving with 1 tablespoon of the Parmesan cheese.

To Make Ahead: Prepare as directed above. Cover and refrigerate. Top with the Parmesan cheese just before serving.

BONUS YEARS DAILY PERCENTAGES
Per serving: Fruits and vegetables 30%; Garlic 100%

NUTRITIONAL ANALYSIS
Per serving: Calories 275, Protein 11g, Total fat 6g, Sat fat 1g, Trans fat 0g,
Cholesterol 4mg, Carbohydrate 47g, Dietary fiber 6g, Sodium 425mg

Sole Poached
in Seafood Court Bouillon

MAKES 4 SERVINGS

This simple poaching recipe will work great with any thinly cut white fish fillet, just choose the freshest one the next time you are at the market.

¾ cup julienned fennel bulb (3 ounces)
¾ cup julienned carrots (3 ounces)
¾ cup julienned zucchini (3 ounces)
¾ cup julienned yellow summer squash (3 ounces)
1 recipe Seafood Court Bouillon (recipe follows)
4 (5- to 6-ounce) skinless pieces petrale sole or flounder
kosher salt and freshly ground black pepper, to taste
2 teaspoons arrowroot dissolved in 2 teaspoons cold water
1 to 2 tablespoons butter, chilled, cut into pieces (optional)
minced fresh flat-leaf parsley, for garnish

Spray a nonstick skillet with cooking spray and heat over medium heat. Add the fennel and carrots and sauté for 2 minutes. Add the zucchini and yellow squash and sauté until the vegetables are just tender, 2 to 3 minutes. Transfer to a bowl, cover, and keep warm.

Bring the court bouillon to a simmer in a 12-inch skillet. Place the sole in the skillet and simmer until the sole is just opaque, about 5 minutes. Remove the sole from the skillet and place on a heated plate, cover, and keep warm.

Place the skillet containing the court bouillon over medium-high heat. Boil until reduced to 1 cup, and season with salt and pepper. Whisk in the arrowroot mixture and the butter, piece by piece (if using) to thicken the sauce.

In each of four large rimmed serving plates, place one-fourth of the vegetables, top with a piece of the sole, and spoon one-fourth of the sauce around the vegetables. Garnish with the parsley.

BONUS YEARS DAILY PERCENTAGES

Per serving: Fruits and vegetables 20%; Fish 100%

NUTRITIONAL ANALYSIS

Per serving: Calories 196, Protein 28g, Total fat 2g, Sat fat 0g, Trans fat 0g, Cholesterol 68mg, Carbohydrate 6g, Dietary fiber 2g, Sodium 544mg

Seafood Court Bouillon

The court bouillon can be made ahead of time, refrigerated, and used when needed as a poaching liquid for seafood.

1 tablespoon extra-virgin olive oil
½ cup chopped carrot
½ cup chopped celery
½ cup chopped onion
½ cup chopped fennel
2 cups dry red wine
4 cups water
1 tart green apple, cored and coarsely chopped
3 tablespoons red wine vinegar
1 tablespoon black peppercorns
1 bay leaf
3 whole cloves

Heat a 10-inch nonstick skillet over medium-high heat. Add the olive oil and heat to just below smoking. Add the carrot, celery, onion, and fennel and sauté until the vegetables are softened and just beginning to brown. Add the wine, 2 cups of the water, the apple, and vinegar, peppercorns, bay leaf, and cloves and simmer until the liquid is reduced by half.

Add the remaining 2 cups water and simmer until about 1¼ cups of liquid remain. Strain the liquid and reserve.

Almond Rice Pilaf

MAKES 4 (¾-CUP) SERVINGS

Toasting the almonds and rice adds a real nuttiness to the dish.
By lightly sautéing the rice, the individual grains are guaran-
teed to remain separate and to fluff up beautifully.

½ cup slivered almonds
1 tablespoon canola or grapeseed oil
⅓ cup finely chopped onion
1 cup long-grain white rice
1¾ cups low-sodium chicken broth

Heat the almonds in a dry, heavy skillet over medium heat until lightly toasted, stirring frequently, about 5 minutes. Or place the almonds on a baking sheet and toast in a 375-degree oven for 10 minutes, stirring at least once.

Heat the oil in a 3-quart saucepan over medium heat. Add the onion and sauté for about 1 minute. Add the rice and sauté until the rice just begins to change color but is not actually brown, about 5 minutes. Add the broth and almonds, and bring to a low boil. Reduce the heat to very low, cover, and cook until the rice is tender, about 20 minutes. Remove from the heat. Let the rice rest for 5 minutes, uncover, and fluff before serving.

BONUS YEARS DAILY PERCENTAGES
Per serving: Nuts 25%

NUTRITIONAL ANALYSIS
Per serving: Calories 321, Protein 8g, Total fat 13g, Sat fat 1g, Trans fat 0g, Cholesterol 2mg, Carbohydrate 42g, Dietary fiber 2g, Sodium 51mg

STEAMED BROCCOLI

BONUS YEARS DAILY PERCENTAGES

Per ½-cup serving: Fruits and vegetables 20%

NUTRITIONAL ANALYSIS

Per ½-cup serving: Calories 22, Protein 2g, Total fat 0g, Sat fat 0g, Cholesterol 0mg, Carbohydrate 4g, Dietary fiber 2g, Sodium 21mg

PEAR

BONUS YEARS DAILY PERCENTAGES

Per serving: Fruits and vegetables 20%

NUTRITIONAL ANALYSIS

Per serving: Calories 98, Protein 1g, Total fat 1g, Sat fat 0g, Trans fat 0g, Cholesterol 0mg, Carbohydrate 25g, Dietary fiber 4g, Sodium 1mg

RED WINE

NUTRITIONAL ANALYSIS

Per 5 ounces: Calories 106, Protein 0g, Total fat 0g, Sat fat 0g, Trans fat 0g, Cholesterol 0mg, Carbohydrate 2g, Dietary fiber 0g, Sodium 7mg

DARK CHOCOLATE

NUTRITIONAL ANALYSIS

Per 2 ounces: Calories 302, Protein 3g, Total fat 16g, Sat fat 10g, Trans fat 0g, Cholesterol 0mg, Carbohydrate 36g, Dietary fiber 2g, Sodium 9mg

NUTS

NUTRITIONAL ANALYSIS

Per ½ ounce: Calories 84, Protein 2g, Total fat 7g, Sat fat 1g, Trans fat 0g, Cholesterol 0mg, Carbohydrate 3g, Dietary fiber 1g, Sodium 2mg

DAY 20: FRIDAY

Breakfast

Ricotta-Fruit Breakfast Parfait
BONUS YEARS POINTS: FRUITS AND VEGETABLES 40%;
NUTS 25%
CALORIES: 407

Lunch

Spanish-Style Chickpea Salad
BONUS YEARS POINTS: FRUITS AND VEGETABLES 40%;
GARLIC 75%
CALORIES: 600

Dinner

Pan-Roasted Salmon
with Shanghai Red Sauce
½ cup cooked soba noodles
BONUS YEARS POINTS: FRUITS AND VEGETABLES 20%;
FISH 100%; GARLIC 50%
CALORIES: 352

5 ounces wine
BONUS YEARS POINTS: WINE 100%
CALORIES: 106

Snacks

2 ounces dark chocolate
BONUS YEARS POINTS: CHOCOLATE 100%
CALORIES: 302

1½ ounces unsalted dry-roasted
or natural nuts
BONUS YEARS POINTS: NUTS 75%
CALORIES: 253

DAY'S TOTAL BONUS YEARS POINTS: WINE 100%; CHOCOLATE 100%;
FRUITS AND VEGETABLES 100%; FISH 100%; GARLIC 125%; NUTS 100%
TOTAL CALORIES: 2,190

Ricotta-Fruit Breakfast Parfait

MAKES 1 SERVING

1 fresh peach (4 ounces), peeled and diced (about ½ cup)
½ cup fresh raspberries
½ cup part-skim ricotta cheese
1 tablespoon honey
½ teaspoon ground cinnamon, preferable Saigon
2 tablespoons pistachios

Layer half of the peach and raspberries in a glass dish. Top with half of the ricotta. Drizzle the ricotta with half of the honey and sprinkle with half of the cinnamon. Repeat with a layer of the remaining fruit and top with the remaining ricotta, honey, and cinnamon. Sprinkle with the pistachios.

BONUS YEARS DAILY PERCENTAGES
Per serving: Fruits and vegetables 40%; Nuts 25%

NUTRITIONAL ANALYSIS
Per serving: Calories 407, Protein 19g, Total fat 17g, Sat fat 7g, Trans fat 0g,
Cholesterol 38mg, Carbohydrate 49g, Dietary fiber 9g, Sodium 156mg

Spanish-Style Chickpea Salad

MAKES 4 (1¼-CUP) SERVINGS

Chickpeas and roasted bell peppers are often used in Spanish appetizers (tapas, or little plates). Here we use them to get some delicious Bonus Years points.

¾ cup dried chickpeas, or 1 (16-ounce) can chickpeas, drained
   and rinsed
½ cup diced roasted red bell pepper (2 ounces) (see page 378)
1 cup diced unpeeled hothouse or English cucumber
   (4 ounces)
1 cup diced red onion (4 ounces)
½ pound 96% fat-free, lower-sodium ham or smoked
   turkey, diced
¼ cup chopped flat-leaf parsley (optional)
kosher salt and freshly ground black pepper, to taste
¾ cup Roasted Garlic-Shallot Vinaigrette (recipe follows) or
   other low-fat Mediterranean-style dressing

If using the dried chickpeas, soak them overnight in cold water to cover. Drain the chickpeas and add enough fresh water to cover by about 2 inches. Bring to a boil; reduce the heat, cover and simmer until the beans are tender, about 40 minutes. Drain the beans.

Combine the beans with the remaining ingredients, except the dressing; cover, and refrigerate. When ready to serve, remove the salad from the refrigerator, add the dressing, and divide among four plates.

To Make Ahead: Refrigerate the bean mixture and dressing separately up to 1 day. Toss together just before serving.

BONUS YEARS DAILY PERCENTAGES

Per serving: Fruits and vegetables 40%; Garlic 75%

NUTRITIONAL ANALYSIS

Per serving: Calories 600, Protein 22g, Total fat 37g, Sat fat 6g, Trans fat 0g, Cholesterol 25mg, Carbohydrate 45g, Dietary fiber 8g, Sodium 850mg

Roasted Garlic-Shallot Vinaigrette

MAKES ABOUT 1 CUP

*This can be used as a basic salad dressing, served over steamed
vegetables, or as a base for other sauces (see Stovetop-Grilled
Swordfish in Basil-Tomato Vinaigrette, page 308).*

2 medium shallots (about 2½ ounces), unpeeled
4 large cloves garlic, unpeeled
5 tablespoons white wine vinegar
1 tablespoon freshly squeezed lemon juice
3 tablespoons extra-virgin olive oil
kosher salt, to taste
⅛ teaspoon freshly ground black pepper
1 tablespoon Dijon mustard
½ cup low-sodium chicken broth
1 teaspoon arrowroot dissolved in 2 teaspoons water

Preheat the oven to 400 degrees. Place the shallots and garlic in a
small baking dish. Cover with aluminum foil and roast for 35 to
45 minutes, or until soft. Squeeze the shallots and garlic out of their
skins into a blender. Add the vinegar, lemon juice, olive oil, salt, pepper, and mustard and blend until pureed.

Bring the broth to a simmer in a small saucepan over low heat,
then whisk in the dissolved arrowroot. Add the thickened broth to the
blender and mix with the garlic-shallot puree.

BONUS YEARS DAILY PERCENTAGES

Per serving: Garlic 100%

NUTRITIONAL ANALYSIS

Per ¼ cup: Calories 122, Protein 1g, Total fat 11g, Sat fat 1g, Trans fat 0g, Cholesterol 1mg, Carbohydrate 5g, Dietary fiber 0g, Sodium 105mg

Pan-Roasted Salmon with Shanghai Red Sauce

MAKES 4 SERVINGS

We grill the salmon, which adds a smoky touch. Then it is quickly braised in a red wine sauce with oven-roasted mushrooms, adding a touch of meatiness to the dish. These techniques ensure a dish that goes well with red wine. The reduced wine and the acidity of the vinegar help to cut the richness of the salmon.

Salmon is a delicate fish. If you cooked it all the way through on the stovetop, you might burn it on the outside. Finishing it off in the oven guarantees a nice crisp exterior with a moist and succulent interior.

A Nero d'Avola or a California Pinot Noir would go great with this dish.

4 ounces fresh shiitake mushrooms, stems removed

1 tablespoon plus 1 teaspoon canola oil

2 tablespoons plus 1 cup water

1 cup chopped onion

4 cloves garlic, minced

2 tablespoons minced fresh ginger

2 cups dry red wine

⅔ cup dry sherry or Chinese rice wine

½ cup low-sodium soy sauce

2 tablespoons Chinese dark soy sauce or regular soy sauce

6 tablespoons light brown sugar

¼ cup Chinese black vinegar or balsamic vinegar

¼ teaspoon Asian chili sauce

20 broccoli florets (about 8 ounces)

4 (6-ounce) pieces salmon

freshly ground black pepper, to taste

chopped fresh chives, for garnish

Preheat the oven to 350 degrees. Combine the mushrooms, the 1 teaspoon oil, and the 2 tablespoons water in a small ovenproof dish. Cover and bake for 25 minutes. Remove from the oven and re-serve. Leave the oven on.

Meanwhile, heat the 1 tablespoon oil in a medium saucepan over medium heat. Add the onion and sauté for about 3 minutes. Add the garlic and ginger and sauté, stirring occasionally, until the onion is soft; do not burn the garlic. Add the red wine, the 1 cup water, sherry, soy sauces, sugar, vinegar, and chili sauce and simmer until the sauce is reduced by half, about 25 minutes. Add the mushrooms, transfer the wine sauce to a large ovenproof skillet, and set aside.

Bring a large pot of water to a boil. Prepare a large bowl of ice and water. Add the broccoli to the boiling water and drain after 1 minute. Immediately transfer the broccoli to the ice water to stop the cooking. Drain and reserve.

Spray a ridged stovetop grill pan with cooking spray and place over medium heat. Season the salmon with pepper. Arrange the salmon on the grill pan and cook for 3 minutes. It should be nicely marked. Add the salmon to the wine sauce and transfer to the oven. Bake the salmon for about 7 minutes, or until cooked through.

To serve, place a piece of salmon in the center of each of four plates. Spoon ¼ cup of the wine sauce and one-fourth of the mush-rooms around each piece of salmon. Garnish the salmon with the chives. Arrange 5 broccoli florets around the edge of each plate.

BONUS YEARS DAILY PERCENTAGES

Per serving: Fruits and vegetables 20%; Fish 100%; Garlic 50%

NUTRITIONAL ANALYSIS

Per serving: Calories 466, Protein 40g, Total fat 11g, Saturated fat 2g, Trans fat 0g, Cholesterol 77mg, Carbohydrate 15g, Dietary fiber 1g, Sodium 656mg

COOKED SOBA NOODLES

NUTRITIONAL ANALYSIS

Per ½ cup: Calories 56, Protein 3g, Total fat 0g, Sat fat 0g, Trans fat 0g, Cholesterol 0mg, Carbohydrate 12g, Dietary fiber 0g, Sodium 34mg

RED WINE

NUTRITIONAL ANALYSIS

Per 5 ounces: Calories 106, Protein 0g, Total fat 0g, Sat fat 0g, Trans fat 0g, Cholesterol 0mg, Carbohydrate 2g, Dietary fiber 0g, Sodium 7mg

DARK CHOCOLATE

NUTRITIONAL ANALYSIS

Per 2 ounces: Calories 302, Protein 3g, Total fat 16g, Sat fat 10g, Trans fat 0g, Cholesterol 0mg, Carbohydrate 36g, Dietary fiber 2g, Sodium 9mg

NUTS

NUTRITIONAL ANALYSIS

Per 1½ ounces: Calories 253, Protein 7g, Total fat 22g, Sat fat 3g, Trans fat 0g, Cholesterol 0mg, Carbohydrate 11g, Dietary fiber 4g, Sodium 5mg

DAY 21: SATURDAY

Breakfast

Ricotta–Whole Wheat Pancakes
with Fresh Fruit
BONUS YEARS POINTS: FRUITS AND VEGETABLES 15%
CALORIES: 394

Lunch

Veggie Burrito
BONUS YEARS POINTS: FRUITS AND VEGETABLES 55%;
GARLIC 100%
CALORIES: 270

Dinner

Penne with Sausage, Bell Peppers,
and Sun-Dried Tomato Wine Sauce
Mixed Baby Greens with Roasted
Garlic Vinaigrette (1½ recipes,
page 112)
BONUS YEARS POINTS: FRUITS AND VEGETABLES 100%;
GARLIC 65%
CALORIES: 697

5 ounces wine
BONUS YEARS POINTS: WINE 100%
CALORIES: 106

Snacks

2 ounces dark chocolate
BONUS YEARS POINTS: CHOCOLATE 100%
CALORIES: 302

2 ounces unsalted dry-roasted
or natural nuts
BONUS YEARS POINTS: NUTS 100%
CALORIES: 337

DAY'S TOTAL BONUS YEARS POINTS: WINE **100%**; CHOCOLATE **100%**;
FRUITS AND VEGETABLES **170%**; GARLIC **165%**; NUTS **100%**
TOTAL CALORIES: **2,106**

Ricotta–Whole Wheat Pancakes with Fresh Fruit

MAKES ABOUT 8 (5-INCH) PANCAKES; 4 SERVINGS

¾ cup plus 2 tablespoons unbleached all-purpose flour
¾ cup white whole wheat or regular whole wheat flour
2 teaspoons baking powder
1 tablespoon sugar
pinch kosher salt
1½ cups fat-free milk
1 cup part-skim ricotta cheese
2 tablespoons canola oil
1 teaspoon vanilla extract
2 egg whites
2 cups chopped fresh fruits of your choice, such as peaches,
   berries, bananas, and mangoes
maple syrup (optional)

Combine the flours, baking powder, sugar, and salt in a medium bowl. Beat the milk, ricotta cheese, oil, and vanilla in another medium bowl until smooth.

Beat the egg whites in a small bowl until stiff but not dry. Pour the milk mixture into the dry ingredients, and stir just until combined. Fold in the egg whites.

Preheat a griddle or large skillet over medium heat. Spray with nonstick cooking spray. For each pancake, pour about ⅓ cup batter onto griddle. Cook until bubbles form in pancakes and edges start to dry. Turn and cook until lightly browned on bottoms. Serve with fruit and syrup (if using).

BONUS YEARS DAILY PERCENTAGES

Per serving: Fruits and vegetables 15%

NUTRITIONAL ANALYSIS

Per serving: Calories 394, Protein 17g, Total fat 12g, Sat fat 3g, Trans fat 0g, Cholesterol 27mg, Carbohydrate 57g, Dietary fiber 5g, Sodium 489mg

Veggie Burrito

MAKES 4 SERVINGS

---

1 large tomato (14 ounces), cored and roughly chopped

1 zucchini (about 6 ounces), cut into ¼-inch dice (1 cup)

1 yellow summer squash (about 6 ounces), cut into ¼-inch
   dice (1 cup)

2 large red bell peppers (12 ounces total), roasted (see page
   378), peeled, and diced, or 1 (12-ounce) jar roasted red bell
   peppers, drained and diced

4 cloves garlic, thinly sliced

4 teaspoons taco seasoning

kosher salt and freshly ground black pepper, to taste

4 large (10-inch) spinach or whole wheat tortillas

½ cup low-fat sour cream

½ cup grated low-fat cheddar cheese

Combine the vegetables, garlic, and taco seasoning in a large bowl. Season with salt and pepper; toss to combine.

Heat the tortillas in a microwave on high power for about 30 seconds. Place one-fourth of the vegetables in each softened tortilla, roll up, and top with 2 tablespoon each of the sour cream and the cheese.

To Make Ahead: Cover and refrigerate the vegetable mixture until ready to eat. Heat the tortillas, add the vegetable mixture, roll up, and top with the sour cream and cheese.

BONUS YEARS DAILY PERCENTAGES

Per serving: Fruits and vegetables 55%; Garlic 100%

NUTRITIONAL ANALYSIS

Per serving: Calories 270, Protein 11g, Total fat 8g, Sat fat 3g, Trans fat 0g, Cholesterol 15mg, Carbohydrate 38g, Dietary fiber 5g, Sodium 563mg

Penne with Sausage, Bell Peppers, and Sun-Dried Tomato Wine Sauce

MAKES 5 CUPS SAUCE; 6 SERVINGS

This recipe makes a great basic marinara sauce, which can be used with any Italian dish that calls for a tomato sauce. It works great with pasta. If possible, make this a day ahead of time and keep it in the refrigerator. The sauce tastes best after the flavors have had time to meld.

Choose an Italian red wine, such as a Chianti or Nero d'Avola.

SUN-DRIED TOMATO WINE SAUCE

1½ tablespoons extra-virgin olive oil
1 large onion (8 to 10 ounces), roughly chopped
1 large carrot (about 5 ounces), peeled and roughly chopped
2 celery stalks, roughly chopped
4 cloves garlic, chopped
1 teaspoon fennel seed
½ teaspoon dried oregano
½ teaspoon dried basil
⅛ to ¼ teaspoon red pepper flakes, or to taste
1 cup Chianti wine
1 (28-ounce) can no-salt-added tomatoes, roughly chopped
⅓ cup dry-packed, sun-dried tomatoes, reconstituted
   according to package directions in ½ cup water
1 cup low-sodium chicken broth
kosher salt and freshly ground black pepper, to taste

6 large Italian turkey sausages
2 large red bell peppers (12 ounces total), roasted (see
   page 378), peeled, and cut into strips, or 1 (12-ounce) jar
   roasted red bell peppers, drained and cut into strips

1 pound penne or rigatoni pasta, cooked al dente

chopped fresh flat-leaf parsley, for garnish

Make the sauce: Heat the oil in a 4-quart saucepan over medium heat. Add the onion, carrot, and celery and sauté until softened, about 5 minutes. Add the garlic and sauté for 1 minute. Add the fennel seed, oregano, basil, and pepper flakes and cook for 2 minutes.

Add the wine and simmer until reduced by half. Add the canned tomatoes with their juice, sun-dried tomatoes with their liquid, and the broth. Simmer until reduced by half, about 1 hour. Season with salt and pepper. Transfer to a food processor and process until coarsely pureed; the sauce should be chunky. (The sauce can be made ahead, cooled, and refrigerated for up to 2 days.)

Place the sausages in a skillet with about ¼ inch of water. Simmer until the water has evaporated. Cook the sausages until lightly browned. Cut the sausages into ½-inch-thick slices.

Add the sausage and bell peppers to the sauce. Heat until hot. Add the cooked penne and thoroughly mix to coat the penne with the sauce. Divide among 6 bowls. Garnish with the parsley.

BONUS YEARS DAILY PERCENTAGES

Per serving: Fruits and vegetables 65%; Garlic 65%

NUTRITIONAL ANALYSIS

Per serving: Calories 583, Protein 29g, Total fat 14g, Sat fat 4g, Trans fat 0g, Cholesterol 51mg, Carbohydrate 80g, Dietary fiber 7g, Sodium 667mg

Dr. Chef's Note

Try to match the shape of the pasta with that of the cut vegetables and meats. I like to prepare my pasta Italian style, al dente, tender yet still firm to the bite, not mushy. Undercook the pasta slightly, because it will continue to cook after it is mixed with the hot sauce.

RED WINE

NUTRITIONAL ANALYSIS

Per 5 ounces: Calories 106, Protein 0g, Total fat 0g, Sat fat 0g, Trans fat 0g,
Cholesterol 0mg, Carbohydrate 2g, Dietary fiber 0g, Sodium 7mg

DARK CHOCOLATE

NUTRITIONAL ANALYSIS

Per 2 ounces: Calories 302, Protein 3g, Total fat 16g, Sat fat 10g, Trans fat 0g,
Cholesterol 0mg, Carbohydrate 36g, Dietary fiber 2g, Sodium 9mg

NUTS

NUTRITIONAL ANALYSIS

Per 2 ounces: Calories 337, Protein 10g, Total fat 29g, Sat fat 4g, Trans fat 0g,
Cholesterol 0mg, Carbohydrate 14g, Dietary fiber 5g, Sodium 7mg

DAY 22: SUNDAY

Breakfast

Southwestern Omelet
with Pico de Gallo
BONUS YEARS POINTS: FRUITS AND VEGETABLES 25%;
GARLIC 100%
CALORIES: 232

Lunch

Moroccan Vegetable Couscous
Medley
½ cup light vanilla ice cream mixed
with 1 ounce mini chocolate chips
and 1 ounce sliced almonds
BONUS YEARS POINTS: CHOCOLATE 50%; FRUITS AND
VEGETABLES 60%; GARLIC 100%; NUTS 60%
CALORIES: 766

Dinner

Duck Breasts with
Port and Fig Sauce
Spinach and Arugula Sauté
½ cup cooked wild rice
BONUS YEARS POINTS: FRUITS AND VEGETABLES 70%;
GARLIC 150%; NUTS 25%
CALORIES: 711

5 ounces wine
BONUS YEARS POINTS: WINE 100%
CALORIES: 106

Snacks

1 ounce dark chocolate
BONUS YEARS POINTS: CHOCOLATE 50%
CALORIES: 151

½ ounce unsalted dry-roasted
or natural nuts
BONUS YEARS POINTS: NUTS 25%
CALORIES: 84

DAY'S TOTAL BONUS YEARS POINTS: WINE 100%; CHOCOLATE 100%;
FRUITS AND VEGETABLES 155%; GARLIC 350%; NUTS 100%
TOTAL CALORIES: 2,008

Southwestern Omelet with Pico de Gallo

MAKES 2 SERVINGS

---

1 green onion, thinly sliced on the diagonal

2 cloves garlic, thinly sliced

½ cup mixed fresh vegetables, such as red and green bell peppers, jicama, and yellow squash, cut into ¼-inch dice

8 ounces egg substitute, or 4 eggs, beaten

kosher salt and freshly ground black pepper, to taste

2 teaspoons extra-virgin olive oil

Pico de Gallo (recipe follows)

Spray a 10-inch nonstick skillet with cooking spray. Add the onion and sauté for about 2 minutes. Add the garlic and vegetables and sauté until they are crisp-tender, about 3 minutes. Remove from the skillet and reserve.

Season the egg substitute with salt and pepper. Lightly beat with a fork. Heat the skillet over medium-high heat. Add the oil and heat until it begins to shimmer. Add the egg substitute, vigorously shake the skillet, and stir the eggs. When they just begin to set, use a spatula to lift the edge and allow the liquid egg substitute that remains to flow around the edge. Use the spatula to again loosen the edge and to shape. Let the omelet cook for about 15 seconds; only a small amount of liquid should be remaining in the center. Add the sautéed vegetables along the lower two-thirds of the omelet. Shake the pan and use the spatula to loosen the omelet. Fold the upper third of the omelet over the vegetables, slide the omelet onto the plate, and fold over the remaining two-thirds of the omelet. Divide into two servings. Serve with Pico de Gallo.

BONUS YEARS DAILY PERCENTAGES

Per serving: Fruits and vegetables 5%; Garlic 100%

NUTRITIONAL ANALYSIS

Per serving: Calories 187, Protein 15g, Total fat 9g, Sat fat 1g, Trans fat 0g, Cholesterol 1mg, Carbohydrate 11g, Dietary fiber 3g, Sodium 232mg

Pico de Gallo

MAKES ABOUT 2 CUPS; 4 SERVINGS

3 Roma tomatoes (9 ounces total), seeds removed and
coarsely chopped

½ cup coarsely chopped red onion (2 ounces)

⅓ cup diced unpeeled hothouse or English cucumber
(1¼ ounces)

1 serrano chili, seeds removed and finely minced

1¾ tablespoons freshly squeezed lime juice

¾ tablespoon extra-virgin olive oil

kosher salt and freshly ground black pepper, to taste

Gently mix all the ingredients in a bowl. Cover and let stand for at least an hour before serving. Refrigerate any leftovers.

BONUS YEARS DAILY PERCENTAGES

Per serving: Fruits and vegetables 20%

NUTRITIONAL ANALYSIS

Per serving: Calories 45, Protein 0g, Total fat 6g, Sat fat 0g, Trans fat 0g,
Cholesterol 0mg, Carbohydrate 5g, Dietary fiber 1g, Sodium 5mg

Moroccan Vegetable
Couscous Medley

MAKES 6 CUPS; 4 SERVINGS

---

*This hearty vegetarian main dish is as filling as it is delicious.
It can also be served as a side dish. The condiments add just the
right touch of heat and spice to keep you coming back for more.*

1½ tablespoons extra-virgin olive oil

1½ teaspoons ground cumin

1 tablespoon sweet paprika, preferably smoked Spanish
   paprika

1½ cups sliced red onion (about 6 ounces)

1 medium zucchini (4 ounces), cut into ¼-inch dice (about
   1 cup)

1 medium yellow summer squash (4 ounces), cut into ¼-inch
   dice (about 1 cup)

1 cup diced, peeled eggplant (about 4 ounces)

1 cup diced carrots (about 4 ounces)

1 small red bell pepper (4 ounces), cut into ¼-inch dice
   (1 cup)

4 cloves garlic, thinly sliced

2 tablespoons tomato paste

1 medium tomato (7 to 8 ounces), coarsely chopped (1 cup)

1¼ cups dry couscous prepared according to package
   directions (2½ cups cooked couscous)

kosher salt and freshly ground black pepper, to taste

¼ cup minced flat-leaf parsley

¼ cup chopped mint

Heat the oil in a 12-inch skillet over medium heat. Add the cumin
and paprika and sauté for about 30 seconds. Add the onion and

sauté for 2 minutes. Add the zucchini, yellow squash, eggplant, carrots, and bell pepper and sauté for 4 minutes. Add the garlic and sauté for 2 to 3 minutes. Add the tomato paste and tomato and sauté for 2 minutes, stirring to mix them into the vegetables.

Add the warm couscous, and thoroughly mix. Season with salt and pepper, and fold in the chopped herbs. Divide among four plates.

BONUS YEARS DAILY PERCENTAGES

Per serving: Fruits and vegetables 60%; Garlic 100%

NUTRITIONAL ANALYSIS

Per serving: Calories 334, Protein 10g, Total fat 6g, Sat fat 1g, Trans fat 0g, Cholesterol 0mg, Carbohydrate 59g, Dietary fiber 8g, Sodium 39mg

½ CUP LIGHT VANILLA ICE CREAM MIXED WITH 1 OUNCE MINI CHOCOLATE CHIPS AND ¾ OUNCE SLICED ALMONDS

BONUS YEARS DAILY PERCENTAGES

Per serving: Chocolate 50%; Nuts 100%

NUTRITIONAL ANALYSIS

Per serving: Calories 390, Protein 8g, Total fat 21g, Sat fat 7g, Trans fat 0g, Cholesterol 5mg, Carbohydrate 41g, Dietary fiber 4g, Sodium 52mg

Duck Breasts with Port and Fig Sauce

MAKES 4 SERVINGS

This makes an elegant "three-star" pan-roasted dish. An initial sear in the skillet produces a fond *(the browned and caramelized bits of meat stuck to the skillet), which forms the basis of a delicious sauce when deglazed with the port, vinegar, and figs. Meanwhile, the beautifully browned duck is finished off in the oven, ensuring it will be moist and tender. This is another basic technique which can be applied to an endless number of sauces and cuts of meat.*

Choose an Australian Shiraz or California Zinfandel to match the jammy flavor of the port used in the sauce.

½ cup dry red wine
2½ tablespoons extra-virgin olive oil
2 cloves garlic, crushed
¼ cup minced onion
¼ teaspoon dried thyme
4 (5- to 6-ounce) deboned duck breasts, skin removed
1½ cups ruby port
3 tablespoons minced shallot
½ cup low-sodium chicken broth
8 dried figs, quartered
2 teaspoons balsamic vinegar
1 teaspoon arrowroot mixed with 2 teaspoons water
kosher salt and freshly ground black pepper, to taste

Combine the red wine, 1 tablespoon of the oil, the garlic, onion, and thyme in a bowl. Add the duck and marinate in the refrigerator for 1 to 2 hours.

Place the port in a small saucepan over low heat and simmer until reduced by half.

Preheat the oven to 350 degrees. Remove the duck from the marinade and pat dry with paper towels. Heat the remaining 1½ tablespoons oil in a 12-inch nonstick skillet over medium heat to just below smoking. Add the duck and reduce the heat to very low. Cook for 3 minutes, turn over, and cook for 3 minutes. Transfer the duck to a baking pan and roast for 8 to 10 minutes, or until the duck is just pink in the middle. Remove from the oven, cover, and keep warm.

Meanwhile, remove all but about 2 teaspoons of fat from the skillet. Add the shallot to the skillet and sauté until it is softened, 2 to 3 minutes. Stir in the reduced port, scraping up the browned bits from the bottom of the skillet. Add the broth, figs, and vinegar and simmer until the liquid is reduced to about ½ cup. Stir in the arrowroot mixture. Season with salt and pepper.

Slice the duck on the diagonal and transfer a duck breast to each of four plates. Spoon the sauce over and around the duck.

BONUS YEARS DAILY PERCENTAGES
Per serving: Fruits and vegetables 20%; Garlic 50%

NUTRITIONAL ANALYSIS
Per serving: Calories 426, Protein 31g, Total fat 11g, Sat fat 3g, Trans fat 0g, Cholesterol 109mg, Carbohydrate 40g, Dietary fiber 1g, Sodium 109mg

Spinach and Arugula Sauté

MAKES 4 SERVINGS

---

18 ounces fresh baby spinach

6 ounces fresh arugula

1 tablespoon plus 1 teaspoon extra-virgin olive oil

2 medium shallots, minced

¾ cup coarsely chopped fresh tomatoes

4 cloves garlic, coarsely chopped

2 tablespoons red wine vinegar

2 teaspoons balsamic vinegar

kosher salt and freshly ground black pepper, to taste

½ cup pine nuts, toasted (see page 159)

Bring a large pot of water to a boil. Remove any large stems from the spinach and arugula. Add the spinach and arugula to the water and let stand until bright green, about 30 seconds. Drain and rinse the spinach and arugula under cold running water to stop the cooking. Drain well and place on paper towels. Squeeze out all the water.

Heat the oil in a nonstick skillet over medium heat to just below smoking. Add the shallots and sauté until softened, 1 to 2 minutes. Add the tomatoes and sauté for 1 minute. Add the garlic and sauté until it is just cooked through but not browned, 30 seconds to 1 minute.

Add the spinach and arugula, tossing to coat with the oil, garlic, and shallots until hot. Add the vinegars and season with salt and pepper. Add the pine nuts and toss to combine.

BONUS YEARS DAILY PERCENTAGES

Per serving: Fruits and vegetables 50%; Garlic 100%; Nuts 25%

NUTRITIONAL ANALYSIS

Per serving: Calories 202, Protein 10g, Total fat 14g, Sat fat 2g, Trans fat 0g, Cholesterol 0mg, Carbohydrate 14g, Dietary fiber 5g, Sodium 119mg

Dr. Chef's Note

Water-blanching the arugula and spinach before sautéing them guarantees evenly cooked greens.

COOKED WILD RICE

NUTRITIONAL ANALYSIS

Per ½ cup: Calories 83, Protein 3g, Total fat 0g, Sat fat 0g, Trans fat 0g, Cholesterol 0mg, Carbohydrate 17g, Dietary fiber 1g, Sodium 2mg

RED WINE

NUTRITIONAL ANALYSIS

Per 5 ounces: Calories 106, Protein 0g, Total fat 0g, Sat fat 0g, Trans fat 0g, Cholesterol 0mg, Carbohydrate 2g, Dietary fiber 0g, Sodium 7mg

DARK CHOCOLATE

NUTRITIONAL ANALYSIS

Per 1 ounce: Calories 151, Protein 1g, Total fat 8g, Sat fat 5g, Trans fat 0g, Cholesterol 0mg, Carbohydrate 18g, Dietary fiber 1g, Sodium 5mg

DAY 23: MONDAY

Breakfast

⅔ cup high-fiber cereal with ½ cup raspberries and ½ cup fat-free milk

BONUS YEARS POINTS: FRUITS AND VEGETABLES 15%

NUTRITIONAL ANALYSIS: CALORIES 188, PROTEIN 8G, TOTAL FAT 1G, SAT FAT 0G, TRANS FAT 0G, CHOLES-TEROL 2MG, CARBOHYDRATE 42G, DIETARY FIBER 7G, SODIUM 173MG

Lunch

Green Bean, Berry, and Spinach Salad

BONUS YEARS POINTS: FRUITS AND VEGETABLES 35%; NUTS 50%

CALORIES: 394

Dinner

Cod Iberia
Steamed new potatoes with parsley
Creamy Chocolate Rice Pudding

BONUS YEARS POINTS: FRUITS AND VEGETABLES 55%; FISH 100%; GARLIC 100%; CHOCOLATE 25%

CALORIES: 587

5 ounces wine

BONUS YEARS POINTS: WINE 100%

CALORIES: 106

Snacks

1½ ounces dark chocolate

BONUS YEARS POINTS: CHOCOLATE 100%

CALORIES: 302

1 ounce unsalted dry-roasted or natural nuts

BONUS YEARS POINTS: NUTS 50%

CALORIES: 168

DAY'S TOTAL BONUS YEARS POINTS: WINE 100%; CHOCOLATE 100%; FRUITS AND VEGETABLES 105%; FISH 100%; GARLIC 100%; NUTS 100%

TOTAL CALORIES: 1,481

Green Bean, Berry, and Spinach Salad

MAKES 4 SERVINGS

1 cup thinly sliced red onion (4 ounces)

4 ounces green beans, preferably thin haricot vert (French green beans), cut into 1-inch lengths (about 1 cup), or drained canned green beans

8 cups fresh spinach (6 ounces), washed and spun dry

8 ounces mixed raspberries, blueberries, and strawberries (about 2 cups)

1 cup chopped walnuts (4 ounces)

½ cup Raspberry Vinaigrette (recipe follows)

Soak the onion in ice water for about 20 minutes and drain.

Bring a pot of water to a boil. Prepare a bowl of ice and water. Add the beans to the boiling water and drain after 1 minute. Immediately transfer the beans to the ice water to stop the cooking. Drain.

Add the spinach, onion, and green beans to a large bowl and toss to combine. Divide among four plates. Top with the berries and nuts, and drizzle with the dressing.

To Make Ahead: Wash and dry the spinach, soak the onion, blanch the green beans (if using fresh ones), and prepare the dressing. Refrigerate separately and combine all ingredients just before eating.

BONUS YEARS DAILY PERCENTAGES

Per serving: Fruits and vegetables 35%; Nuts 50%

NUTRITIONAL ANALYSIS

Per serving: Calories 394, Protein 9g, Total fat 33g, Sat fat 3g, Trans fat 0g, Cholesterol 0mg, Carbohydrate 19g, Dietary fiber 10g, Sodium 80mg

Raspberry Vinaigrette

MAKES ABOUT 1 CUP

½ cup low-sodium chicken broth
1 teaspoon arrowroot dissolved in 1 teaspoon cold water
2 tablespoons extra-virgin olive oil
¼ cup raspberry vinegar
1 teaspoon honey
1 teaspoon Dijon mustard
kosher salt and freshly ground black pepper, to taste

Heat the broth and arrowroot mixture in a small saucepan over medium heat until thickened. Whisk all the ingredients together in a small bowl and refrigerate.

NUTRITIONAL ANALYSIS

Per 2 tablespoons: Calories 40, Protein 0g, Total fat 3g, Sat fat 0g, Trans fat 0g, Cholesterol 0mg, Carbohydrate 2g, Dietary fiber 0g, Sodium 20mg

Cod Iberia

MAKES 4 SERVINGS

———————

The smoky sweet Spanish paprika adds some real zing to the recipe, but any good-quality paprika can be substituted for it.

2 tablespoons extra-virgin olive oil
1 teaspoon sweet smoky Spanish paprika (available in specialty markets), or any good-quality sweet paprika
1 medium yellow onion (about 6 ounces), coarsely chopped
1 small red bell pepper (about 4 ounces), coarsely chopped
1 small green bell pepper (about 4 ounces), coarsely chopped
4 large cloves garlic, thinly sliced
2 medium tomatoes (about 1 pound), cored and coarsely chopped
1 tablespoon red wine vinegar
3 sprigs parsley, coarsely chopped
2 whole bay leaves
1 cup low-sodium chicken broth or good fish stock
kosher salt and freshly ground black pepper, to taste
4 (5- to 6-ounce) cod fillets

Heat 1 tablespoon of the oil in a 12-inch skillet over medium heat. Add the paprika, onion, and bell peppers and sauté for about 5 minutes. Add the garlic and sauté for about 2 minutes. Add the tomatoes, vinegar, parsley, bay leaves, and broth. Bring to a simmer, reduce heat, cover, and cook until the sauce just begins to thicken, 20 to 25 minutes. Season the sauce with salt and pepper.

Preheat the oven to 350 degrees. After the sauce has been cooking about 15 minutes, season the cod with salt and pepper. Add the remaining 1 tablespoon oil to an ovenproof 12-inch nonstick skillet over medium heat and heat until the oil is just below smoking. Add the cod, reduce the heat to low, and brown the cod for 3 minutes on each side. Pour the thickened vegetable sauce over the cod, and transfer to the oven. Roast for 6 to 8 minutes, or until the cod is opaque. Remove from the oven and divide the cod and the sauce among four plates.

BONUS YEARS DAILY PERCENTAGES
Per serving: Fruits and vegetables 55%; Fish 100%; Garlic 100%

NUTRITIONAL ANALYSIS
Per serving: Calories 243, Protein 28g, Total fat 9g, Sat fat 1g, Trans fat 0g, Cholesterol 62mg, Carbohydrate 13g, Dietary fiber 3g, Sodium 116mg

STEAMED NEW POTATOES WITH PARSLEY
NUTRITIONAL ANALYSIS
Per ½-cup serving: Calories 80, Protein 3g, Total fat 0g, Sat fat 0g, Trans fat 0g, Cholesterol 0mg, Carbohydrate 20g, Dietary fiber 2g, Sodium 30mg

Creamy Chocolate Rice Pudding

For an elegant presentation, line four ramekins or custard cups with aluminum foil, leaving the ends extending over the edges. Divide the pudding among the cups. Cover and refrigerate until chilled. Turn out the cups onto dessert plates and remove the foil. Surround with fresh orange segments sprinkled with chopped pistachios.

½ cup Arborio rice

1 cup boiling water

2 cups fat-free milk

¼ cup sugar

1 teaspoon vanilla extract

1 tablespoon freshly grated orange zest

2 ounces semisweet or bittersweet chocolate

2 tablespoons orange liqueur, such as Grand Marnier
  (optional)

Combine the rice and boiling water in a medium saucepan. Bring to a simmer over medium heat. Simmer, stirring occasionally, until most of the water is absorbed. Meanwhile heat the milk over low heat just until hot. Add the milk, ½ cup at a time, to the rice and simmer, stirring constantly, until the milk is absorbed. Add the sugar, vanilla, and orange zest with the last addition of milk. The rice should be tender by the time all the milk is used. If not, add additional boiling water and cook until the mixture is creamy and the rice tender but slightly firm and the pudding is the desired consistency. The total cooking time should be about 40 minutes. Remove from the heat and add the chocolate and orange liqueur (if using). Stir until the chocolate is melted. Serve warm or chilled.

To Make Ahead: Make as directed. Divide among four serving dishes, cover, and refrigerate. Serve chilled or bring to room temperature before serving.

BONUS YEARS DAILY PERCENTAGES

Per serving: Chocolate 25%

NUTRITIONAL ANALYSIS

Per serving: Calories 264, Protein 8g, Total fat 4g, Sat fat 3g, Trans fat 0g, Cholesterol 2mg, Carbohydrate 49g, Dietary fiber 1g, Sodium 67mg

Dr. Chef's Note

Arborio rice should never be rinsed before cooking. The starch coating adds the creamy consistency to the finished dish.

RED WINE

NUTRITIONAL ANALYSIS

Per 5 ounces: Calories 106, Protein 0g, Total fat 0g, Sat fat 0g, Trans fat 0g, Cholesterol 0mg, Carbohydrate 2g, Dietary fiber 0g, Sodium 7mg

DARK CHOCOLATE

NUTRITIONAL ANALYSIS

Per 1½ ounces: Calories 227, Protein 2g, Total fat 12g, Sat fat 7g, Trans fat 0g, Cholesterol 0mg, Carbohydrate 27g, Dietary fiber 2g, Sodium 7mg

NUTS

NUTRITIONAL ANALYSIS

Per 1 ounce: Calories 168, Protein 5g, Total fat 14g, Sat fat 2g, Trans fat 0g, Cholesterol 0mg, Carbohydrate 7g, Dietary fiber 2g, Sodium 3mg

DAY 24: TUESDAY

Breakfast

Berry Yogurt Cup
1 slice whole wheat bread, toasted,
with 1 tablespoon nut butter
BONUS YEARS POINTS: FRUITS AND VEGETABLES 50%;
NUTS 50%
CALORIES: 477

Lunch

Caesar Salad Wrap
BONUS YEARS POINTS: FRUITS AND VEGETABLES 10%;
FISH 60%
CALORIES: 284

Dinner

Braised Szechuan Chicken Thighs
Asian-Style Vegetable Stir-fry
½ cup steamed brown rice
BONUS YEARS POINTS: FRUITS AND VEGETABLES 30%;
GARLIC 100%
CALORIES: 922

5 ounces wine
BONUS YEARS POINTS: WINE 100%
CALORIES: 106

Snacks

2 ounces dark chocolate
BONUS YEARS POINTS: CHOCOLATE 100%
CALORIES: 302

1 ounce unsalted dry-roasted
or natural nuts
BONUS YEARS POINTS: NUTS 50%
CALORIES: 168

1 apple
BONUS YEARS POINTS: FRUITS AND VEGETABLES 20%
CALORIES: 80

DAY'S TOTAL BONUS YEARS POINTS: WINE 100%; CHOCOLATE 100%;
FRUITS AND VEGETABLES 110%; FISH 60%; GARLIC 100%; NUTS 100%
TOTAL CALORIES: 2,339

Berry Yogurt Cup

MAKES 1 SERVING

1 cup mixed fresh or thawed frozen berries
½ cup fat-free berry yogurt
2 tablespoons dried cranberries or currants
2 tablespoons chopped pecans, preferably toasted (see page 159)

Combine the mixed berries and yogurt in a small bowl. Sprinkle the cranberries and pecans over the top.

BONUS YEARS DAILY PERCENTAGES

Per serving: Fruits and vegetables 50%; Nuts 25%

NUTRITIONAL ANALYSIS

Per serving: Calories 313, Protein 7g, Total fat 11g, Sat fat 1g, Trans fat 0g, Cholesterol 2mg, Carbohydrate 50g, Dietary fiber 10g, Sodium 59mg

WHOLE WHEAT BREAD

NUTRITIONAL ANALYSIS

Per slice: Calories 69, Protein 3g, Total fat 1g, Sat fat 0g, Trans fat 0g, Cholesterol 0mg, Carbohydrate 13g, Dietary fiber 2g, Sodium 147mg

NUT BUTTER (SUCH AS ALMOND OR PEANUT)

BONUS YEARS DAILY PERCENTAGES

Per tablespoon: Nuts 25%

NUTRITIONAL ANALYSIS

Per tablespoon: Calories 95, Protein 4g, Total fat 8g, Sat fat 1g, Trans fat 0g, Cholesterol 0mg, Carbohydrate 3g, Dietary fiber 1g, Sodium 74mg

Caesar Salad Wrap

MAKES 4 SERVINGS

1 (12-ounce) can water-pack tuna, drained and shredded, or
 2 chicken breasts, cooked and shredded
1 small head romaine lettuce (about 5½ ounces), shredded
 (about 4 cups)
2 green onions, cut into thin rings (green and white parts)
¼ cup low-fat prepared Caesar salad dressing
¼ cup freshly grated Parmesan cheese
kosher salt and freshly ground black pepper, to taste
4 large (9- to 10-inch) tortillas

Add the tuna and lettuce to a large bowl and toss to thoroughly combine. Add the green onions, salad dressing, and cheese, and mix. Season with salt and pepper.

Heat each of the tortillas in a microwave oven on high for about 20 seconds to soften them. Place 1 cup of the salad across the bottom of each tortilla; the salad should not quite touch the edge. Roll the tortilla tightly over the salad filling, then fold in the two sides and continue rolling until the filling is completely wrapped.

To Make Ahead: Prepare the salad and refrigerate until ready to eat. Heat the tortillas, add the salad, and roll up.

BONUS YEARS DAILY PERCENTAGES
Per serving: Fruits and vegetables 10%; Fish 60%
NUTRITIONAL ANALYSIS
Per serving: Calories 284, Protein 28g, Total fat 6g, Sat fat 2g, Trans fat 0g, Cholesterol 29mg, Carbohydrate 28g, Dietary fiber 1g, Sodium 831mg

Braised Szechuan Chicken Thighs

MAKES 4 SERVINGS

---

*The chicken thighs will be meltingly tender after braising in
this typical Chinese wine sauce. Traditionally, this type of dish
is made in a clay sandy pot, which are very reasonable in price
and can be purchased in many Asian markets. The braise can
be served tableside in the clay pot and makes an elegant presentation, sure to wow friends and family.*

*Serve a fruity red wine with low amounts of tannin, such as
a simple Australian Shiraz or a Pinot Noir.*

8 chicken thighs (about 2 pounds), skin removed and fat
  trimmed
½ cup unbleached all-purpose flour
2 tablespoons canola oil
2 green onions (green and white parts), sliced into ¼-inch
  rings
4 cloves garlic, minced
2 tablespoons minced fresh ginger
1 to 2 teaspoons Asian chili paste, or other hot sauce to taste
3 tablespoons hoisin sauce
1 cup dry red wine
2 to 4 tablespoons low-sodium soy sauce
¼ cup low-sodium chicken broth
2 teaspoons arrowroot or cornstarch mixed with 2 teaspoons
  cold water
1 teaspoon sesame oil
2 tablespoons minced green onion, for garnish

Preheat the oven to 350 degrees. Dredge the chicken thighs in the flour and shake off any excess. Heat 1 tablespoon of the canola oil to just below smoking in a 12-inch ovenproof skillet. Turn the heat to low, add four of the chicken thighs, and cook until chicken is nicely browned, about 4 minutes on each side. Don't move the chicken as it is browning on each side. Remove the chicken from the skillet. Add the remaining 1 tablespoon oil and heat to below smoking; cook the remaining chicken thighs. Remove the chicken from the skillet and set aside.

Heat the fat remaining in the skillet. Add the sliced green onions and sauté for about 1 minute. Add the garlic and ginger and sauté for 1 minute. Stir in the chili paste and heat for 1 minute. Stir in the hoisin sauce, thoroughly mix, and heat for 1 minute. Add the wine and simmer until reduced by half. Add the soy sauce and broth, bring to a simmer, and add the chicken thighs. Cover the skillet and transfer to the oven. Cook about 50 minutes, or until the chicken is very tender.

Remove the skillet from the oven, and place over low heat. Whisk in the arrowroot mixture and sesame oil and cook, stirring, until thickened. Divide the chicken and sauce among four plates. Garnish with the minced green onion.

BONUS YEARS DAILY PERCENTAGES
Per serving: Garlic 100%

NUTRITIONAL ANALYSIS
Per serving: Calories 700, Protein 43g, Total fat 43g, Sat fat 10g, Trans fat 0g, Cholesterol 191mg, Carbohydrate 23g, Dietary fiber 1g, Sodium 733mg

Asian-Style Vegetable Stir-fry

1 (1-pound) package fresh vegetable stir-fry mix
1 teaspoon canola oil
2 green onions (white and pale green parts), minced
  (1 tablespoon)
½ tablespoon minced fresh ginger
1 large clove garlic, minced
½ cup low-sodium chicken broth
1 tablespoon low-sodium soy sauce
1 tablespoon dry sherry or Chinese rice wine
2 teaspoons cornstarch dissolved in 1 tablespoon cold water
kosher salt and freshly ground black pepper, to taste

Bring a large pot of water to a boil. Prepare a large bowl of ice and water. Add the stir-fry mix to the boiling water and drain after 1 minute. Immediately transfer the vegetables to the ice water to stop the cooking. Drain the vegetables and set aside.

Heat the oil in a large skillet over medium heat. Add the green onions and sauté for 1 minute. Add the ginger and garlic and sauté for 2 to 3 minutes; be careful not to burn the garlic. Add the broth, soy sauce, and sherry and bring to a simmer.

Add the vegetables and stir to combine. Add the cornstarch mixture, stir to mix thoroughly, and cook until the vegetables are hot and the sauce thickens and lightly coats the vegetables. Season with salt and pepper.

BONUS YEARS DAILY PERCENTAGES

Per serving: Fruits and vegetables 30%

Per serving: Calories 114, Protein 4g, Total fat 3g, Sat fat 0g, Trans fat 0g, Cholesterol 0mg, Carbohydrate 17g, Dietary fiber 1g, Sodium 728mg

STEAMED BROWN RICE

Per ½ cup: Calories 108, Protein 2g, Total fat 0g, Sat fat 0g, Trans fat 0g, Cholesterol 0mg, Carbohydrate 22g, Dietary fiber 2g, Sodium 5mg

RED WINE

Per 5 ounces: Calories 106, Protein 0g, Total fat 0g, Sat fat 0g, Trans fat 0g, Cholesterol 0mg, Carbohydrate 2g, Dietary fiber 0g, Sodium 7mg

DARK CHOCOLATE

Per 2 ounces: Calories 302, Protein 3g, Total fat 16g, Sat fat 10g, Trans fat 0g, Cholesterol 0mg, Carbohydrate 36g, Dietary fiber 2g, Sodium 9mg

NUTS

Per 1 ounce: Calories 168, Protein 5g, Total fat 14g, Sat fat 2g, Trans fat 0g, Cholesterol 0mg, Carbohydrate 7g, Dietary fiber 2g, Sodium 3mg

APPLE

BONUS YEARS DAILY PERCENTAGES

Per apple: Fruits and vegetables 20%

Per serving: Calories 80, Protein 0g, Total fat 0g, Sat fat 0g, Trans fat 0g, Cholesterol 0mg, Carbohydrate 22g, Dietary fiber 5g, Sodium 0mg

DAY 25: WEDNESDAY

Breakfast

Strawberry-Banana-Soy Smoothie
BONUS YEARS POINTS: FRUITS AND VEGETABLES 30%
CALORIES: 215

5 ounces wine
BONUS YEARS POINTS: WINE 100%
CALORIES: 100

Lunch

Creamy Roasted Carrot–Miso Soup
Crusty bread
1 pear
BONUS YEARS POINTS: FRUITS AND VEGETABLES 50%
CALORIES: 509

Snacks

2 ounces dark chocolate
BONUS YEARS POINTS: CHOCOLATE 100%
CALORIES: 302

1½ ounces unsalted dry-roasted
or natural nuts
BONUS YEARS POINTS: NUTS 75%
CALORIES: 253

Dinner

Stovetop-Grilled Swordfish in
Basil-Tomato Vinaigrette
½ cup steamed broccoli
¾ cup Almond Rice Pilaf
(page 262)
BONUS YEARS POINTS: FRUITS AND VEGETABLES 35%;
FISH 100%; GARLIC 100%; NUTS 25%
CALORIES: 662

DAY'S TOTAL BONUS YEARS POINTS: WINE 100%; CHOCOLATE 100%;
FRUITS AND VEGETABLES 115%; FISH 100%; GARLIC 100%; NUTS 100%
TOTAL CALORIES: 2,047

Strawberry-Banana-Soy Smoothie

MAKES 2 SERVINGS

1 frozen peeled medium banana, cut into chunks
1 cup fresh or frozen strawberries (about 8 ounces)
½ cup soft silken tofu
1 cup fat-free soymilk
2 tablespoons strawberry syrup, or sugar, to taste
1 teaspoon vanilla extract

Combine the banana, strawberries, tofu, and ½ cup of the milk in a blender. Blend until smooth. Add the remaining milk, syrup, and vanilla and blend until combined. Pour into two glasses and serve.

BONUS YEARS DAILY PERCENTAGES
Per serving: Fruits and vegetables 30%
NUTRITIONAL ANALYSIS
Per serving: Calories 215, Protein 8g, Total fat 5g, Sat fat 1g, Trans fat 0g, Cholesterol 0mg, Carbohydrate 36g, Dietary fiber 5g, Sodium 23mg

Variation

Fat-free yogurt and fat-free milk can be substituted for the tofu and soymilk.

Creamy Roasted Carrot–Miso Soup

MAKES 4 SERVINGS

*The miso adds a wonderfully sublime taste and is rich in soy.
You can't ask for a healthier or more flavorful creamed soup.
The Arborio rice adds a touch of creaminess. This recipe works
equally well warm or as a chilled soup in the summer.*

1 pound baby carrots, coarsely chopped
½ large onion (about 5 ounces), sliced into half rings
3¼ cups low-sodium chicken broth
2 tablespoons uncooked Arborio rice
6 ounces silken Japanese tofu
1½ tablespoons red or brown Japanese miso
kosher salt, to taste
⅛ to ¼ teaspoon ground white pepper
1 tablespoon chopped dill

Preheat the oven to 400 degrees. Place the carrots and onion in an ovenproof dish, spray with cooking spray, and roast for 40 minutes. Then add the carrots, onion, broth, and rice to a 4-quart saucepan, and bring to a low boil. Reduce the heat and simmer for 20 minutes.

Add the tofu and miso to a blender and puree. Add the rice and vegetable mixture and blend until smooth. Return the puree to the saucepan, bring to a simmer, stirring, and season with salt and pepper. Sprinkle with the dill.

To Make Ahead: Prepare the soup as directed above, except transfer the puree to a bowl instead of heating in a saucepan. Cover and refrigerate for up to 2 days. Heat before serving, or serve chilled, sprinkled with the dill.

BONUS YEARS DAILY PERCENTAGES

Per serving: Fruits and vegetables 30%

NUTRITIONAL ANALYSIS

Per serving: Calories 148, Protein 8g, Total fat 5g, Sat fat 1g, Trans fat 0g, Cholesterol 3mg, Carbohydrate 19g, Dietary fiber 15g, Sodium 440mg

CRUSTY BREAD

NUTRITIONAL ANALYSIS

Per 1 slice: Calories 263, Protein 8g, Total fat 3g, Sat fat 0g, Trans fat 0g, Cholesterol 0mg, Carbohydrate 50g, Dietary fiber 3g, Sodium 584mg

PEAR

BONUS YEARS DAILY PERCENTAGES

Per serving: Fruits and vegetables 20%

NUTRITIONAL ANALYSIS

Per serving: Calories 98, Protein 1g, Total fat 1g, Sat fat 0g, Trans fat 0g, Cholesterol 0mg, Carbohydrate 25g, Dietary fiber 4g, Sodium 1mg

Stovetop-Grilled Swordfish in Basil-Tomato Vinaigrette

MAKES 4 SERVINGS

Firm white fish fillets, such as swordfish and shark, will grill perfectly on a ridged stovetop grill pan without having to be finished off in the oven. More delicate fish such as salmon steaks or fillets will tend to burn on the outside if you try to cook them all the way through on the ridged pan, so completing the cooking in the oven (pan roasting) is often the best way to prepare these items.

1 cup Roasted Garlic-Shallot Vinaigrette (page 268) or other
   Mediterranean-style vinaigrette
¼ cup tightly packed chopped fresh basil (about ⅔ ounce)
¾ cup seeded, diced fresh tomatoes
¾ teaspoon chopped garlic
kosher salt and freshly ground black pepper, to taste
4 (6-ounce) swordfish, shark, or marlin steaks

Thoroughly mix the vinaigrette with the basil, tomatoes, garlic, salt, and pepper. Marinate the fish in the vinaigrette mixture for 45 minutes. Remove the fish from the marinade, reserving the marinade, and pat dry with paper towels.

Preheat a ridged grill pan over medium heat. (Or use an outdoor grill.) Add the fish and grill for about 4 minutes per side, turning the fillets a quarter turn after 2 minutes on a side to mark them.

Bring the reserved marinade to a boil and ladle over the grilled fish to serve.

BONUS YEARS DAILY PERCENTAGES

Per serving: Fruits and vegetables 5%; Fish 100%; Garlic 100%

NUTRITIONAL ANALYSIS

Per serving: Calories 319, Protein 33g, Total fat 17g, Sat fat 3g, Trans fat 0g, Cholesterol 62mg, Carbohydrate 6g, Dietary fiber 0g, Sodium 209mg

STEAMED BROCCOLI

BONUS YEARS DAILY PERCENTAGES

Per ½-cup serving: Fruits and vegetables 20%

NUTRITIONAL ANALYSIS

Per ½-cup serving: Calories 22, Protein 2g, Total fat 0g, Sat fat 0g, Cholesterol 0mg, Trans fat 0g, Carbohydrate 4g, Dietary fiber 2g, Sodium 21mg

RED WINE

NUTRITIONAL ANALYSIS

Per 5 ounces: Calories 106, Protein 0g, Total fat 0g, Sat fat 0g, Trans fat 0g, Cholesterol 0mg, Carbohydrate 2g, Dietary fiber 0g, Sodium 7mg

DARK CHOCOLATE

NUTRITIONAL ANALYSIS

Per 2 ounces: Calories 302, Protein 3g, Total fat 16g, Sat fat 10g, Trans fat 0g, Cholesterol 0mg, Carbohydrate 36g, Dietary fiber 2g, Sodium 9mg

NUTS

NUTRITIONAL ANALYSIS

Per 1½ ounces: Calories 253, Protein 7g, Total fat 22g, Sat fat 3g, Trans fat 0g, Cholesterol 0mg, Carbohydrate 11g, Dietary fiber 4g, Sodium 5mg

DAY 26: THURSDAY

Breakfast

¾ cup fat-free berry yogurt mixed
with 2 tablespoons slivered almonds,
½ cup high-fiber cereal, and ½ cup
raspberries or strawberries

BONUS YEARS POINTS: FRUITS AND VEGETABLES 15%;
NUTS 25%
NUTRITIONAL ANALYSIS: CALORIES 283, PROTEIN 12G,
TOTAL FAT 9G, SAT FAT 1G, TRANS FAT 0G,
CHOLESTEROL 4MG, CARBOHYDRATE 41G,
DIETARY FIBER 6G, SODIUM 314MG

Lunch

Mushroom-Walnut Salad with
Roquefort Vinaigrette
Whole wheat roll

BONUS YEARS POINTS: FRUITS AND VEGETABLES 20%;
NUTS 50%
CALORIES: 494

Dinner

Sicilian Poached Chicken Breasts
Italian Potato Salad
½ cup steamed spinach

BONUS YEARS POINTS: FRUITS AND VEGETABLES 45%;
GARLIC 100%
CALORIES: 476

5 ounces wine

BONUS YEARS POINTS: WINE 100%
CALORIES: 106

Snacks

2 ounces dark chocolate

BONUS YEARS POINTS: CHOCOLATE 100%
CALORIES: 302

½ ounce unsalted dry-roasted
or natural nuts

BONUS YEARS POINTS: NUTS 25%
CALORIES: 84

1 orange

BONUS YEARS POINTS: FRUITS AND VEGETABLES 20%
CALORIES: 65

DAY'S TOTAL BONUS YEARS POINTS: WINE 100%; CHOCOLATE 100%;
FRUITS AND VEGETABLES 105%; GARLIC 100%; NUTS 100%

TOTAL CALORIES: 1,810

Mushroom-Walnut Salad with Roquefort Vinaigrette

MAKES 4 SERVINGS

10 ounces button or cremini mushrooms, quartered
1 cup chopped walnuts
1½ cups chopped unpeeled red apple (1 medium apple)
Roquefort Vinaigrette (recipe follows)
9 leaves Boston or Bibb lettuce, washed and dried
9 radicchio leaves, washed and dried

Thoroughly mix the mushrooms, walnuts, and apple with the vinaigrette in a medium bowl. Cut a leaf of the lettuce and a leaf of the radicchio into thin strips. Toss with the mushroom mixture.

To serve: Arrange two of the lettuce leaves and two of the radicchio leaves into a round nest shape on each of four plates. Spoon the mushroom mixture into each salad nest.

BONUS YEARS DAILY PERCENTAGES
Per serving: Fruits and vegetables 20%; Nuts 50%

NUTRITIONAL ANALYSIS
Per serving: Calories 419, Protein 11g, Total fat 36g, Sat fat 5g, Trans fat 0g, Cholesterol 7mg, Carbohydrate 19g, Sodium 194mg

Roquefort Vinaigrette

MAKES ABOUT ¾ CUP

6 tablespoons thickened reduced-sodium chicken broth
   (see Dr. Chef's Note, page 113)
2 tablespoons walnut or extra-virgin olive oil
3 tablespoons sherry vinegar
½ teaspoon Dijon mustard
1 tablespoon minced shallot
2 tablespoons crumbled Roquefort cheese
kosher salt and freshly ground black pepper, to taste

Place all the ingredients in a jar with a lid. Shake to combine. You may refrigerate for up to 3 days if making ahead. Bring to room temperature before using.

NUTRITIONAL ANALYSIS

Per 2 tablespoons: Calories 59, Protein 1g, Total fat 5g, Sat fat 1g, Trans fat 0g, Cholesterol 2mg, Carbohydrate 2g, Dietary fiber 0g, Sodium 59mg

WHOLE WHEAT ROLL

NUTRITIONAL ANALYSIS

Per roll: Calories 75, Protein 2g, Total fat 1g, Sat fat 0g, Trans fat 0g, Cholesterol 0mg, Carbohydrate 14g, Dietary fiber 2g, Sodium 135mg

Sicilian Poached Chicken Breasts

MAKES 4 SERVINGS

The brining and the poaching guarantee a succulent and juicy entrée. If you have any leftover veggies, chop them up into small dice and just add them to the tomato and wine sauce.

The tangy flavors of this dish would be complemented by a Valpolicella or simple Chianti wine.

4 (5- to 6-ounce) boneless, skinless chicken breasts,
    preferably brined (see page 376) for 2 hours
1 tablespoon olive oil
4 cloves garlic, thinly sliced
3 medium anchovy fillets, mashed
½ cup dry white wine, such as Sauvignon Blanc
1 (14.5-ounce) can Italian-style plum tomatoes, coarsely
    chopped and juice reserved
½ cup pitted black olives, coarsely chopped
kosher salt and freshly ground black pepper, to taste
3 tablespoons chopped flat-leaf parsley, for garnish

Rinse the chicken under cold water and pat dry.
Preheat the oven to 350 degrees. Heat the oil in a 12-inch oven-proof skillet over medium heat. Add the garlic and anchovies and cook about 30 seconds, dissolving the anchovies in the oil. Add the wine and simmer until reduced by half. Add the tomatoes, tomato juice, and olives. Simmer for 5 minutes. Add the chicken, cover, and transfer to the oven. Cook for about 15 minutes, or until the chicken is just cooked through. Place one breast on each of four plates. Season the sauce with salt and pepper, and divide the sauce evenly over the chicken; garnish with the parsley.

BONUS YEARS DAILY PERCENTAGES

Per serving: Fruits and vegetables 25%; Garlic 100%

NUTRITIONAL ANALYSIS

Per serving: Calories 256, Protein 35g, Total fat 7g, Sat fat 1g, Trans fat 0g, Cholesterol 84mg, Carbohydrate 7g, Dietary fiber 2g, Sodium 467mg

Italian Potato Salad

MAKES 4 SERVINGS

This is a variation of the classic German potato salad. The flavor of the warmed vinaigrette will permeate the just-cooked and still-hot potatoes.

1½ pounds new red potatoes
4 slices turkey bacon, cut into small dice
¼ cup minced onion
1 recipe Roasted Garlic Vinaigrette (page 113) or other low-fat Italian vinaigrette
2 teaspoons arrowroot dissolved in 2 teaspoons water
2 tablespoons chopped flat-leaf parsley

Place the potatoes in a saucepan and cover with water. Bring to a boil; reduce the heat and simmer until the potatoes are just tender, about 25 minutes. Drain the potatoes and allow to cool to the point where they can be handled. Cut into bite-size pieces (the potatoes must be served warm).

Meanwhile, cook the bacon in a skillet over medium-low heat until brown. Add the onion and sauté until just tender. Add the vinaigrette and bring to a low simmer; stir in the arrowroot mixture and simmer until the sauce is just thickened. Pour the sauce over the warm potatoes and mix thoroughly. Sprinkle with the parsley and serve warm.

NUTRITIONAL ANALYSIS

Per serving: Calories 209, Protein 10g, Total fat 7g, Sat fat 1g, Trans fat 0g, Cholesterol 13mg, Carbohydrate 31g, Dietary fiber 3g, Sodium 325mg

STEAMED SPINACH

BONUS YEARS DAILY PERCENTAGES

Per ½-cup serving: Fruits and vegetables 20%

NUTRITIONAL ANALYSIS

Per ½-cup serving: Calories 11, Protein 1g, Total fat 0g, Sat fat 0g, Trans fat 0g, Cholesterol 0mg, Carbohydrate 2g, Dietary fiber 1g, Sodium 96mg

ORANGE

BONUS YEARS DAILY PERCENTAGES

Per serving: Fruits and vegetables 20%

NUTRITIONAL ANALYSIS

Per serving: Calories 65, Protein 1g, Total fat 0g, Sat fat 0g, Trans fat 0g, Cholesterol 0mg, Carbohydrate 16g, Dietary fiber 2g, Sodium 1mg

RED WINE

NUTRITIONAL ANALYSIS

Per 5 ounces: Calories 106, Protein 0g, Total fat 0g, Sat fat 0g, Trans fat 0g, Cholesterol 0mg, Carbohydrate 2g, Dietary fiber 0g, Sodium 7mg

DARK CHOCOLATE

NUTRITIONAL ANALYSIS

Per 2 ounces: Calories 302, Protein 3g, Total fat 16g, Sat fat 10g, Trans fat 0g, Cholesterol 0mg, Carbohydrate 36g, Dietary fiber 2g, Sodium 9mg

NUTS

NUTRITIONAL ANALYSIS

Per ½ ounce: Calories 84, Protein 2g, Total fat 7g, Sat fat 1g, Trans fat 0g, Cholesterol 0mg, Carbohydrate 3g, Dietary fiber 1g, Sodium 2mg

DAY 27: FRIDAY

Breakfast

Scrambled Egg Burrito
1 orange
BONUS YEARS POINTS: FRUITS AND VEGETABLES 20%
CALORIES: 359

Lunch

Lentil and Sausage Stew
BONUS YEARS POINTS: FRUITS AND VEGETABLES 85%;
GARLIC 100%
CALORIES: 429

Dinner

Broiled Miso-Glazed Salmon with
Soba Noodles
Steamed Broccoli, Asian Style
BONUS YEARS POINTS: FRUITS AND VEGETABLES 40%;
FISH 100%
CALORIES: 590

5 ounces wine
BONUS YEARS POINTS: WINE 100%
CALORIES: 106

Snacks

2 ounces dark chocolate
BONUS YEARS POINTS: CHOCOLATE 100%
CALORIES: 302

2 ounces unsalted dry-roasted
or natural nuts
BONUS YEARS POINTS: NUTS 100%
CALORIES: 337

DAY'S TOTAL BONUS YEARS POINTS: WINE 100%; CHOCOLATE 100%;
FRUITS AND VEGETABLES 145%; FISH 100%; GARLIC 100%; NUTS 100%
TOTAL CALORIES: 2,123

Scrambled Egg Burrito

MAKES 1 SERVING

½ cup egg substitute, or 2 eggs, lightly beaten
2 tablespoons reduced-fat or fat-free cream cheese, cut into
   small pieces
kosher salt and freshly ground black pepper, to taste
1 (about 7-inch) 100% whole wheat tortilla, warmed
Salsa, to taste

Combine the egg substitute and cream cheese in a medium bowl.
Season with salt and black pepper.

Spray a small nonstick skillet with cooking spray and place over
medium heat. Add the egg mixture and cook, stirring gently, until the
egg mixture is set. Pour the egg mixture into the center of the tortilla.
Top with salsa. Fold up one side, then roll to enclose the filling.

NUTRITIONAL ANALYSIS

Per serving: Calories 294, Protein 22g, Total fat 13g, Sat fat 5g, Trans fat 0g,
Cholesterol 0mg, Carbohydrate 21g, Dietary fiber 4g, Sodium 520mg

ORANGE

BONUS YEARS DAILY PERCENTAGES

Per serving: Fruits and vegetables 20%

NUTRITIONAL ANALYSIS

Per serving: Calories 65, Protein 1g, Total fat 0g, Sat fat 0g, Trans fat 0g,
Cholesterol 0mg, Carbohydrate 16g, Dietary fiber 2g, Sodium 1mg

Lentil and Sausage Stew

MAKES 4 (1½-CUP) SERVINGS

—————

French green lentils, or lentilles vertes, *are available in spe-cialty markets. They are much meatier than the standard brown or red lentils and won't break down when cooked. They make a perfect complement to the sausage.*

1 tablespoon extra-virgin olive oil
1 tablespoon Italian seasoning
1 large onion (8 to 9 ounces), coarsely diced
1 medium carrot (about 4 ounces), diced
3 stalks celery (about 4 ounces), diced
1 bunch Swiss chard (about 9 ounces), preferably the red
    variety, woody stalks removed and coarsely chopped and
    the leaves coarsely chopped (about 8 cups)
4 cloves garlic, thinly sliced
4½ cups low-sodium chicken broth
1 (about ¾-pound) smoked ham hock (optional)
1 cup lentils, preferably the green French variety
1 (14.5-ounce) can diced no-salt-added tomatoes
1 bay leaf
12 ounces Italian turkey sausage (sweet or hot to your taste),
    cut into ½-inch-thick slices
kosher salt and freshly ground black pepper, to taste

Heat the oil in a heavy, 4-quart saucepan over medium heat. Add the Italian seasoning and sauté for about 30 seconds. Add the onion, carrot, celery, and Swiss chard stems and sauté, stirring occasionally, for 5 minutes. Add the garlic and sauté for 2 minutes. Add the broth and ham hock (if using), and simmer for 45 minutes.

Add the lentils, tomatoes with their juices, and bay leaf and simmer about 15 minutes.

Add the sausage and Swiss chard leaves, and simmer until the lentils are tender, about 15 minutes. Remove the ham hock (if used). Remove the bay leaf. Season the soup with salt and pepper. Divide among four soup bowls.

To Make Ahead: Prepare as directed above. Transfer to a large heatproof bowl, cover, and refrigerate for up to 3 days, or freeze in individual portions for up to 1 month. Thaw in the refrigerator or microwave. Reheat before serving.

BONUS YEARS DAILY PERCENTAGES

Per serving: Fruits and vegetables 85%; Garlic 100%

NUTRITIONAL ANALYSIS

Per serving: Calories 429, Protein 32g, Total fat 15g, Sat fat 4g, Trans fat 0g, Cholesterol 55mg, Carbohydrate 45g, Dietary fiber 11g, Sodium 867mg

Broiled Miso-Glazed Salmon with Soba Noodles

MAKES 4 SERVINGS

Broiling for 7 minutes guarantees a beautiful dark caramelized crust. Finish cooking the salmon in a 375-degree oven, similar to pan roasting, but in this recipe with the initial sear under the broiler instead of in the skillet.

Serve a light fruity red wine with earthy tones, such as an Oregon or California Pinot Noir with this dish.

2 tablespoons red or dark brown miso paste
2 tablespoons mirin (rice wine) or dry sherry
1 tablespoon light brown sugar
1 tablespoon low-sodium chicken broth
1 tablespoon unseasoned rice vinegar
1 tablespoon freshly squeezed lime juice
1 tablespoon Asian sesame oil
4 (5- to 6-ounce) salmon fillets (about 1 inch thick)

1 medium red onion (6 ounces), cut into thin semicircles
10 ounces moderately thin asparagus, woody ends removed, peeled, and cut into 1-inch-long pieces
6 ounces Japanese soba noodles, or thin dried wheat noodles, or angel hair pasta cooked according to package directions
1 tablespoon low-sodium soy sauce, or to taste
1 tablespoon Asian sesame oil

Thoroughly combine the miso, mirin, sugar, broth, vinegar, lime juice, and oil in a large glass dish. Add the salmon and turn to coat with the miso mixture. Marinate the salmon at room temperature for 30 minutes, or 1 hour in the refrigerator.

Meanwhile, prepare the noodles: Place the onion in a bowl of cold water for about 20 minutes, remove, and spin the onion dry.

Bring a pot of water to a boil. Prepare a bowl of ice and water. Add the asparagus to the boiling water and drain after 1 minute. Immediately transfer the asparagus to the ice water to stop the cooking. Drain the asparagus.

Toss the noodles with the asparagus and onion. Thoroughly mix in the soy sauce and oil and set aside.

Preheat the broiler. Remove the salmon from the marinade, and place on a broiler rack. Broil about 4 inches from the heat source for 7 minutes. Turn off the broiler, close the oven door, and turn the oven temperature to 375 degrees. Cook for 2 to 3 minutes; the salmon should be just cooked through. For added flavor, brush some of the remaining marinade over the salmon halfway through broiling.

Divide the soba noodles among four plates and top each with a salmon fillet.

BONUS YEARS DAILY PERCENTAGES

Per serving: Fruits and vegetables 20%; Fish 100%

NUTRITIONAL ANALYSIS

Per serving: Calories 548, Protein 38g, Total fat 23g, Sat fat 5g, Trans fat 0g, Cholesterol 94mg, Carbohydrate 48g, Sodium 588mg

Steamed Broccoli, Asian Style

MAKES 4 SERVINGS

In preparing low-fat dishes, it is really important to use the freshest ingredients to add flavor. Fresh orange juice makes this dressing really zing; it is worth the little extra effort to juice your own.

¾ pound broccoli florets (about 6 cups)
1½ tablespoons freshly squeezed orange juice
1 tablespoon low-sodium soy sauce
1 tablespoon unseasoned rice vinegar
½ tablespoon mirin (rice wine)
¾ teaspoon Asian sesame oil
freshly ground black pepper, to taste
¾ teaspoon sesame seeds, toasted

Steam the broccoli florets over boiling water for 3 minutes. Remove from the steamer and place in a large bowl.

Meanwhile, mix together the orange juice, soy sauce, vinegar, mirin, and oil in a small bowl.

Add the orange juice mixture to the broccoli, tossing to thoroughly coat the florets, and season with pepper. Toss with the toasted sesame seeds and serve.

BONUS YEARS DAILY PERCENTAGES
Per serving: Fruits and vegetables 20%

NUTRITIONAL ANALYSIS
Per serving: Calories 42, Protein 3g, Total fat 1g, Sat fat 0g, Trans fat 0g, Cholesterol 0mg, Carbohydrate 6g, Dietary fiber 0g, Sodium 156mg

RED WINE

NUTRITIONAL ANALYSIS

Per 5 ounces: Calories 106, Protein 0g, Total fat 0g, Sat fat 0g, Trans fat 0g, Cholesterol 0mg, Carbohydrate 2g, Dietary fiber 0g, Sodium 7mg

DARK CHOCOLATE

NUTRITIONAL ANALYSIS

Per 2 ounces: Calories 302, Protein 3g, Total fat 16g, Sat fat 10g, Trans fat 0g, Cholesterol 0mg, Carbohydrate 36g, Dietary fiber 2g, Sodium 9mg

NUTS

NUTRITIONAL ANALYSIS

Per 2 ounces: Calories 337, Protein 10g, Total fat 29g, Sat fat 4g, Trans fat 0g, Cholesterol 0mg, Carbohydrate 14g, Dietary fiber 5g, Sodium 7mg

DAY 28: SATURDAY

Breakfast

Baked Spinach and
Smoked Salmon Frittata
BONUS YEARS POINTS: FRUITS AND VEGETABLES 20%;
FISH 20%
CALORIES: 198

Lunch

Black Bean Chili
BONUS YEARS POINTS: FRUITS AND VEGETABLES 20%;
GARLIC 100%
CALORIES: 230

Dinner

Curried Jamaican Mango Pork
Island Slaw
Chocolate-Cinnamon
Bread Pudding
BONUS YEARS POINTS: FRUITS AND VEGETABLES 65%;
GARLIC 65%; NUTS 50%; CHOCOLATE 50%
CALORIES: 919

5 ounces wine
BONUS YEARS POINTS: WINE 100%
CALORIES: 106

Snacks

1 ounce dark chocolate
BONUS YEARS POINTS: CHOCOLATE 100%
CALORIES: 302

1 ounce unsalted dry-roasted
or natural nuts
BONUS YEARS POINTS: NUTS 50%
CALORIES: 168

DAY'S TOTAL BONUS YEARS POINTS: WINE 100%; CHOCOLATE 100%;
FRUITS AND VEGETABLES 105%; FISH 20%; GARLIC 165%; NUTS 100%
TOTAL CALORIES: 1,668

Baked Spinach and Smoked Salmon Frittata

This brunch entrée is easier to cook than a traditional frittata because it is baked in the oven. Another time, serve it as a summer lunch with a green salad or as a light supper dish.

1 tablespoon canola oil
1 cup diced red bell pepper (5 ounces)
½ cup diced onion (2 ounces)
1 cup packed fresh baby spinach (2 ounces)
1¼ cups egg substitute, or 5 eggs, lightly beaten
¼ cup fat-free milk
kosher salt and freshly ground black pepper, to taste
1 teaspoon finely chopped fresh tarragon, or ¼ teaspoon dried
  tarragon
3 ounces smoked salmon, finely chopped
½ cup shredded reduced-fat, reduced-sodium Swiss cheese,
  such as Alpine Lace (2 ounces)
1 cup diced fresh tomatoes, drained

Preheat the oven to 425 degrees. Spray a 9-inch nonstick pie pan with cooking spray.

Heat the oil in a medium skillet over medium-low heat. Add the bell pepper and onion and sauté, stirring occasionally, until softened, about 5 minutes. Stir in the spinach and cook until wilted.

Beat the egg substitute, milk, salt, pepper, and tarragon in a medium bowl. Stir in the salmon, cheese, and the spinach mixture. Pour the mixture into the prepared pan.

Bake for about 20 minutes, or until the frittata is set in the center. Cut into 4 wedges and serve warm. Garnish each serving with ¼ cup of the tomatoes.

BONUS YEARS DAILY PERCENTAGES

Per serving: Fruits and vegetables 20%; Fish 20%

NUTRITIONAL ANALYSIS

Per serving: Calories 198, Protein 19g, Total fat 10g, Sat fat 3g, Trans fat 0g, Cholesterol 16mg, Carbohydrate 8g, Dietary fiber 2g, Sodium 612mg

Black Bean Chili

MAKES 4 (1-CUP) SERVINGS

―――――――

―――

This is a great make-ahead lunch. The flavors will meld overnight and make for a very hearty meal.

1 large red onion (about 10 ounces), chopped
2 stalks celery (4 ounces), chopped into ¼-inch dice (¾ cup)
1 medium carrot (4 ounces), cut into ¼-inch dice (¾ cup)
6 ounces mushrooms, stems removed and chopped
   (about 2 cups)
4 cloves garlic, minced
1 medium zucchini (6 ounces), cut into ¼-inch dice (1 cup)
2 cups cooked black beans, or 1 (15-ounce) can black beans,
   rinsed and drained
1 (14.5-ounce) can chopped tomatoes, preferably
   Mexican style
1 large red bell pepper (preferably roasted, see page 378),
   chopped (1 cup)
1 large green bell pepper (preferably roasted, see page 378),
   chopped (1 cup)
1 to 1½ tablespoons chili powder
2 teaspoons ground cumin (preferably toasted before being
   ground, see page 378)
1 tablespoon good-quality balsamic vinegar
kosher salt and freshly ground black pepper, to taste
3 tablespoons chopped cilantro, for garnish

Spray a 4-quart saucepan with cooking spray. Add the onion, celery, and carrot and sauté over medium heat for about 7 minutes. Add the mushrooms and sauté for 2 minutes. Add the garlic and cook for 2 minutes.

Add the zucchini, beans, tomatoes with their juices, bell peppers, chili powder, cumin, and vinegar. Simmer for 20 minutes. Season with salt and pepper. Divide among four bowls and garnish with the cilantro.

To Make Ahead: Prepare as directed above. Transfer to a large heatproof bowl, cover, and refrigerate for up to 3 days, or freeze in individual portions for up to 1 month. Thaw in the refrigerator or microwave. Reheat before serving and garnish with the cilantro.

BONUS YEARS DAILY PERCENTAGES

Per serving: Fruits and vegetables 20%; Garlic 100%

NUTRITIONAL ANALYSIS

Per serving: Calories 230, Protein 12g, Total fat 1g, Sat fat 0g, Trans fat 0g, Cholesterol 0mg, Carbohydrate 46g, Dietary fiber 14g, Sodium 77mg

Curried Jamaican Mango Pork

Jamaican cooking is very eclectic, using ingredients from all over the world to complement its own cuisine. In that tradition, this recipe uses soy sauce, curry powder, and tomatoes to create a melange of international flavors.

1½ pounds pork tenderloin, preferably brined (see page 376) for 3 to 4 hours in the refrigerator

1 tablespoon canola or grapeseed oil

1 large onion (about 8 ounces), cut into ¼-inch-thick slices (about 2 cups sliced onion)

1 red bell pepper (about 6 ounces), cut into ½-inch squares

1 green bell pepper (about 6 ounces), cut into ½-inch squares

1 tablespoon no-salt-added tomato paste

1 tablespoon Madras (Indian) curry powder, or your favorite curry mixture

1 teaspoon jerk seasoning

4 cloves garlic, minced

½ cup low-sodium soy sauce

½ cup dry sherry or Chinese rice wine

1 (14.5-ounce) can no-salt-added tomatoes

1 (11.5-ounce) can mango nectar (1½ cups)

1½ tablespoons light brown sugar

12 ounces russet baking potatoes, peeled and cut into ½-inch cubes

2 cups mango slices

Rinse the pork and pat dry. Cut the pork into ½-inch cubes. Preheat the oven to 350 degrees. Heat the oil in a large oven-proof skillet over medium heat. Add the onion and sauté for 5 minutes. Add the bell peppers and sauté for 3 minutes. Add the pork and garlic and sauté for 3 minutes. Add the tomato paste, curry powder, jerk seasoning, and garlic and sauté for 3 minutes, being careful not to burn the garlic and stirring to thoroughly combine all the ingredients.

Add the soy sauce, sherry, tomatoes with their juices, nectar, sugar, and potatoes. Bring to a simmer. Transfer to the oven and bake, uncovered, for 25 minutes. Remove from the oven and stir in the mango slices. Simmer until the sauce is slightly thickened, about 10 minutes.

BONUS YEARS DAILY PERCENTAGES

Per serving: Fruits and vegetables 40%; Garlic 65%

NUTRITIONAL ANALYSIS

Per serving: Calories 363, Protein 29g, Total fat 7g, Sat fat 1g, Trans fat 0g, Cholesterol 74mg, Carbohydrate 46g, Dietary fiber 5g, Sodium 877mg

Variation

Substitute peach nectar and 2 cups sliced peaches (about 3 medium peaches, 1 pound) for the mango nectar and mango slices.

Island Slaw

MAKES 4 (1-CUP) SERVINGS

———

3 cups shredded green cabbage (4 ounces)
3 cups shredded red cabbage (4 ounces)
1 small red bell pepper (4 ounces), cut into ⅛-inch-thick slices
1 cup shredded peeled carrots (2 ounces)
⅓ cup minced green onions (white and pale green parts)
1 cup chopped walnuts (4 ounces)
½ cup Basic Creamy Salad Dressing (recipe follows)
2 tablespoons cider vinegar
2 tablespoons light brown sugar
1½ teaspoons freshly squeezed lime juice
½ teaspoon jerk seasoning

Combine the cabbages, bell pepper, carrots, green onions, and walnuts in a salad bowl.

Whisk the dressing, vinegar, brown sugar, lime juice, and jerk seasoning together in a small bowl. Add the dressing to the mixed vegetables, toss to combine, and refrigerate for about 30 minutes before serving.

BONUS YEARS DAILY PERCENTAGES

Per serving: Fruits and vegetables 25%; Nuts 50%

NUTRITIONAL ANALYSIS

Per serving: Calories 301, Protein 8g, Total fat 20g, Sat fat 2g, Trans fat 0g, Cholesterol 16mg, Carbohydrate 27g, Dietary fiber 7g, Sodium 140mg

Basic Creamy Salad Dressing

This makes a wonderfully sweet and creamy base for salad dressings. It has less than half a gram of fat per two tablespoons, with almost no saturated fat.

5 ounces firm silken tofu
½ cup fat-free mayonnaise
½ cup low-fat buttermilk

Place all the ingredients in a blender and blend until pureed.

NUTRITIONAL ANALYSIS

Per 2 tablespoons: Calories 17, Protein 1g, Total fat 0g, Sat fat 0g, Trans fat 0g,
Cholesterol 1mg, Carbohydrate 2g, Dietary fiber 0g, Sodium 104mg

Chocolate-Cinnamon Bread Puddings

MAKES 4 SERVINGS

My favorite way to serve this is to bake the pudding in teacups, top each warm serving with a dollop of marshmallow creme, and serve the cups with their saucers. It's almost like eating hot chocolate with a spoon, but even better—comfort food without guilt.

⅓ cup sugar
¼ cup unsweetened cocoa powder (not Dutch processed)
1¼ teaspoons ground cinnamon
dash hot chili powder, or to taste
1½ cups fat-free milk
½ cup egg substitute or 2 eggs, beaten
1 teaspoon vanilla extract
4 thin slices raisin or other firm bread (about 4 ounces), cut
   into about ½-inch squares
4 tablespoons large bittersweet or semisweet chocolate chips
   or chunks

Combine the sugar, cocoa, cinnamon, and chili powder in a medium bowl. Add a little of the milk and stir to make a thin paste. Whisk in the remaining milk and egg substitute. Whisk in the vanilla. Add the bread and stir to coat. Cover and refrigerate for at least 30 minutes or overnight, stirring occasionally.

Preheat the oven to 325 degrees. Spray 4 (6-ounce) ramekins or custard cups with cooking spray. Divide the bread mixture among the prepared ramekins. Top each with 1 tablespoon of the chocolate chips. Arrange the ramekins in a 9-inch-square pan. Add enough boiling water to come about halfway up the sides. Bake for about

35 minutes, or until a knife inserted in an area without chips comes out clean. Cool slightly and serve warm.

To Make Ahead: The bread and milk mixture can be refrigerated overnight or 8 hours before baking. The baked puddings can be covered, refrigerated, and warmed in a microwave before serving.

BONUS YEARS DAILY PERCENTAGES

Per serving: Chocolate 50%

NUTRITIONAL ANALYSIS

Per serving: Calories 255, Protein 10g, Total fat 5g, Sat fat 2g, Trans fat 0g, Cholesterol 2mg, Carbohydrate 47g, Dietary fiber 3g, Sodium 255mg

RED WINE

NUTRITIONAL ANALYSIS

Per 5 ounces: Calories 106, Protein 0g, Total fat 0g, Sat fat 0g, Trans fat 0g, Cholesterol 0mg, Carbohydrate 2g, Dietary fiber 0g, Sodium 7mg

DARK CHOCOLATE

NUTRITIONAL ANALYSIS

Per 1 ounce: Calories 151, Protein 2g, Total fat 8g, Sat fat 5g, Trans fat 0g, Cholesterol 0mg, Carbohydrate 18g, Dietary fiber 2g, Sodium 5mg

NUTS

NUTRITIONAL ANALYSIS

Per 1 ounce: Calories 168, Protein 5g, Total fat 14g, Sat fat 2g, Trans fat 0g, Cholesterol 0mg, Carbohydrate 7g, Dietary fiber 2g, Sodium 3mg

DAY 29: SUNDAY

Breakfast

Broccoli Strata
½ cup orange and grapefruit
segments
BONUS YEARS POINTS: FRUITS AND VEGETABLES 35%;
GARLIC 50%
CALORIES: 240

Lunch

White Bean Salad
with Fennel and Feta
Mediterranean Dried Fruit
BONUS YEARS POINTS: FRUITS AND VEGETABLES 40%;
NUTS 25%
CALORIES: 701

Dinner

Baked Trout
Broiled Tomatoes
Oven-Roasted Fingerling Potatoes
(page 155)
Individual Chocolate Trifle
BONUS YEARS POINTS: CHOCOLATE 25%; FRUITS AND
VEGETABLES 45%; FISH 100%; GARLIC 100%
CALORIES: 770

5 ounces wine
BONUS YEARS POINTS: WINE 100%
CALORIES: 106

Snacks

1½ ounces dark chocolate
BONUS YEARS POINTS: CHOCOLATE 75%
CALORIES: 227

1½ ounces unsalted dry-roasted
or natural nuts
BONUS YEARS POINTS: NUTS 75%
CALORIES: 253

DAY'S TOTAL BONUS YEARS POINTS: WINE 100%; CHOCOLATE 100%;
FRUITS AND VEGETABLES 120%; FISH 100%; GARLIC 150%; NUTS 100%

TOTAL CALORIES: 2,297

Broccoli Strata

————

Because the strata should be refrigerated overnight before baking, it makes preparing brunch even easier. Just add some fresh fruit and freshly brewed coffee and you are ready to eat.

6 ounces broccoli florets, chopped

3 slices whole wheat bread, cut into 1-inch cubes

½ cup diced red bell pepper

1 cup fat-free milk

1 cup egg substitute, or 4 eggs, beaten

¼ cup minced fresh chives

2 cloves garlic, roasted

½ teaspoon dry mustard

pinch freshly grated nutmeg

¼ teaspoon salt

freshly ground black pepper, to taste

½ cup shredded reduced-fat, reduced-salt Swiss cheese, such as Alpine Lace

2 to 4 tablespoons freshly grated Parmesan cheese

Bring a pot of water to a boil. Prepare a bowl of ice and water. Add the broccoli to the boiling water and drain after 1 minute. Immediately transfer the broccoli to the ice water to stop the cooking. Drain the broccoli and finely chop.

Spray a 9-inch-square baking dish with cooking spray. Arrange the bread cubes in the dish. Sprinkle the bell pepper and broccoli over the bread cubes. Combine the milk, egg substitute, chives, garlic, mustard, nutmeg, salt, and pepper in a medium bowl. Stir in the cheeses. Pour over the bread and vegetables. Cover with aluminum foil and refrigerate overnight.

Preheat the oven to 350 degrees. Bake, covered, for about 40 minutes, or until the center is set.

BONUS YEARS DAILY PERCENTAGES

Per serving: Fruits and vegetables 15%; Garlic 50%

NUTRITIONAL ANALYSIS

Per serving: Calories 202, Protein 18g, Total fat 7g, Sat fat 3g, Trans fat 0g, Cholesterol 14mg, Carbohydrate 17g, Dietary fiber 3g, Sodium 448mg

ORANGE AND GRAPEFRUIT SEGMENTS

BONUS YEARS DAILY PERCENTAGES

Per ½-cup serving: Fruits and vegetables 20%

NUTRITIONAL ANALYSIS

Per ½-cup serving: Calories 38, Protein 1g, Total fat 0g, Sat fat 0g, Trans fat 0g, Cholesterol 0mg, Carbohydrate 10g, Dietary fiber 2g, Sodium 0mg

White Bean Salad
with Fennel and Feta

MAKES 4 SERVINGS

2 tablespoons extra-virgin olive oil

3 tablespoons cider vinegar

½ teaspoon ground cumin

2 cloves garlic, minced

3½ cups canned or cooked dried cannellini beans, drained

1 (9-ounce) fennel bulb, fronds removed and bulb diced

2 Roma tomatoes, diced

1 large green bell pepper (6 ounces), diced

4 ounces reduced-fat feta cheese, crumbled

kosher salt and freshly ground black pepper, to taste

Whisk the oil, vinegar, cumin, and garlic in a large bowl. Add the beans, fennel, tomatoes, bell pepper, and feta and toss gently to combine. Season with salt and pepper.

Let stand at room temperature for 30 minutes for flavors to blend.

To Make Ahead: Prepare as directed above. Cover and refrigerate. For the best flavor, bring to room temperature before serving.

BONUS YEARS DAILY PERCENTAGES

Per ½-cup serving: Fruits and vegetables 20%

NUTRITIONAL ANALYSIS

Per ½-cup serving: Calories 330, Protein 16g, Total fat 11g, Sat fat 3g, Trans fat 0g, Cholesterol 10mg, Carbohydrate 32g, Dietary fiber 12g, Sodium 407mg

Mediterranean Dried Fruit

MAKES 4 SERVINGS

1 (8-ounce) package mixed dried fruit

1 cinnamon stick

grated fresh zest and juice of 1 medium orange (about ½ cup juice)

¼ cup water

2 tablespoons sugar

½ cup low-fat sour cream

½ cup plain low-fat yogurt

¼ cup orange liqueur, such as triple sec or Grand Marnier

1 tablespoon honey

½ cup chopped walnuts (2 ounces), toasted (see page 159)

Place the fruit, cinnamon stick, orange zest, juice, and water in a small saucepan. Bring to a simmer. Add the sugar and stir until dissolved. Cover and simmer for about 15 minutes. Transfer the fruit to a bowl, cover, and refrigerate until it is cool.

In a small bowl, combine the sour cream, yogurt, liqueur, and honey. Mix the fruit with the yogurt sauce. Serve immediately or refrigerate for up to 8 hours. To serve, divide the fruit among four plates and top with the walnuts.

BONUS YEARS DAILY PERCENTAGES

Per serving: Fruits and vegetables 20%; Nuts 25%

NUTRITIONAL ANALYSIS

Per serving: Calories 371, Protein 6g, Total fat 10g, Sat fat 1g, Trans fat 0g, Cholesterol 0mg, Carbohydrate 61g, Dietary fiber 6g, Sodium 73mg

Baked Trout

MAKES 4 SERVINGS

This is another easy-to-prepare and delicious Bonus Years seafood dinner. Start with really fresh trout and bake it until it is opaque and begins to flake.

1½ pounds skinless trout fillets
kosher salt and freshly ground black pepper, to taste
½ cup dry white wine, such as Sauvignon Blanc
¼ cup freshly squeezed lemon juice
4 cloves garlic, chopped
2 green onions (green and white parts), thinly sliced
6 ounces button mushrooms, thinly sliced

Preheat the oven to 375 degrees. Spray a baking pan large enough to hold the trout in one layer with cooking spray. Season the trout with salt and pepper. Arrange the trout in the prepared baking pan. Spoon the wine and lemon juice over the trout. Top with the garlic, green onions, and mushrooms.

Bake for 15 to 20 minutes, or until the trout is opaque. To serve, place a trout fillet on each of four dinner plates, and top with one-fourth of the mushrooms and the pan juices.

BONUS YEARS DAILY PERCENTAGES
Per serving: Fish 100%; Garlic 100%

NUTRITIONAL ANALYSIS
Per serving: Calories 276, Protein 37g, Total fat 9g, Sat fat 3g, Trans fat 0g, Cholesterol 100mg, Carbohydrate 5g, Dietary fiber 1g, Sodium 64mg

Broiled Tomatoes

½ cup dry fine bread crumbs
½ cup freshly grated Parmesan cheese
½ tablespoon dried oregano
½ tablespoon dried basil
4 medium tomatoes, cut in half horizontally
kosher salt and freshly ground black pepper,
   to taste
3 tablespoons Dijon mustard
minced flat-leaf parsley, for garnish

Preheat the broiler. Cover a baking sheet with aluminum foil and spray the foil with cooking spray. Mix the bread crumbs, Parmesan cheese, oregano, and basil in a small bowl.

Season the tomatoes with salt and pepper and lightly spread about 2 teaspoons of the mustard on each half. Sprinkle a thin coating of the bread crumb mixture on top of each of the tomato halves. Coat each tomato half with cooking spray. Place the tomatoes on the prepared baking sheet. Broil about 4 inches from the heat for 4 to 5 minutes, or until the topping is nicely browned and the tomatoes are cooked through.

Remove from the oven and garnish with the parsley.

BONUS YEARS DAILY PERCENTAGES

Per serving: Fruits and vegetables 30%

NUTRITIONAL ANALYSIS

Per serving: Calories 127, Protein 7g, Total fat 4g, Sat fat 2g, Trans fat 0g, Cholesterol 8mg, Carbohydrate 14g, Dietary fiber 1g, Sodium 578mg

Individual Chocolate Trifles

MAKES 4 SERVINGS

Use the fresh fruits that are in season for this easy dessert.

1½ cups thinly sliced strawberries, or other fresh fruit
2 tablespoons sugar, or to taste
12 thin trans fat–free chocolate wafers, crushed (about 1 cup)
1 recipe Chocolate Mousse (page 139), without nuts
plain fat-free yogurt (optional)

Toss the strawberries with the sugar in a medium bowl. Spread about ¼ cup of the berries in each of four small glass dessert dishes. Sprinkle each with about 2 tablespoons of the crushed cookies. Spoon one-fourth of the mousse over the crumbs in each dish. Top with the remaining crumbs and the remaining berries. Cover and chill for up to 8 hours. Top with each serving with a small dollop of yogurt (if using).

BONUS YEARS DAILY PERCENTAGES

Per serving: Fruits and vegetables 15%; Chocolate 25%

NUTRITIONAL ANALYSIS

Per serving: Calories 257, Protein 9g, Total fat 6g, Sat fat 3g, Trans fat 1g, Cholesterol 10mg, Carbohydrate 24g, Dietary fiber 3g, Sodium 259mg

RED WINE

NUTRITIONAL ANALYSIS

Per 5 ounces: Calories 106, Protein 0g, Total fat 0g, Sat fat 0g, Trans fat 0g, Cholesterol 0mg, Carbohydrate 2g, Dietary fiber 0g, Sodium 7mg

DARK CHOCOLATE

NUTRITIONAL ANALYSIS

Per 1½ ounces: Calories 227, Protein 2g, Total fat 12g, Sat fat 7g, Trans fat 0g, Cholesterol 0mg, Carbohydrate 27g, Dietary fiber 2g, Sodium 7mg

NUTS

NUTRITIONAL ANALYSIS

Per 1½ ounces: Calories 253, Protein 7g, Total fat 22g, Sat fat 3g, Trans fat 0g, Cholesterol 0mg, Carbohydrate 11g, Dietary fiber 4g, Sodium 5mg

DAY 30: MONDAY

Breakfast

½ whole wheat bagel with
2 tablespoons nut butter
1 cup low-sodium vegetable juice
cocktail
BONUS YEARS POINTS: FRUITS AND VEGETABLES 20%;
NUTS 50%
CALORIES: 320

Lunch

Roasted Vegetable Soup
Crusty bread
BONUS YEARS POINTS: FRUITS AND VEGETABLES 65%;
GARLIC 100%
CALORIES: 379

Dinner

Jamaican Snapper
Corn and Sweet Pepper Sauté
in Broth
½ cup steamed brown rice
BONUS YEARS POINTS: FRUITS AND VEGETABLES 25%;
FISH 100%
CALORIES: 371

5 ounces wine
BONUS YEARS POINTS: WINE 100%
CALORIES: 106

Snacks

2 ounces dark chocolate
BONUS YEARS POINTS: CHOCOLATE 100%
CALORIES: 302

1 ounce unsalted dry-roasted
or natural nuts
BONUS YEARS POINTS: NUTS 50%
CALORIES: 168

DAY'S TOTAL BONUS YEARS POINTS: WINE 100%; CHOCOLATE 100%;
FRUITS AND VEGETABLES 110%; FISH 100%; GARLIC 100%; NUTS 100%
TOTAL CALORIES: 1,646

WHOLE WHEAT BAGEL

NUTRITIONAL ANALYSIS

Per ½ bagel: Calories 72, Protein 3g, Total fat 1g, Sat fat 0g, Trans fat 0g, Cholesterol 0mg, Carbohydrate 15g, Dietary fiber 2g, Sodium 148mg

NUT BUTTER (SUCH AS ALMOND OR PEANUT)

BONUS YEARS DAILY PERCENTAGES

Per 2 tablespoons: Nuts 50%

NUTRITIONAL ANALYSIS

Per 2 tablespoons: Calories 188, Protein 8g, Total fat 16g, Sat fat 3g, Trans fat 0g, Cholesterol 0mg, Carbohydrate 6g, Dietary fiber 2g, Sodium 148mg

LOW-SODIUM VEGETABLE JUICE COCKTAIL

BONUS YEARS DAILY PERCENTAGES

Per 8 ounces: Fruits and vegetables 20%

NUTRITIONAL ANALYSIS

Per 8 ounces: Calories 60, Protein 2g, Total fat 0g, Sat fat 0g, Trans fat 0g, Cholesterol 0mg, Carbohydrate 11g, Dietary fiber 2g, Sodium 140mg

Roasted Vegetable Soup

MAKES 6 CUPS; 4 SERVINGS

The soup can be served immediately, topped with a bit of cheese for garnish, but I often make this the night before and bring it to work the next day. It really tastes wonderful if the flavors are allowed to blend overnight. Serve with toasted, crusty bread.

1 onion (about 6 ounces), cut into thick slices
1 yellow summer squash (5 to 6 ounces), cut into ½-inch dice (about 1 cup)
1 medium carrot (about 4 ounces), cut into ½-inch dice
1 medium red potato, cut into ½-inch dice
4 ounces broccoli florets, cut into small pieces (about 2 cups)
4 ounces cauliflower florets, cut into small pieces (about 2 cups)
kosher salt and freshly ground black pepper, to taste
1 teaspoon extra-virgin olive oil
4 large cloves garlic, thinly sliced
1½ teaspoons Italian seasoning
4 cups low-sodium vegetable stock or chicken broth
1 (14.5-ounce) can Italian stewed tomatoes, drained
generous pinch cayenne pepper
grated low-fat Parmesan cheese, for garnish

Preheat the oven to 400 degrees. Place the onion, squash, carrot, potato, broccoli, and cauliflower in a roasting pan in a single layer. Coat the vegetables with cooking spray and season with salt and pepper. Roast the vegetables for about 35 minutes, or until lightly browned.

Meanwhile, heat the oil in a 4-quart saucepan over medium heat. Add the garlic and Italian seasoning and sauté for about 30 seconds;

be sure not to burn the garlic. Add the stock and tomatoes and simmer for about 10 minutes. Add the roasted vegetables and simmer for 15 minutes. Taste for seasoning and add the cayenne and salt and pepper as needed. Ladle into bowls and top with Parmesan cheese.

To Make Ahead: Prepare as directed above. Transfer to a large heatproof bowl, cover, and refrigerate for up to 3 days. Reheat before serving and top with Parmesan cheese.

BONUS YEARS DAILY PERCENTAGES

Per serving: Fruits and vegetables 65%; Garlic 100%

NUTRITIONAL ANALYSIS

Per serving: Calories 116, Protein 5g, Total fat 2g, Sat fat 0g, Trans fat 0g, Cholesterol 0mg, Carbohydrate 22g, Dietary fiber 5g, Sodium 313mg

CRUSTY BREAD

NUTRITIONAL ANALYSIS

Per slice: Calories 263, Protein 8g, Total fat 3g, Sat fat 0g, Trans fat 0g, Cholesterol 0mg, Carbohydrate 50g, Dietary fiber 3g, Sodium 584mg

Jamaican Snapper

This is a quick way to easily prepare a medium- or firm-textured fish. Season one side with a spicy rub and then oven-roast it. Serve it with an appropriate vegetable side dish and you have a quick, delicious, and healthy Bonus Years dinner.

4 (5- to 6-ounce) skinless red snapper fillets
2 tablespoons jerk seasoning
1 tablespoon canola or grapeseed oil

Preheat the oven to 375 degrees. Season one side of each of the fillets with ½ tablespoon of the jerk seasoning. Heat the oil in a 12-inch nonstick skillet over medium heat. Add the fillets, seasoned side down, and cook over medium-low heat for 4 minutes.

Transfer the fillets, seasoned side down, to the oven and roast for 7 to 10 minutes. The snapper should be juicy and just opaque. Remove from the oven and serve.

BONUS YEARS DAILY PERCENTAGES
Per serving: Fish 100%

NUTRITIONAL ANALYSIS
Per serving: Calories 172, Protein 29g, Total fat 5g, Sat fat 1g, Trans fat 0g, Cholesterol 52mg, Carbohydrate 0g, Dietary fiber 0g, Sodium 91mg

Corn and Sweet Pepper Sauté in Broth

MAKES 4 SERVINGS

½ cup chopped red onion (2 ounces)

1¾ cups fresh corn cut from about 3 ears, or 9 ounces frozen corn

½ green bell pepper (2 ounces), cut into ¼-inch dice

½ red bell pepper (2 ounces), cut into ¼-inch dice

¼ cup low-sodium chicken broth

1 tablespoon freshly squeezed lime juice

kosher salt and freshly ground black pepper, to taste

Lightly spray a 12-inch nonstick with cooking spray. Heat over medium heat. Add the onion and sauté for about 1 minute. Add the corn and bell peppers and cook for 2 minutes, stirring to allow the vegetables to begin to caramelize. Add the broth, a few tablespoons at a time, to prevent burning. Stir the vegetables; continue to add the broth and sauté until the vegetables are just crisp-tender, about 3 minutes. Stir in the lime juice, season with salt and pepper, and serve.

BONUS YEARS DAILY PERCENTAGES

Per serving: Fruits and vegetables 25%

NUTRITIONAL ANALYSIS

Per serving: Calories 91, Protein 3g, Total fat 1g, Sat fat 0g, Trans fat 0g, Cholesterol 0mg, Carbohydrate 21g, Dietary fiber 3g, Sodium 12mg

STEAMED BROWN RICE

NUTRITIONAL ANALYSIS

Per ½-cup serving: Calories 108, Protein 2g, Total fat 0g, Sat fat 0g, Trans fat 0g, Cholesterol 0mg, Carbohydrate 22g, Dietary fiber 2g, Sodium 5mg

RED WINE

NUTRITIONAL ANALYSIS

Per 5 ounces: Calories 106, Protein 0g, Total fat 0g, Sat fat 0g, Trans fat 0g, Cholesterol 0mg, Carbohydrate 2g, Dietary fiber 0g, Sodium 7mg

DARK CHOCOLATE

NUTRITIONAL ANALYSIS

Per 2 ounces: Calories 302, Protein 3g, Total fat 16g, Sat fat 10g, Trans fat 0g, Cholesterol 0mg, Carbohydrate 36g, Dietary fiber 2g, Sodium 9mg

NUTS

NUTRITIONAL ANALYSIS

Per 1 ounce: Calories 168, Protein 5g, Total fat 14g, Sat fat 2g, Trans fat 0g, Cholesterol 0mg, Carbohydrate 7g, Dietary fiber 2g, Sodium 3mg

CHAPTER 8

The Bonus Years Food Pantry

The first step to getting your Bonus Years is to shop smarter. And smart shopping means stocking your kitchen with the ingredients that make it easy to prepare Bonus Years meals that are as delicious as they are healthy. Most of the following ingredients can be found easily at any one of your larger supermarkets, but some, such as fish sauce or miso, may require a trip to a local Asian market or health food store. Be bold! Although the names may sound strange, they will soon become as familiar as salt and pepper. It's the Bonus Years Rx for a happy and healthy kitchen.

Anchovy fillets: Salt-cured small Mediterranean fish, they are often used in dressings and sauces.

Arrowroot: A white starchy powder, similar to cornstarch, it is used to thicken stocks and sauces, and is typically available in most supermarket and health food stores. Liquids need not be as hot when thickened with arrowroot as compared to cornstarch or flour, and the cooking time to thicken is less. Also, arrowroot does not cause thickened liquids to become cloudy or starchy tasting. It thus produces more elegant-appearing and -tasting sauces and stocks. Arrowroot should be mixed with a little cold water to form a liquidy paste before being used as a thickener.

Artichokes, canned in water: They make an upscale addition to salads and Mediterranean fare and a quick substitute for fresh artichokes.

Barley, pearl: An easy-to-prepare grain, it has a wonderful chewy texture.

Beans: Have on hand a wide variety of dried and canned beans, including white kidney, navy, northern, garbanzo (chickpeas), black, and red kidney beans. Always rinse and drain canned dried beans before using, to freshen the flavor and remove some of the sodium. No-salt-added canned beans in several varieties are available at natural foods stores. Freshly cooked dried beans have a better flavor and texture, and you can control the amount of salt they contain. Both cooked and canned dried beans are high in protein, fiber, and iron.

Bulgur wheat: Derived from whole wheat berries that have been cooked, dried, and cracked, it is quick and easy to cook. Best known for its use in Middle Eastern tabbouleh, it is also great in pilafs.

Buttermilk: Despite its name, buttermilk can be very low in fat (1 percent fat buttermilk). It makes an excellent base for dressings (see Basic Creamy Salad Dressing, page 333) and can be used to coat meats and seafood before oven frying.

Chilies: There are a practically unlimited number of dried and fresh chilies now commonly available in American markets. Even chilies of the same type can differ markedly in their spiciness, so each recipe must be individually taste tested. Two commonly used chilies are the jalapeño and the mild green chili, sometimes called Anaheim. Both are available fresh and canned.

Chili oil, Asian: Available in Asian markets, this is a very spicy red-tinted oil made by infusing red chilies in hot oil. A little goes a long way, so be careful when adding it to stir-fries and sauces.

Chili paste, Asian: A spicy, hot sauce, it is made from small dried chilies that are thickened with soybeans.

Chipotles in adobo sauce: These are smoked, dried jalapeño chilies canned in a spicy tomato sauce. They add a wonderful smoky flavor to Mexican sauces and stews.

Chocolate: The chocolate must be dark and contain at least 60 percent cocoa solids (70 percent is even better); bittersweet baker's chocolate is a typical example. Dark chocolate has a high level of the plant antioxidants flavonols, which are critical to lowering blood pressure. European dark chocolates typically are darker and richer in these antioxidants but also more expensive. Milk chocolate, which contains significant amounts of sugar and milk products, is much lower in flavonols and is not part of the Bonus Years plan.

Cocoa powder, unsweetened: Unsweetened cocoa powder (not the sweetened mix that is sold for making hot chocolate) can be substituted for dark chocolate. Two tablespoons of cocoa powder is equal to one ounce of dark chocolate. Do not use Dutch processed chocolate powder, which is treated with alkali to remove the acids normally found in pure cocoa powder; this also destroys the antioxidants.

Cooking oils: Canola oil and extra-virgin olive oil are two staples for healthy cooking. They are both high in monounsaturated fats and have high smoking temperatures, so they are stable under intense heat. I use canola oil when stir-frying and olive oil when I want that Mediterranean flavor. Sometimes I use grapeseed oil, as it has a relatively high smoking point and is good for sautéing or stir-frying.

Couscous: Actually a pasta, not a grain, couscous is made from durum wheat. This North African specialty is quick to prepare and is versatile.

Cumin seed: Toasted and ground, this spice adds real punch to Mexican and Middle Eastern cooking.

Fish sauce: Salty, anchovy-based Thai or Vietnamese sauce, not reproducible by other condiments, adds a unique pungency to dishes. It is used as commonly in these cuisines as is soy sauce in Chinese and Japanese cooking.

Flours: Unbleached all-purpose flour is made from a blend of low- and high-gluten wheat and is used for general baking. Whole wheat flour contains the germ and bran, which are removed when milling all-purpose flour, and has a higher nutritional content, including fiber. Made from a special variety of wheat, white whole wheat flour is creamy white instead of the tan color of regular whole wheat flour, yet it has all the nutrients of whole wheat. The flavor is much milder than that of regular whole wheat flour.

Garlic: Always keep fresh garlic on hand.

Ginger root: Don't substitute dried ginger for the fresh. Usually peeled and grated before using, fresh ginger root should be stored loosely wrapped in paper, in the crisper drawer of the refrigerator. Grated fresh ginger can be tightly wrapped and frozen.

Herbs: Always have dried basil, oregano, marjoram, rosemary, and thyme available. If a recipe calls for fresh herbs and they are not available, substitute one-third as much of the dried variety.

Hoisin sauce: This spicy, sweet Chinese condiment adds a deep, reddish brown color to quick braises (hence the name "Chinese red cooking") and flavor to dips and sauces.

Juice concentrates, frozen: Use frozen orange- or apple-juice concentrate as a natural sweetener for dressings, sauces, and desserts.

Lemongrass: A fibrous plant with long grasslike leaves, it is sold in long stalks in Asian markets. The bottom six to eight inches are chopped or sliced and added to sauces and soups to impart a delicate lemony fragrance. Remove the lemongrass before serving. Use the fresh variety in cooking. Dried lemongrass should only be used in teas.

Mirin: A sweet Japanese rice wine, mirin is used only in cooking to flavor vinaigrettes and sauces.

Miso: Used as a flavoring for soups and sauces, miso is a Japanese soybean paste. Shiro miso is a dark yellow variety with a mellow taste. Sendai miso has a dark, reddish brown color with a stronger, more pungent taste.

Mushrooms: Regular cultivated white button mushrooms, brown mushrooms, and portobellos are available almost everywhere. Coarsely chopped, they add meatiness to stir-fries, salads, sandwiches, and pasta dishes whether served raw, roasted, or sautéed. Shiitake, for Asian dishes, and porcini, which add a Mediterranean accent, are among my favorite dried mushrooms. Dried mushrooms are usually first rehydrated in hot water; the soaking liquid itself makes a great base for a sauce or soup. Dried mushrooms can also be pulverized to a powder in a coffee grinder, and the resulting powder can be added directly to soups or sauces as a flavoring or used as a rub on fish and meats before searing them.

Mustard, Dijon: A pale yellow mustard with a clean, sharp, flavor, it is a favorite in sauces and dressings.

Nuts: Purchase raw or dry-roasted unsalted nuts. All are low in saturated fat and are cholesterol free. Almonds, walnuts, pecans, hazelnuts, and peanuts are among my favorites. Some companies are now offering portion-control packets containing one ounce of nuts, a great way to snack and get your Bonus Points.

Oyster sauce: A thick, brown salty Chinese condiment, it is made from oyster extract and serves as a basis for many sauces.

Pasta: Choose from among the endless Italian and Asian varieties, matching the shape of the pasta to your sauce. Dried pasta is ideal for making quick one-pot or skillet meals by adding it to sauce, some veggies, and a bit of meat or fish. The new whole-grain pastas, especially those imported from Italy, are quite delicious and a major departure from the heavy, leaden whole-grain pasta of the past. They also contain a fair amount of heart-healthy fiber, so do try them. Count on two to three ounces of dried pasta per person.

Ramen noodles are a type of Asian dried pasta that goes great in salads. The ramen noodles sold in most regular markets as part of a soup mix are high in sodium, calories, and fat (they are deep-fried). Health food stores offer a baked variety that is every bit as tasty without all the fat and calories.

Peppercorns: Peppercorns come in black, white, and green varieties. Freshly ground whole peppercorns provide much more flavor than pre-ground pepper.

Plum sauce: This sweet, tart Chinese condiment is often used in barbecue and dipping sauces.

Polenta: The signature cornmeal porridge from northern Italy makes an elegant side dish. I prefer freshly made, soft polenta to the firm kind that is available in plastic-wrapped rolls.

Rice: Keep a variety of rices on hand. Use Arborio, a short-grain Italian rice, in risotto. Basmati rice, from northern India, is a long-grain rice with a unique nutty flavor, ideal as an accompaniment to Indian-inspired dishes. Brown rice has more fiber and nutrients than traditional white rice. Wild rice, not really a rice at all, is a grass seed with a rich nutty flavor and chewy texture.

Roasted bell peppers: These are sold in jars and are a great addition to salads, sandwiches, pasta, and southwestern-style dishes. The jarred peppers are usually red. If you have the time to roast your own, also prepare yellow, orange, or green bell peppers to add extra color and flavor to a variety of dishes.

Sesame oil, Asian: Oil made from toasted white sesame seeds and found in Asian markets and some supermarkets. A teaspoon or two is often used at the end of cooking to flavor stir-fries. Don't confuse this with unflavored sesame oil found in health food stores and used as a cooking oil.

Sour cream: The dairy industry has done a great job in making low-fat and nonfat varieties of sour cream that are great in sauces and as toppings. If adding to a hot sauce, stir in a little arrowroot to thicken and prevent the sour cream from breaking.

Soy sauces: Unless otherwise indicated, use the regular supermarket variety, such as Kikkoman; for those on sodium-restricted diets, use Kikkoman light. Dark soy sauce has added molasses, giving it a darker and thicker appearance and sweeter taste. It is less salty, thicker, and more full-bodied in flavor than regular soy sauce, adds a great deal of color to dishes, and is traditionally used in Chinese "red cooking" or braises. Dark soy sauce can be purchased in Asian markets. Also found in Chinese markets is thin soy sauce. Sometimes called light soy sauce, it is lighter in color than regular soy sauce but is actually saltier. Don't confuse it with *reduced-sodium* light soy sauce. Mushroom soy sauce, also available in Asian markets, is made by adding the flavorings of Chinese straw mushrooms to soy sauce. It produces a deeper, more rounded-tasting soy sauce.

Stir-fry or vegetables mixes: Available in plastic pouches in the refrigerated produce section of most markets, these mixes are a combination of fresh-cut, cleaned vegetables, such as broccoli, carrots, cauliflower, and snow peas or sugar snap peas. Usually sold in 12-ounce to 1-pound packages, they are perfect for a dinner for four.

Tofu: Custardlike cakes made from soybean curd, this true Booster food comes in many varieties. Chinese firm tofu is used in stir-fries, and Japanese silken tofu is for dressings, soups, and desserts.

Tomato products: Canned tomato products are convenient to use and often have better flavor than some fresh tomatoes from the supermarket. No-salt-added products, such as canned tomatoes and tomato sauce, allow you to control the amount of salt in your recipes.

Turmeric: A bitter and pungent spice, it adds an intense yellow-orange color to Caribbean and Indian dishes.

Vinegars: Balsamic vinegar, a pungent, sweet, dark Italian variety, adds a sophisticated mellowness to dressings and sauces. Cider vinegar is a tart, fruity, caramel-colored vinegar made from apples. It is used in relishes, chutney, and salad dressings. White vinegar, the standard one in pickles, is used when a very strong flavor is required. Wine vinegars, pungent and tart, are staples for salads and dressings. Rice wine vinegar, commonly called rice vinegar, is made from fermented rice and has a mild, sweet flavor, making it excellent in salads.

Yogurt: Plain low-fat and nonfat yogurts make a great base for sauces, dressings, and toppings.

CHAPTER 9

Cooking Up the Bonus Years

A s someone who savors each and every meal, I wouldn't follow an eating plan if the food didn't taste good, and I don't expect you to, either. At the same time, as a physician, I hear a little voice whispering in my ear, "Ralph, it's not just about tasting great, it's also about health."

Fortunately, healthy food and food that tastes good are not a contradiction in terms. If properly prepared, healthy food can taste great. You just have to know the right way to cook it.

It all comes down to the proper cooking technique. In the pages that follow, I share a few of the basics that show how to prepare your Bonus Years foods so that they taste as good as they are good for you. These techniques include braising, brining, broiling, broth sautéing, oven-frying, oven roasting, pan roasting, poaching, stir-frying, and stovetop grilling. They don't require a lot of skill and can be done in virtually any kitchen.

Furthermore, like you, I have a busy life. After a long day at work, I want to be able to put meals together quickly and easily. And that's exactly what learning these techniques can do for you too.

A word to the novice chef: don't be intimidated by the thought of cooking. Even if you can barely boil water or scramble an egg, the most inexperienced of cooks will find these techniques are simple enough.

Cooking well requires more than good technique: quality ingredients are essential. The most pristine, glistening block of tuna can turn to leather within minutes if subjected to unregulated heat. And the best chef in the world can't resurrect a fillet of dull, muddy brown halibut.

Overcooking Is the Biggest Mistake

Overcooking is probably the most common error made in the kitchen, whether it is by the home cook or professional chef. Fortunately, with a simple primer on basic techniques, patience in the kitchen, and a little practice, you can guarantee meals that will sparkle with their freshness and succulence. The rate at which foods cook reflects their differing structures. Cuts of meat that come from much-used muscles, such as the legs, tend to be tougher and require more cooking time but are more flavorful. In cattle, chuck roast from the shoulder area versus a tender filet mignon from the loin is a good example. With poultry, thighs and legs can be compared to the chicken breast. Chuck steaks will take considerably longer to cook than a filet mignon, just as chicken thighs and legs require more cooking time than the breast, which explains why chuck roasts and chicken thighs and legs do well with a long braise, while a filet mignon or boneless chicken breast is better prepared with a quick grilling.

Because fish live in water and don't need strong muscles for support against gravity, their meat is much more tender and delicate with much less connective tissue than that of land animals. This is why cooking times for seafood must be very carefully monitored to guard against overcooking.

Cooking Methods

There are three main cooking methods: dry heat, moist heat, and a combination of moist and dry cooking. Some dry heat techniques (e.g., grilling, broiling, and baking) are done without the addition of fats; others, such as sautéing and stir-frying, rely on some oil to lightly coat the food while cooking. All dry heat cooking forms a seal around the food, which dramatically adds to the texture and taste.

Moist heat methods transfer heat through steam or a cooking liquid, such as water, stock, or sauce and include poaching, steaming, and en papillote (placing food with a small amount of liquid in parchment paper or foil package and finishing off in the oven). Because foods cooked with moist heat techniques don't form an initial seal, they lack the rich color and crust produced with dry heat methods.

Braising and stewing represent the most popular combination cooking methods, using both dry and moist heat techniques. There is usually an initial sauté or sear in a small amount of fat, then the food is transferred to a pot, immersed in liquid, covered, and finished off over low heat on the stovetop or in the oven.

Because dry heat cooking methods are done at high temperatures without added moisture, foods prepared with these techniques can dry out easily. One way to protect meats, poultry, and seafood is to add moisture by brining (see page 376) the food before cooking. Meats that are naturally tender, or with lots of internal fat marbling, do well with dry heat methods, but unfortunately the fat is often highly saturated and so these cuts do not represent a good, healthful choice. Leaner cuts, such as pork tenderloin or boneless, skinless chicken breasts, turn out well under high, dry heat if cooked quickly, and they are excellent when brined first.

The thickness of the meat is also a consideration when cooking with dry heat. If too thick, the food may require so much time to cook completely through that the outside crusts will burn first. Professional chefs often get around this by pan roasting, which uses a combination of two dry heat techniques: an initial sauté or a sear in a hot pan and then finishing off in the oven under high heat (roasting). Lean cuts, such as boneless, skinless chicken breasts or pork tenderloin, which don't have a great deal of extra moisture or fat, also often benefit from pan roasting, as do many fish fillets. Whether the item is thick or lean, pan roasting it assures moist and tender results with a beautifully seared crust. Richer, thinner cuts of meat (one inch or less) are often easy to cook with dry heat methods because they can be entirely cooked through when grilled or broiled by the time their outer surfaces are nicely browned and crusty. Pounding meats to a uniform thickness is one way to speed up cooking times and ensure that the outside will not burn before the meat is fully cooked.

Steaming works well with many vegetables and fish because they are relatively low in fat. Because it adds moisture, steaming makes foods very tender. Although, if overcooked, even steamed foods can dry out, in general steaming is a way to ensure a succulent, flavorful dish. Steamed foods also retain a high proportion of their nutrients, making this an especially healthful cooking alternative. Adding a flavorful sauce over fish before steaming is a particularly elegant way to prepare seafood. The steamed liquids from the fish will meld perfectly with the sauce.

Finally, poaching is another desirable moist heat method to prepare delicate, tender seafood or white poultry. Adding broth or stock (seafood, vegetable, or chicken), wine, vegetables, and herbs to the poaching liquid is a great way to enhance the flavor.

Braising less-tender cuts of meat, such as bottom round, short ribs, and chuck roasts, adds flavor and moisture through a combination of dry and moist heat techniques: prolonged simmering in a flavored liquid after an initial sear. Low-fat fish fillets and boneless, skinless chicken breasts can also be short-braised (see Braising, below) in a flavored cooking liquid after they have been initially sautéed in a hot pan. Both braising and short pan-roasting use a two-step technique of dry and then moist cooking. Unlike red meats or chicken thighs, which require a long braise of an hour or more, the more delicate fish and chicken breasts may only require ten to twenty minutes of simmering in the braising liquid.

BRAISING

Braised Szechuan Chicken Thighs (page 300)
Curried Jamaican Mango Pork (page 330)

Braising uses a combination of dry and moist heat techniques to prepare dishes unique in their tenderness and depth of flavor. This requires two steps: first, evenly brown the meat in a small amount of fat, and then finish it off in a covered pot with liquid, either in the oven or over low heat on the stovetop. The limitless variations of braising liquids, such as wine, stock, broth, and juice, make for endless flavoring possibilities and explain why braising is a popular cooking technique.

Braises can be short, thirty to sixty minutes, or long, greater than an hour. Longer braises work well for less-tender cuts of meat like beef top round, beef chuck steak, and chicken legs, which have a great deal of connective tissue (collagen) between their muscle fibers. With long, slow cooking, the collagen will melt and turn into gelatin, making the meat remarkably tender and flavorful. These cuts often require two to three hours of cooking time and are usually done in the oven at 275 to 300 degrees, to allow uniform and stable heat to surround the pot. Short braising is best suited to more tender foods, such as skinless chicken breasts, seafood, and more delicate vegetables. Here the braising liquid is used to impart flavor to the final dish but not to tenderize. These short braises require more frequent checking of the liquid to ensure that the food is not overcooked and are often done on the stovetop where it is easier to monitor. Heartier vegetables, such as cabbage and fennel, and root vegetables, such as potatoes, parsnips, and turnips, do well with shorter braises, often requiring only thirty minutes to an hour. An added bonus of this technique is that the braising liquid absorbs the flavors of the meat and vegetables to produce a deeply rich and textured sauce.

WATER-BLANCHING

Asian Salad with Tangy Miso Dressing (page 120)
Asian-Style Vegetable Stir-fry (page 302)
Crab Salad with Creamy Dressing (page 143)
Italian Pasta Vegetable Salad (page 258)
Pan-Roasted Salmon with Shanghai Red Sauce (page 270)
Ramen Noodle Salad with Balsamic Cilantro Vinaigrette (page 238)
Spanish-Style Chickpea Salad (page 266)
Spinach and Arugula Sauté (page 288)
Velvet Chicken (page 193)
Warm Asian-Style Shrimp Salad (page 161)

Water-blanching is used to precook meats, poultry, and vegetables by placing them in boiling hot water for one to two minutes. After vegetables are heated in the boiling water, they are transferred immediately to an ice-water bath to halt the cooking process, which helps them retain their crispiness and vibrant color. This technique is particularly useful when stir-frying because it allows the water-blanched vegetables to be quickly and evenly cooked in the wok. Water-blanching also removes the raw taste from vegetables added to salads while still maintaining their crisp texture.

"Velvet" chicken is a favorite dish in many Chinese restaurants. The secret is to first marinate strips or cubes of chicken in a cornstarch mixture for a few minutes, then water-blanch the chicken in a pot of boiling water before adding it to the wok. Soy sauce or wine added to the cornstarch marinade will add flavor as well as aid in tenderizing the chicken. This technique can also be used for thinly sliced cuts of beef, such as eye of round or flank steak, that are not naturally tender. After water-blanching, they can be quickly finished off by stir-frying, sautéing, or heating in a sauce.

STIR-FRYING

Asian-Style Vegetable Stir-fry (page 302)
Three-Pepper and Beef Stir-fry (page 207)
Velvet Chicken (page 193)

My first professional culinary experience was in a Chinese restaurant, so it is no surprise that I am a big fan of stir-frying. When properly done, there is no better way of preparing food. Unfortunately, intense heat, a key element to successful stir-frying, is usually not available in the typical American kitchen. Most conventional home ranges, whether gas or electric, only produce a fraction of the heat of the Chinese firepots found in Asian restaurants. Standard wok recipes call for stir-frying all the meat and vegetables at once. That's fine when you have the large burners of a commercial restaurant, but it will produce soggy and flavorless food on a home stove, which is why it is so common to hear people say no matter how closely they follow the recipes, they just don't taste authentic. Not to worry: if you cook the meat and vegetables separately, as discussed below, you can produce authentic-tasting Asian dishes at home. With a little planning and patience you too can become a master "woker."

Woks traditionally have a rounded bottom, designed to fit snugly into a cylindrical firepot. This shape works poorly on our flat stovetops, because so little of the rounded bottom actually comes into contact with the heat. So it is best to use a flat-bottomed wok on the stove to maximize heat conduction. Wok size is also important. For home use, a 14-inch wok works well. If not available, a 12-inch nonstick skillet or cast-iron skillet that is fully seasoned works equally well. High heat is absolutely essential for proper stir-frying; the oil used must have a high smoking point. Canola or grapeseed oil is an excellent choice. Either one withstands high heat, and also has no intrinsic flavor to interfere with the Asian condiments. For this reason, the distinctive taste of olive oil won't do when stir-frying Asian dishes. To maintain high heat, it is important not to stir-fry too much in the wok when initially cooking raw meats and vegetables. This means stir-frying less than about one pound of meat or seafood at a time (less than about four ounces per person for four people, a very healthy choice). Accompany the meat or seafood with about one and a half to two pounds of chopped vegetables (three to four cups), which will fit into a standard-size home wok.

Preparation for stir-frying meats and seafood begins with cutting them into small, uniform-size pieces according to the recipe's directions, which is important to allow quick and even cooking.

The wok or skillet should be heated until very hot. Drizzle a teaspoon or so of oil into the center of the wok, rolling it around to coat the lower sides of the wok. Heat the oil until it just begins to shimmer and then add meat or seafood, stir, and toss in the wok until completely opaque, two to three minutes. Remove the meat and seafood from the wok and set aside.

Now, cooking the vegetables can be a bit tricky because the cooking times vary significantly. So I usually first water-blanch (see page 365) the denser vegetables, such as cauliflower, broccoli, carrots, and green beans, giving them a crunchy bite and intensifying their colors. You can do this step hours ahead of time and keep the water-blanched vegetables, thoroughly drained, in the refrigerator. The more tender vegetables, such as squash, zucchini, and mushrooms, are done after only a couple of minutes in the wok.

The final step again requires reheating the wok and adding a teaspoon of oil. This intense heat allows the flavor of the condiments and aromatics to permeate the cooking oil and, ultimately, the entire sauce. Add the ginger, garlic, and green onions as directed in the recipe and stir-fry for about ten seconds, tossing constantly to avoid burning. Then add the Asian aromatics, such as oyster, hoisin, or chili sauce, mix thoroughly with the ginger and garlic, and then add the broth and the rest of the liquid ingredients. Bring to a low boil and simmer for a minute or so before adding the reserved vegetables, meat, or seafood. Simmer for a few more minutes, until all the ingredients are hot. Thicken the sauce with dissolved cornstarch, and the dish is ready to serve.

Although this technique may sound cumbersome, with a little practice you can complete the steps in six to eight minutes. Organization is the key. Do all of the mincing, chopping, and blanching ahead of time. Arrange the ingredients in bowls next to the stove in the order of their use, ready to be stir-fried in an instant. Once the wok is fired up and the oil is hot, there is no time to fumble around looking for this spice or that sauce.

SAUTÉING

Cod Iberia (page 293)
Farfalle with Monkfish, Mushrooms, and Fennel (page 185)
Jamaican Snapper (page 350)
Sautéed Halibut with Roasted Brussels Sprouts and Mushrooms
in Red Wine Pan Sauce (page 153)
Sonoran Turkey Cutlets in Tequila-Lime Sauce (page 163)

The term *sauté* comes from the French word for "jump," and in classical cooking it means to quickly prepare food in a small amount of hot fat. Four boneless, skinless chicken breasts or fish fillets are typically sautéed in 2 tablespoons of oil or butter, which is about 28 grams of fat. Even if we cook with a healthy, monounsaturated oil, such as olive or canola oil, that is still over 250 calories. An easy way to reduce the calories and fat is to sauté in a heavy-bottomed, high-quality nonstick skillet, which can uniformly distribute high heat. Heat the skillet over medium heat for a few minutes, and then add a tablespoon of oil and heat the oil until it begins to shimmer. Turn the heat down to low, and place four seasoned fish fillets, skin side down, in the skillet. It is very important to not move the fish for the initial cooking period. Let it cook for three to four minutes; the fillets should be golden brown if skinless and have a nice crisp crust if the skin is left on. Now turn the fillets over, and if they are thin (less than half an inch thick) they can be finished off by cooking for another three minutes on the stovetop.

If you are preparing thicker fillets, you may wish to complete the cooking in a preheated 375-degree oven for six to ten minutes. Either way, you will have a moist and beautifully golden brown fish fillet. With boneless, skinless chicken breasts, I often like to pound them to a uniform thickness of about half an inch to speed up the cooking if I don't want to finish them off in the oven.

When cooking fish fillets or boneless chicken breasts, sprinkle the fish or chicken with paprika as another way to ensure a beautiful golden crust without a lot of fat.

Broth Sautéing of Vegetables

Corn and Sweet Pepper Sauté in Broth (page 351)

Often when sautéing vegetables, you can eliminate the fat by cooking them in broth, or "sweating" them. Begin by lightly coating a nonstick skillet with cooking spray and then placing it over medium heat for a couple of minutes. Add the sliced vegetables and sauté, periodically adding a few tablespoons of broth as needed to prevent burning and sticking. It is important that the pan not be too small and that not too much broth is added at one time, as this will prevent the caramelization of the vegetable's natural sugars. Many vegetables can be prepared in five to seven minutes using this technique.

A special note about onions: because they have more sugar than any other vegetable, onions can require from fifteen to twenty minutes over low heat to become fully caramelized, but taking the time to properly caramelize them is worth it. When fully caramelized, they add a richness and depth of flavor, which can transform a dish from bland to spectacular. If you don't have the time to be in the kitchen while the onions are sautéing, consider oven-roasting them.

Stovetop Grilling

Pan-Grilled Salmon with Frisée Salad Lyonnaise (page 136)
Pan-Grilled Shiitake Chicken Breasts (page 145)
Steak and Chickpea Salad (page 246)
Stovetop-Grilled Swordfish in Basil-Tomato Vinaigrette (page 308)

In Italy, they call it *graticola,* a ridged, square-shaped skillet with a long handle. Stovetop grilling is indispensable for Italian home-style cooking, and it is for the Dr. Chef's healthy kitchen as well. While an authentic Italian *graticola* may not be readily available, practically every camping or hardware store has ridged cast-iron skillets (usually about 10 inches in diameter) as well as the much larger rectangular ridged griddles. And they are every bit as good as their Italian namesakes. What makes them so terrific? By preheating the ridged skillet or griddle until it is smoking hot, it is possible to quickly prepare grilled chicken, meats, seafood, and vegetables as succulent and tasty as those served in the finest restaurants. There are quite a number of ridged skillets with nonstick coatings that have recently come on the market, and are two or three times as expensive as the cast iron variety. Cast iron is the best because it is able to reach and maintain very high temperatures that are evenly distributed across the cooking surface. When I discuss stovetop grilling in the recipes in this book, it means using cast iron. When using a ridged cast-iron skillet or griddle, preheat for about ten minutes on medium-high heat until the skillet is just smoking, then brush a thin film of oil on the top of the ridges. There will be a little smoke, so be sure there is ample ventilation. Firm fish such as swordfish, tuna, and halibut can be grilled in four to five minutes on each side per inch of thickness. After two minutes of grilling on a side, I rotate the fish a quarter turn (ninety degrees) to add professional-looking crosshatching to the fish.

Boneless, skinless chicken breasts are best done with an additional step, as in pan roasting. It takes about twelve minutes total grilling time for a typical half chicken breast weighing five or six ounces. With the intense heat of stovetop grilling the outside of the chicken breast would become tough and dry. To avoid this, I grill a chicken breast for three minutes on each side, and then finish it off in a preheated 375-degree oven for seven to eight minutes. The chicken breast will be perfectly grilled on the outside (not burnt or dry) and moist on the inside.

Salmon fillets also work best when pan roasted, but starting on the stovetop grill. I typically grill a five- to six-ounce fillet three minutes on each side and then complete the cooking in a preheated 375-degree oven for about eight minutes. The outside of the salmon will have a wonderful crispiness and the inside will have that sweet tenderness that defines great grilled salmon. Often I like to brine (see page 376) chicken breasts and salmon before cooking to ensure their moistness and tenderness.

Relatively thin seafood fillets with the skin on, such as red snapper, can also be easily done on the stovetop grill. The fish is first grilled on one side for two minutes, then turned and grilled for another minute.

PAN ROASTING

Cod Iberia (page 293)
Duck Breasts with Port and Fig Sauce (page 286)
Jamaican Snapper (page 350)
Oven-Roasted Pork Chops with Sun-Dried Cherry Wine Sauce (page 230)

Pan-Grilled Salmon with Frisée Salad Lyonnaise (page 136)
Pan-Grilled Shiitake Chicken Breasts (page 145)
Pan-Roasted Pork Tenderloin with Apples (page 114)
Pan-Roasted Salmon with Shanghai Red Sauce (page 270)
Sautéed Halibut with Roasted Brussels Sprouts and Mushrooms
in Red Wine Pan Sauce (page 153)
Sear-Roasted Sea Bass with Olives, Capers, and Tomatoes (page 253)
Steak and Chickpea Salad (page 246)

Ever wonder how restaurants get their meats and seafood to form such a crispy brown outer crust with a moist and tender interior? Pan roasting is the secret. It is a simple technique that involves searing food on the stovetop to give a great crust and finishing it off in a preheated oven. The stovetop cooking may be done in a regular flat skillet or a ridged griddle that is oven safe— without wooden or plastic handles (see Stovetop Grilling, page 369). Take the food out of the refrigerator and let it come to room temperature so it can be cooked quickly. If using a flat skillet, cover with a thin film of oil and heat it over medium-high heat to just below smoking. If the oil isn't hot enough, the food will stick to the skillet; if too hot and smoking, the crust will burn. Once in the skillet, cook the food for about three minutes without moving, to allow a nice crust to form. Then turn the food over and place the pan in a preheated oven for five to ten minutes to complete cooking it through. The result: a golden crust on the outside and moist and tender meat on the inside. It is usually best to use thicker cuts of meat (greater than about ¾ inch) when pan roasting so that the food doesn't cook too quickly and dry out.

Depending on the dish, the main item may be removed from the skillet, covered, and kept warm (this allows the juices to redistribute), and the pan drippings used to make a sauce. First sauté shallots, garlic, and/or onions in the leftover drippings to add a flavor base. Then add wine, vinegar, and/or broth and scrape up (deglaze) the browned bits, called fond, stuck to the bottom of the skillet into the sauce to capture all the flavors of the initial sear. However, do not add acidic ingredients to a cast-iron skillet, because they will leach the iron and give the sauce a metallic taste. Typically, you would heat the sauce for another few minutes to reduce and then finish off with herbs and seasonings. You may want to whisk in a bit of dissolved arrowroot at the end of cooking to add some body and sheen to the final sauce.

Pan roasting also complements stovetop grilling done on a ridged cast-iron surface (see Stovetop Grilling, page 369). Poultry, such as boneless, skinless chicken breasts, and more delicate fish, such as salmon, easily burn on the exterior if cooked on a smoking-hot grill until completely done. By finishing the meats and seafood off in an oven, you can guarantee a perfectly grilled crust with a succulent and moist interior. Timing is critical, so follow the recipes closely and you won't be disappointed!

OVEN ROASTING

Creamy Roasted Carrot–Miso Soup (page 306)

Oven-Roasted Fingerling Potatoes (page 155)

Roasted Mushrooms and Asparagus (page 202)

Roasted Mushrooms with Onions (page 138)

Roasted Root-Vegetable Puree with Horseradish (page 175)

Roasted Vegetable Soup (page 348)

Salsa Snapper (page 123)

Sautéed Halibut with Roasted Brussels Sprouts and Mushrooms in Red Wine Pan Sauce (page 153)

Turkey Breast with Cranberry-Apple Relish (page 172)

In the past, the word *roast* would invariably conjure up an image of roast beef or leg of lamb. And while roasting meats still provides delicious fare, vegetables and fish definitely reign supreme in today's healthy oven. That's because roasting is an easy way to cook, using the natural juices of the food rather than a lot of fat to provide flavor. Roasting requires relatively high heat. Vegetables demand the same high, dry heat as traditional roasted meats, 400 to 500 degrees, otherwise food will just steam in its own juices. The high heat of the oven radiates uniformly and so provides for more even cooking than a skillet or pot. In addition, the high heat caramelizes (browns) the sugars on the outer surface of the food while sweetening and deepening the internal flavors. Even bland cauliflower tastes so good you can't resist it after oven roasting. This intensification of flavors is so dramatic that peppers, tomatoes, and garlic are commonly first roasted before being used in dips, sauces, and dressings. It's a great way to boost flavor without adding fat.

Very little fat is needed to properly oven roast. A thin film of cooking spray that covers each item works well. Or if you prefer, about 4 teaspoons of oil should nicely cover about 1½ pounds of vegetables cut into 1¼-inch pieces.

The size of the roasting pan is important: use one that will just hold all of the vegetables in a single layer. If the pan is too small, the caramelization of the outer surface of the vegetables is prevented because the vegetables will begin to steam rather than brown. If the pan is too large, the edges of the pan will tend to get too hot and the vegetables begin to burn. A shallow height (1½ to 2 inches in height) is also preferred, otherwise the pan will act as a steamer and again retard caramelization. Standard 14 x 12 x 2-inch and 12 x 8 x 1½-inch pans work well. First line the pan with aluminum foil to make cleanup easy.

Roasting Vegetables: Cut root vegetables, such as potatoes, carrots, peeled onions, parsnips, and turnips, into 1- to 1¼-inch wedges, coat very lightly with cooking spray or oil, and season with salt and pepper. For added flavor, add whole thyme leaves or finely chopped rosemary to the vegetables. Place in a preheated oven at 425 degrees for about 20 minutes, turn the vegetables over to evenly brown, and continue to roast for about another 20 minutes. If the vegetables appear to be browning too fast, add a tablespoon or so of broth.

Roasting Garlic: Peel off the papery outside layer, then slice off about ½ inch from the top of the garlic head to expose the tip of the cloves. Drizzle the head with cooking spray or oil, wrap in foil, and place in a preheated 425-degree oven for about 30 minutes. The garlic cloves will then be very soft (practically pureed) and you can easily remove them from the skin by pushing up from the root end of the garlic. Roasted garlic is often used in salad dressings; see Roasted Garlic Vinaigrette (page 113).

Fish and Meats: Technically, roasting fish or meats in a hot oven doesn't differ from baking. Roasting has traditionally meant cooking in the open air over a hot fire, often on a spit. This ensures that no moisture surrounds the fish and guarantees a crispy skin. Today, we can get these same results by preparing food in a hot oven. In selecting items to be roasted, choose varieties that are thick and firm with lots of natural oils or moisture, brining if needed, which will help to keep seafood and meats moist and prevent drying out. Leaving the skin on fish fillets will also help to seal in moisture.

Salmon, swordfish, halibut, monkfish, and catfish are some examples of fish that all roast well in the oven.

OVEN FRYING

Oven-Fried Cajun Catfish (page 240)
Toasted Almond and Cumin-Crusted Chicken Breasts (page 128)

Chicken and fish that are crispy on the outside and moist and tender on the inside used to mean deep fried and loaded with fat. Oven frying allows you to re-create that finger-licking-good crust without all those extra calories. The secret is to coat the pieces of fish or poultry with a creamy base, such as plain fat-free yogurt, buttermilk, or beaten egg whites. Keep everything cold so that the creamy base thickly coats the poultry or fish. Roll the coated items over several times in a mixture of seasoned dried crumbs that may be either standard bread crumbs or cereal crumbs, such as cornflakes, or crushed melba toast. Adding ground nuts to the crumb mixture gives an extra crunch plus helps meet your daily dose of this Bonus Years food. Place the thickly coated pieces in a refrigerator for about twenty minutes to allow the coating to set. After misting all sides of the chilled and coated items with cooking spray, placed them on a wire rack that is positioned in the upper third of an oven preheated to 400 degrees. About fifteen minutes later, you can enjoy crunchy and tender chicken or fish. Placing the food on a rack ensures even cooking of both sides of the coated items. The wire rack can be placed on a baking sheet lined with aluminum foil to protect the oven from drippings.

STEAMING

Steamed Salmon Steaks (page 201)

Steaming is as Chinese as the wok, so it's no wonder that I am such a great fan. In fact, the Chinese often use their woks as a base for their steamers. I won't steam a large fish in anything but my wok (it is 24 inches in diameter, so it can hold quite a fish!). Fortunately, steaming is one of the most versatile cooking techniques. Practically any covered pot or skillet can serve as a steamer. Steaming is carried out over boiling water, not in it. A perforated rack separates the food to be steamed from the boiling water below.

The food cooks as it comes into contact with the steam, providing for moist and even heating, and retains its nutrients and flavor because it is cooked in its own natural juices.

Steamed foods remain exceptionally tender and succulent. Place the food to be steamed on a plate or set directly on the perforated rack. I prefer the plate, to save the natural juices, which is essential when preparing food that has been topped with a sauce before cooking. The sauce attains a luxuriant delicate aroma and flavor as it interacts with the steaming food.

Steamers can be purchased as self-contained, stand-alone units designed specifically for steaming or can just as easily be assembled by using a household pot or skillet with a collapsible basket/rack insert. A bamboo steamer that sits on top of a wok works equally well. Also available are sophisticated electrical steamers with built-in screens, which allow for easy addition of herbs and spices to flavor the food; they heat up rapidly and are convenient for preparing vegetables and small whole fish or fillets. The quality of steamed food does not depend on the equipment, so choose what is most convenient.

When done, the flesh of chicken breasts and fish becomes opaque and will easily flake off the bone. A good rule of thumb is ten minutes of steaming for each inch of thickness of the food. I have found that fish is pretty forgiving when it comes to steaming. You are adding moisture, so there is a margin of error to prevent seafood or chicken breasts from drying out.

While you may use any liquid for steaming, remember that stock, wine, or juice adds extra flavor, as does the addition of herbs and spices. As already mentioned, some of the newer electric steamers are specially designed to infuse these flavors.

Before steaming, allow the food to come to room temperature. Avoid uncovering the pot while steaming, but when the cover is removed, lift it so that the steam goes away from you, to prevent injury.

POACHING

Sicilian Poached Chicken Breasts (page 313)
Sole Poached in Seafood Court Bouillon (page 259)

Poaching is a moist heat method especially well suited for more delicate foods like seafood and light-meat poultry. It is ideal for preparing fish fillets or chicken breasts that have little tough connective tissue and can easily fall apart or toughen if exposed to intense heat. By cooking gently in a liquid, foods can be prepared without added fat, retaining their natural moisture and tenderness. To poach, bring a cooking liquid to a minimal simmer (there should be no actual bubbles escaping from the liquid, just some shimmering on the surface) and totally submerge the food. For a small whole fish, a fish fillet, or chicken breast, five to ten minutes is all that is needed.

The poaching liquid should reflect the item being cooked and may include chicken, vegetable, and fish stocks and broths, wine, and juices, along with spices and other seasonings. After you bring the liquid to a very low simmer on the stovetop, submerge the food in the liquid and finish in a preheated oven at 350 degrees for even, uniform cooking. A special poaching pan is not needed, but the pot should be large enough to accommodate the food and liquid as they expand during cooking, but not so large as to require a great deal of extra liquid. Because the poaching liquid can be used as a base for sauces, if too much liquid is used initially for poaching, the flavor of the cooking liquid will be diluted.

It is important that the poaching liquid not be allowed to come to a boil or a more rapid simmer, to avoid overcooking and toughening the food.

BRINING

Oven-Roasted Pork Chops with Sun-Dried Cherry Wine Sauce (page 230)
Pan-Roasted Pork Tenderloin with Apples (page 114)
Sonoran Turkey Cutlets in Tequila-Lime Sauce (page 163)
Turkey Breast with Cranberry-Apple Relish (page 172)

Lean foods, such as chicken or turkey breast, pork tenderloin, and shrimp, are easy to overcook because they have so little fat. A great way to make even the leanest foods juicy and tender is to add moisture *before* cooking through a process called brining. Place the food in a solution prepared with salt and, depending on the recipe, some sugar, spices, and other flavorings for as little as half an hour for shrimp or up to twelve hours for a large turkey.

Brining Solution: For the recipes in this book, add one-quarter cup kosher salt and one-quarter cup sugar to one quart of hot water. Stir until dissolved and let cool to room temperature. The solution must be at room temperature or lower before the meat or poultry is added.

Although there are differences of opinion among food scientists as to all the step-by-step chemical reactions involved in brining, everyone agrees that the final result is that water and salt enter the food, adding moisture and resulting in about a 7 percent increase in weight of the brined food.

In addition, the added salt causes the proteins in the meat to uncoil, trapping water, which helps to prevent the loss of water that normally accompanies cooking. The food becomes incredibly tender and moist, with additional flavorings depending on the other components of the brine.

This technique is so important that I rarely prepare chicken breasts or pork chops or tenderloins without brining them first.

Salmon does well with a short brine, particularly if it is to be prepared with a dry heat method like grilling or broiling.

After the food is brined, rinse it in cold water to remove the excess salt from the surface, then pat dry. Because there is some increase in salt in the meat, it isn't necessary to add salt to the final seasoning, so overall there is not much additional salt added, but the improved tenderness and moistness of the meat is dramatic.

Brining can be done in advance. After brining, rinse the meat in cold water, pat dry with paper towels, and place in a self-sealing plastic bag in the refrigerator for up to 24 hours.

THICKENING BROTH TO REPLACE OIL

Asian-Style Chicken Salad with Peanut Sauce (page 199)

Broiled Tuscan-Style Flank Steak (page 223)

Greek Salad (page 221)

Green Bean, Berry, and Spinach Salad (page 291)

Italian Potato Salad (page 315)

Roasted Garlic Vinaigrette (page 113)

Mushroom-Walnut Salad with Roquefort Vinaigrette (page 311)

Roasted Garlic-Shallot Vinaigrette (page 268)

Stovetop-Grilled Swordfish in Basil-Tomato Vinaigrette (page 308)

Traditionally, salad dressings are prepared with two parts of oil for every one part of vinegar. That can be a lot of fat, even if it is heart-healthy monounsaturated oils. A good substitute is to use thickened broth or stock in place of part of the oil. This gives the same mouthfeel and richness as the original dressing. For example, if a recipe calls for two-thirds cup of oil (about eleven tablespoons) and one-third cup vinegar, I would use eight tablespoons of thickened broth and only three tablespoons of oil with one-third cup vinegar to make 1 cup of dressing. The thickened broth is prepared by bringing half a cup (eight tablespoons) of low-sodium chicken broth to a low simmer in a saucepan, then slowly whisking in one teaspoon of arrowroot that has been dissolved in a very small amount of water. When my recipes for vinaigrettes and dressings call for thickened broth, this is the method that works.

TOASTING SPICES

Toasted Almond and Cumin-Crusted Chicken Breasts (page 128)

Most whole spices need to be crushed, chopped, or ground before using, in order to release their flavor. Their taste can be even further enhanced if the spices are lightly toasted in a *dry* skillet prior to crushing. The heat of toasting causes chemical reactions that concentrate the fragrance and aroma of the whole spices. Cumin, coriander seeds, and Szechuan peppercorns are spices I commonly toast before grinding.

To toast, place about two tablespoons of the spice in an ungreased skillet that has been preheated to medium-high. Heat the spices until they turn somewhat dark and just begin to smoke, three to four minutes. Be sure not to overcook them, or they will burn and be bitter! Also, it is important to constantly shake the skillet to help prevent burning. Once the spices have been properly toasted, remove them from the skillet, cool, and store in a tightly covered container away from heat. The toasted spices then can be ground or crushed as needed.

ROASTING PEPPERS

Roasted Peppers, Fennel, and Artichokes with Baked Polenta (page 177)
Penne with Sausage, Bell Peppers, and Sun-Dried Tomato Wine Sauce
(page 277)

In the Southwest, roasting bell peppers and fresh chilies is as common as toasting bread, and almost as easy. First, thoroughly char the peppers until black on the outside, then place in a sealed plastic bag and allow to "cook" (the trapped heat will steam the peppers and cause the skins to blister). After about thirty minutes, remove the peppers from the plastic bag and peel off the blackened skins. Don't use water to wash off the skins, because that will only remove the peppers' great-tasting roasted oils. (A few bits of blackened skin on the peppers give a rustic and colorful appearance.) Roasted bell peppers and chilies can be frozen for later use—no need to peel before freezing. Freezing will actually make it easier to remove the skins later.

I usually roast the whole bell peppers or chilies directly on a gas grill or gas stovetop, turning them periodically as each side of the pepper is charred. Placing them under a broiler works just as well, especially if you are doing several at a time. And don't limit yourself to just red bell peppers. The green, orange, and yellow varieties roast up just as well and add a lot of color to any dish.

Several of the recipes call for roasted bell peppers. If you are short on time, you can substitute jarred roasted bell peppers, but the flavor is not as fresh, the texture will be softer, and the salt content is higher. If using the jarred product, drain the peppers thoroughly before using.

CHAPTER 10

Fear of "Fishing"

Fear of fish—well, perhaps just of buying, storing, and preparing fish—is easily the greatest barrier to people's eating seafood on a regular basis. In part this is due to geography: many of us live inland and aren't exposed to fresh fish when we are young, and so we never really develop a taste for seafood. But with the advancements in commercial transportation it is now possible for practically everyone to find a wide range of seafood in local markets. I live in the desert in Phoenix, but I am never at a loss when it comes to a selection of fresh fish, from Asian snapper to Dover sole.

Buying Fish

The most common complaint I hear about seafood is that it smells "fishy." Well, if that's the case, it just isn't fresh and will undoubtedly taste worse than it smells. Fresh fish is moist, bright, and glistening, with essentially no smell. It should never appear brown or dried out. The best advice I can give is to get to know a local fish market that you can trust and let the staff guide you to the freshest seafood selections and guarantee your success.

The other complaint that I hear is that fish is expensive. While the cost per pound may seem high, remember that if you are buying fish fillets or steaks, there is very little waste, so the cost per serving is not as expensive as it first appears. Another way to beat the high cost of fresh fish is to buy frozen fish. If you do, check the package for signs that the fish has thawed and been refrozen. Again, sniff the package; if it smells fishy, keep looking.

Fish is generally sold whole or in pieces (fillets and steaks). Fillets refer to meat on one side of the fish. They can either have the skin on or be skinless. Steaks are obtained by cutting crosswise through a section of the fish, with a fillet on the each side of a central bone. Some large fish, like tuna, shark, and swordfish, may first be cut lengthwise into fillets and then crosswise into steaks. Such steaks will not have a central bone.

Fresh fish should be eaten as soon after purchase as possible. If it needs to be stored for a short time, place some ice on the bottom of a flat pan, cover the ice with plastic wrap, and place the fish on top of the wrap. Cover the pan and refrigerate. Be careful that water from the ice doesn't reach the fish by seeping around or through the plastic.

People are often overwhelmed by the myriad of choices available in selecting fish. I would suggest that you begin by choosing a half dozen or so of the most popular types of fish, which are easily available and have a variety of textures and flavors. When you feel comfortable in preparing these, and begin to develop a sense of how best to cook different kinds of fish, you can then easily branch out and become more adventurous.

A good selection would include the following: delicate, mild fillets, such as the commonly available sole and flounder. More medium-textured fillets, including mild-tasting cod and the more moderate-flavored snapper and catfish, are now offered in most markets. Finally, a selection of firm-textured fish could include the milder-tasting sea bass, monkfish, and halibut fillets with more full-flavored steaks, such as swordfish and shark. Salmon is a must on any seafood list because not only it is one of the most popular and readily available fish, but also its high levels of omega-3 fatty acids make it one of the healthiest seafood choices.

Recipes in this book feature many of these selections and should be considered as a springboard for further learning. After you have mastered these recipes and their techniques, you will understand the basic guiding principles to selecting and preparing the most common kinds of fish. These can then be readily applied to other seafood selections, recipes, and cuisines. While the recipes call for a specific fish, often other, similar fish can be easily substituted. For example, a recipe for braised salsa snapper would work equally well with a similar medium-textured fish, such as cod. A grilled shark steak could be substituted for swordfish if the more powerful taste of fresh shark is more to your liking than the milder swordfish. Sautéed monkfish is in one of our featured recipes, but cubed halibut would be just as inviting. Once you feel comfortable preparing a given type of fish with one of the basic techniques, there is no limit to the similar fish and recipes that you can substitute with ease.

Cooking Fish

Ever wonder why the fish in restaurants tastes so great? It is not only the quality of the fish, but also the way it is prepared. The most common mistake in cooking fish and seafood is overcooking. Because fish has generally less fat and connective tissue than meat and poultry, it is particularly easy to dry out. This must always be kept foremost in mind when preparing any kind of fish or seafood. Obviously, thin fillets, such as flounder or sole, cook very quickly. Their delicate texture could never stand up to the high heat of grilling or the prolonged cooking times of braising. Moist heat that adds liquid as the fish cooks is usually preferred. Poaching and steaming are two of the best techniques for this delicate variety of fish.

Medium-textured fish, such as snapper, catfish, and cod, offer a greater range of possibilities. While they may be poached or steamed, it is usually best to take advantage of their more hearty texture and put a nice "sear" on the outside of the fish, adding to the presentation (beautifully browned crust) and providing a nice contrast in texture between the crisp outside and the moist inside. If the fillets are somewhat thin (less than half an inch in thickness), then it is usually possible to sauté them (see page 368) on both sides and completely cook the fish through in about five to seven minutes total cooking time.

Often, it is best to prepare a sauce with the fish, then sear the fish on one side in a nonstick skillet, cover it with the sauce, and finish it off in the oven (a form of both oven roasting and braising), so you don't have to worry about undercooking it on the stovetop. By placing the fish first in the sauce and then in the oven, you have it surrounded with liquid to keep it from drying out. The oven also supplies a more uniform, gentle heat than the high temperature of the burners. When the sauce has lots of veggies, such as tomatoes and onions, this becomes essentially a one-pot meal. If you flavor the sauce with Cajun, Southwestern, or Jamaican seasonings, and then add the appropriate regional vegetables, it becomes easy and quick to prepare an authentic, healthy, and delectably moist fish dinner. We use this method in a number of the recipes. By simply varying the type of fish as well as the other ingredients it becomes a snap to create your own house specialties.

Sturdy steaks, such as swordfish and shark, can take high heat, and are often prepared by grilling or broiling. Grilling, in particular, can give beautiful crosshatch marks to the fish, which add much to their visual appeal. Sea bass, halibut, monkfish, and other firm fish fillets often do well with a combination of initial cooking on the stovetop and then finishing off in the oven, as do medium-textured fish like catfish or snapper. Sautéing firm fillets in a skillet provides the initial sear, but because these are firmer, they can also hold up to an initial grill on a stovetop ridged iron skillet (or other ridged griddle) before they are placed in the oven. As when cooking the more medium-textured catfish or snapper, I often like to prepare a sauce to cover the sea bass or halibut to keep it moist as it is cooking in the oven. This is particularly true of halibut, which has a tendency to dry out somewhat more readily than sea bass or monkfish. Monkfish is particularly hardy and can really stand up to longer braising in the oven (fifteen to twenty minutes), which makes it particularly nice to prepare with a sauce.

If the fish is not to be prepared in a sauce, coating the fish with a dry spice rub is a great way to increase the flavor of a dish. The coated side can then be seared in the skillet for about three minutes to give a well-seasoned and tasty crust, and then the fish is finished off in the oven. Because the rub can burn when it is placed in the fat in a hot skillet, it is important to keep a close watch on the fish as it sears on the stovetop. By completing the cooking in the oven you can carefully control the time the coated rub is exposed to high direct heat in the pan, helping to ensure a crisp and flavorful crust without a burnt taste.

Salmon can be prepared in so many different ways. A firm fish, it takes well to grilling or broiling but also may be steamed, poached, or pan seared. Because of its great versatility and nutritional value, we have included one salmon recipe in each week of the Bonus Years menus.

Cooking Equipment

Fish is rather delicate, so it is important to keep it from sticking to the bottom of the skillet when searing. The pan you use should be heavy and sturdy, to ensure that there is even distribution of heat. That is why I like to use a high-quality nonstick skillet. Less expensive models may look nice, but there will be "hot spots" along the cooking surface, which make for uneven searing.

As far as grilling on the stovetop is concerned, I still vote for the old-fashioned, cast-iron ridged grill pans, which beautifully retain heat, give great grill marks, become nonstick after they have been seasoned (some companies like Lodge are now offering preseasoned skillets), and best of all, are inexpensive.

While stovetop grilling and oven roasting are great ways to prepare restaurant-quality seafood, meats, and poultry, two-sided electric grills offer a good alternative when you're in a hurry. Fast, easy to use, and practically

COOKING FISH

Fish	Texture	Cooking Methods	Tips
Fillets of sole, flounder, and haddock	Delicate, with small tender flakes	Poach, steam, or bake with a sauce surrounding the fish.	Place seasoning, herbs, and spices in the poaching liquid or over the fish before steaming. The sauce adds flavor and protects against drying out when baking.
Fillets of snapper, catfish, cod, trout, and farmed salmon fillets and salmon steaks	Medium, with larger flakes, firmer but still tender	Steam. Sauté (sear) thin (less than ½ inch thick) fillets on both sides. Pan-roast thicker fillets: sear on stovetop for 3 minutes, finish cooking in oven for 7 to 10 minutes.	Before steaming, place a sauce or seasoning over the fish. When pan roasting, use a rub on the fish or top with a sauce before finishing off in the oven at 350 degrees.
Shark steaks, swordfish steaks, sea bass fillets, halibut fillets, monkfish, wild salmon steaks or fillets, and tuna	Firm, larger, more meaty fish	Meaty steaks can be grilled on each side for about 5 minutes. All of these fish can be broiled with a glaze. The fillets can be baked but do really well pan-roasted with an initial sear in a skillet or on a ridged grill pan followed by baking in the oven.	Meaty steaks can be cooked all the way through on a ridged grill pan or grill without fear of burning the surface. Wild salmon steaks and fillets do particularly well grilled. If the salmon steak is thick, cook on the grill or ridged grill pan and finish off in the oven. Don't forget the rub!

foolproof, these grills are a convenient way to quickly prepare your fish and meat entrées with very little mess and cleanup, perfect for a weeknight meal. And to those of you who might feel a bit intimidated by the thought of preparing fish steaks or fillets, these electric grills are a wonderful way get you started in overcoming your fear of "fishing."

Planning a Seafood Dinner

Here are some questions I always ask myself as I select the dishes for the menu.

- What is the theme of the dinner—Asian, Italian, Southwestern, or Cajun, for example? This will help guide the selection of seasonings, vegetables, and sauces.
- Is there a type of seafood that is often prepared with this particular cuisine? Catfish is popular in Cajun cooking, snapper in Mexican fare (think snapper Veracruz). This in turn will guide you in selecting the best cooking method. Medium-textured fish, such as snapper and catfish, can stand up to a hot sear in the skillet, in which case you might first want to apply a Creole or spicy south-of-the-border rub, or if you decide to prepare a sauce, perhaps pan-sear the fish first in a hot skillet and then surround it with an appropriately flavored sauce, which might also contain some regional vegetables. If the fish is more delicate and needs to be poached or steamed, the regional vegetables and the seasonings could be placed in the poaching liquid or around the fish to be steamed. So the type of fish selected not only determines the cooking technique, but also plays a real role in how the seasonings and vegetables of the dish will be presented. Finally, if these specific fish are not available, what other fish with similar thickness, texture, and depth of flavor can be purchased that would allow the same cooking techniques and seasonings to be used?
- What are the regional vegetables associated with the cuisine? Select bok choy or snow peas for Chinese dinners, jicama and corn for Southwestern dishes, and bell peppers and okra for Cajun cooking, for example.

- What flavorings or sauces using authentic local seasonings will be prepared to complement the fish? Can these sauces be easily incorporated with the appropriate regional vegetables?

  Stir-frying is an easy way to add those bonus veggies to your sauces. With dishes including seafood such as shrimp or cubed halibut or swordfish, it may be possible to cook the seafood in the sauce. If preparing a Mediterranean dish with a delicate fish, consider baking the fish covered with a sauce and vegetables. For heartier fish, first sear the seafood in a hot skillet and then finish it off in the oven surrounded by the sauce.

- Will the fish be prepared separately from the sauce and the sauce spooned over or around the fish just before serving? Or will the fish be cooked in the sauce, as in a pan-roasted/braised dish, creating a one-pot meal?

- If the fish is to be pan-seared or grilled, will an appropriate regional spice rub be applied? This is particularly important to increasing the flavor depth of the seafood if the fish is to be cooked separately from the sauce. More hearty fish, which can stand up to the grill or hot sear of the skillet, do well with rubs, so if you decide to use a rub, that will help guide you in your selection of seafood.

Let's look at some specific examples. Perhaps you decide to make a Mediterranean-style dinner. The cooks in Italian seaport cities such as Livorno often prepare seafood with tomatoes, olives, and capers (what could be more Italian!). You could decide to use the traditional snapper, but perhaps your fishmonger says that the sea bass is particularly fresh and inviting. Both snapper and sea bass are relatively mild, sturdy white fish, and both will do well with an initial sear-roast in a hot nonstick skillet to give a nice brown, crunchy crust. Finish the fish off in the oven, smothered in a simple tomato, olive, and caper sauce, and you have a wonderfully light, healthy, and easy-to-prepare seafood meal (see the recipe for Sear-Roasted Sea Bass with Olives, Capers, and Tomatoes, page 253, which shines with the warmth of the Mediterranean).

But maybe the snapper is the best catch of the day, and you opt to do a variation on the Mexican classic snapper Veracruz. Again, just sear-roast the snapper for three minutes as we did with the sea bass, but now finish the fish in the oven with a sauce based on canned Mexican tomatoes and your favorite salsa. You have another quick, easy, and healthy one-pot meal.

If I were going to use the snapper for a N'awlins-inspired dinner, I would probably coat the snapper with a Cajun rub, then pan-sear it in a hot skillet to crust up the spicy seasonings before finishing it seared-side down in a preheated oven to add more crunch and color to the fish. Serve this with a Cajun-inspired vegetable side dish, such as the Cajun Okra-Tomato Braise (page 242) and some rice, and you have your own Mardi Gras.

The above-mentioned recipes use a pan-searing technique, and once you have perfected it, there is an endless variety of simple but elegant seafood dishes that you can create to delight family and friends. Master the other simple techniques of poaching, steaming, and broiling, and you will be a true fish aficionado.

CHAPTER 11

The Bonus Years Lifestyle

The Bonus Years Foods Rx provides you with the tools to live longer and be healthier, but Dr. Franco and I are the first to admit that other factors are also important.

By now you know that men who follow the Bonus Years Foods Rx could gain "on average" 6.4 years of life and women 4.8 years of life. That means that some people will enjoy their full amount of Bonus Years, but others will fall short. I'm often asked, Why do some people fare better on the Bonus Years Diet than others? The answer in a word is *lifestyle*. There are some harmful things you can do to your body from which even the Bonus Years diet can't protect you. (I've mentioned some of these in the previous chapters.) On a positive note, there are many things you can do that will greatly improve the chances of your getting all of your Bonus Years.

Let's get the bad stuff out of the way first. If you smoke, you will forfeit some Bonus Years, but just how many depends on your other risk factors for heart disease. With every puff of smoke, you are negating all the good things that the Bonus Years foods are doing for your arteries. Tobacco is filled with chemicals that are toxic to the delicate lining of the arteries, the endothelium. When you smoke, you increase the oxidation of LDL (bad cholesterol), which promotes the formation of artery-clogging plaque. You are also making your artery walls stiff and less flexible, which will raise your blood pressure. At the same time, your blood is getting stickier and more prone to developing clots. You become a heart attack or stroke waiting to happen, not to mention the fact that you are destroying your lungs and could very well get cancer. If you want your full amount of Bonus Years, don't light up.

If you want to receive the full benefit of the Bonus Years, *do* engage in regular physical activity. Dr. Franco and I agree that as vital as the right diet may be, exercise is an important part of the Bonus Years Diet. And there is strong evidence to support the claim that people who exercise regularly live longer, stay healthier, and are happier than those who are sedentary.

A recent study conducted by Dr. Franco and his research team, which was published in *Archives of Internal Medicine,* showed the results of their examination of the medical records of participants in the Framingham Heart Study, a well-known research project that followed more than 5,200 residents of a Massachusetts town for more than forty years, meticulously gathering data on diet, lifestyle, and overall health.

Similar to his work on the Polymeal, Dr. Franco was the first scientist to calculate the exact benefit of exercise in terms of additional years, or, as we call them, Bonus Years. Based on his analysis of the data, Dr. Franco discovered that people with moderate activity levels can gain 1.3 to 1.5 extra years of life, and those with high physical activity levels can add up to 3.7 years in total life expectancy. Moderate activity was defined as routinely walking for thirty minutes a day, five days a week. More intense exercise was defined as running for thirty minutes, five days a week.

What if you are already following the Bonus Years Foods Rx? Does that mean you can add extra years to your life if you also exercise? Not necessarily, but it still does you a lot of good. Although Dr. Franco's study did not examine the impact of exercise on longevity if you were already on the Bonus Years Diet, he is confident that those who achieve the greatest benefit from the diet will be those who are regularly doing some form of physical activity. And although he can't scientifically prove it yet, he is convinced that exercise is a primary reason why some people on the Bonus Years Diet will max out their full Bonus Years while nonexercisers will not.

No one can dispute that physical activity burns calories and gives you a trimmer, healthier look. And the fact is, if you exercise regularly, you will actually be healthier. Countless studies support the fact that people who exercise on a regular basis feel better, sleep better, and perform better on the job, and they are also reputed to have better sex lives! Even if exercise doesn't buy you more Bonus Years, you'll be better able to enjoy the years you do have.

So along with following the Bonus Years Diet, we strongly recommend that you do some form of cardiovascular exercise (any activity that increases your heart rate, such as walking fast, running, cycling, or jogging) for at least thirty minutes, five days a week. A note of caution: if you have not exercised before, have a heart condition, or are over age forty, do check with your physician before embarking on an exercise program. You don't have to run marathons to benefit from exercise, but you do need to engage in vigorous activity that gives your heart and lungs a good workout. In other words, you need to feel that you are demanding more from your body than usual.

You don't have to join or gym a invest in fancy exercise equipment—unless you want to. Simply taking a brisk walk for thirty minutes every day will do wonders for you, especially if you've been sedentary. If you are a member of a gym, walk on a treadmill or use the elliptical machine for half an hour a day. Indoor cycling on a stationary cycle or riding your bike outdoors is also a great form of exercise. Mix up your activities so you don't get bored. If you have access to a pool, swim laps for half an hour a few days a week and take a brisk walk on other days. Take an aerobics class or even try something like kickboxing. If you do things that you enjoy, you are more likely to stick with your exercise program. And you are more likely to live out your full allotment of Bonus Years.

THE POLYMEAL

Franco, O. H., L. Bonneux, C. de Laet, A. Peters, E. W. Steyerberg, and J. P. Macken-bach. "The Polymeal: a more natural, safer and probably tastier (than the Polypill) strategy to reduce cardiovascular disease by more than 75%." *British Medical Journal*, 2004; 329:1447–1450.

THE BONUS YEARS FOODS

Wine

Castelnuovo, A. D., S. Rotondo, L. Iocoviello, et al. "Meta-Analysis of Wine and Beer Consumption in Relation to Vascular Risk." *Circulation*, 2002; 105:2836–2844.

Dubick, M. A., and S. T. Omaye, Chapter 14: "Modification of Atherogenesis and Heart Disease by Grape Wine and Tea Polyphenols," *Handbook of Nutraceuticals and Functional Foods*, c. 2001 by CRC Press, LLC.

Leikert, J. F., T. R. Rathel, P. Wohlfart, et al. "Red Wine Polyphenols Enhance En-dothelial Nitric Oxide Synthase Expression and Subsequent Nitric Oxide Release from Endothelial Cells." *Circulation*, 2002; 106:1614–1617.

University of Guelph, Ontario, Canada. News Release, April 5, 2004, "Red wine fights cancer, leaves healthy cells alone, new study shows," published by Communications and Public Affairs, (519) 824–4120, ext. 56982 or 53338.

Chocolate

Engler, M. B., M. M. Engler, C. Y. Chen, et al. "Flavonoid-rich dark chocolate improves endothelial function and increases plasma epicatechin concentrations in healthy adults." *Journal of the American College of Nutrition,* 2004 June; 23(3): 197–204.

Fisher, N. D., M. Hughes, M. Gerhard-Herman, and N. K. Hollenberg. "Flavanol-rich cocoa induces nitric-oxide-dependent vasodilation in healthy humans." *J Hypertens,* 2003 December; 21(12):2231–2234.

Hammerstone, J. F., S. A. Lazarus, A. Mitchell, R. Rucker, and H. H. Schmitz. "Identification of procyanidins in cocoa (Theobroma cacao) and chocolate using high-performance liquid chromatography/mass spectometry." *J Agric Food Chem,* 1999; 47:490–496.

Holt, R. R., D. D. Schramm, C. L. Keen, S. A. Lazarus, and H. H. Schmitz. "Chocolate consumption and platelet function." *Journal of the American Medical Association,* 2002; 287:2212.

Karim M., K. McCormick, and T. C. Kappagoda. "Effects of cocoa extracts on endothelium dependent relaxation." *Journal of Nutrition,* 2000; 130(8):2105S–2108S.

Keen, C. L., et al. Abstract presented at symposium during the 2002 Annual Meeting and Science Innovation Exposition of the American Association for the Advancement of Science, Boston, February 2002.

Keen, C. L., R. R. Holt, P. I. Oteiza, C. G. Fraga, and H. H. Schmitz. "Dietary polyphenols and health: proceedings of the 1st International Conference on Polyphenols and Health: Cocoa antioxidants and cardiovascular health." *American Journal of Clinical Nutrition,* January 2005; 81: 1298S–1303S.

Kondo, K., R. Hirano, A. Matsumoto, O. Igarashi, and H. Itakura. "Inhibition of LDL oxidation by cocoa." *The Lancet,* 1996; 348:1514.

Lazarus, S. A., G. E. Adamson, J. F. Hammerstone, and H. H. Schmitz. "High performance liquid chromatography/mass spectrometry analysis of proanthocyanidins in foods and beverages." *J Agric Food Chem,* 1999; 47(9):3693–3701.

Pearson, D. A., T. G. Paglieroni, D. Rein, T. Wun, D. D. Schramm, J. F. Wang, R. R. Holt, R. Gosselin, H. H. Schmitz, and C. L. Keen. "The effects of flavanol-rich cocoa and aspirin on ex vivo platelet function." *Thrombosis Research,* 2002; 106:191–197.

Porter, L. J., Z. Ma, and B. G. Chan. "Cacao procyanidins: major flavonoids and identification of some minor metabolites." *Phytochemistry,* 1991; 30(5):1657–1663.

Rein, D., S. Lotito, R. R. Holt, C. L. Keen, H. H. Schmitz, and C. G. Fraga. "Epicatechin in human plasma: in vivo determination and effect of chocolate consumption on plasma antioxidant capacity." *Journal of Nutrition,* 2000; 130(8):2109S–2114S.

Rein, D., T. G. Paglieroni, T. Wun, D. A. Pearson, H. H. Schmitz, R. Gosselin, and C. L. Keen. "Cocoa inhibits platelet activation and function." *American Journal of Clinical Nutrition,* 2000; 72(1):30–35.

Schroeter, H., C. Heiss, J. Balzer, P. Kleinbongard, C. L. Keen, N. K. Hollenberg, H. Sies, C. Kwik-Uribe, H. H. Schmitz, and M. Kelm. "Epicatechin mediates beneficial effects of flavonol-rich cocoa on vascular function in humans." *Proceedings of the National Academy of Sciences of the United States of America*, 2006; 108: 1024–1029. Online publication: www.pnas.org/papbyrecent.shtml.

Steinberg, F., M. Bearden, and C. L. Keen. "Cocoa and chocolate flavonoids: Implications for cardiovascular health." *Journal of the American Dietetic Association*, 2003. Vol. 3:2:215–223.

Wan, Y., J. A. Vinson, T. D. Etherton, J. Proch, S. A. Lazarus, and P. M. Kris-Ehterton. "Effects of cocoa powder and dark chcocolate on LDL oxidative susceptibility and prostaglandin concentrations in humans," *American Journal of Clinical Nutrition*, November 2001; Vol. 74; 5, 596–602.

http://lpi.oregonstate.edu/infocenter/phytochemicals/flavonoids/index.html Oregon State University, Linus Pauling Institute.

Want, J. F., D. D. Schramm, R. R. Holt, J. L. Ensunsa, C. G. Fraga, H. H. Schmitz, and C. L. Keen. "A dose-response effect from chocolate consumption on plasma epicatechin and oxidative damage." *Journal of Nutrition*, 2000; 130(8):2115S–2119S.

Fruit and Vegetables

Aviram, M., and L. Dornfeld. "Pomegranate juice consumption for three years by patients with carotid artery stenosis reduces common carotid intima-media thickness, blood pressure and LDL oxidation." *Clinical Nutrition*, 23 (June 2004): 423–433.

Hu, F. B. "Plant-based foods and prevention of cardiovascular disease: an overview." *American Journal of Clinical Nutrition*, 2003; 78(supplement): 544S–551S.

John, J. H., S. Ziebland, P. Yudkin, et al. "Effects of fruit and vegetable consumption on plasma antioxidant concentrations and blood pressure: a randomized controlled trial." *The Lancet*, 2002; 359:1969–1974.

Liu, H. R. "Health benefits of fruit and vegetables are from additive and synergistic combinations of phytochemicals." *American Journal of Clinical Nutrition*, 2003; 78(suppl): 517s–520s.

Mennen, L., R. Walker, C. Bennetau-Pelissero, and A. Scalbert. "Risks and safety of polyphenol consumption." *American Journal of Clinical Nutrition*, 2005; 81(suppl): 326S–329S.

Prior, R. "Fruits and vegetables in the prevention of cellular oxidative damage." *American Journal of Clinical Nutrition*, 2003; 78(suppl):570s–578s.

Spedding, G., A. Ratty, and E. Middleton, Jr. "Inhibition of reverse transcriptases by flavonoids." *Antiviral Research* 1989; 12(2):99–110.

Stanner, S. A., J. Hughes, C. N. Kelly, et al. "A review of the epidemiological evidence for the 'antioxidant hypothesis.'" *Public Health Nutrition*, 2004; 7(3):407–422.

Fish

Albert, C. M., H. Campos, M. J. Stampfer, P. M. Ridker, et al. "Blood levels of long-chain n-3 fatty acids and the risk of sudden death." *New England Journal of Medicine*, 2002; 346:1113–1118.

Bucher, H. C., P. Hengstler, C. Schindler, et al. "N-3 polyunsaturated fatty acids in coronary heart disease: a meta-analysis of randomized controlled trials." *The American Journal of Medicine*, 2002; 112:298–304.

Connor, W. E. "Importance of n-3 fatty acids in health and disease." *American Journal of Clinical Nutrition*, 2000; 71(1 Suppl): 171S–175S.

DeFilippis, A. P., and L. Sperling. "Understanding omega-3s." *American Heart Journal*, March 2006; 151(3): 564–570.

De Lorgeril, M., and P. Salen. "Fish and n-3 fatty acids for the prevention and treatment of coronary heart disease: nutrition is not pharmacology." *The American Journal of Medicine*, 2002; 112:316–319.

Kris-Etherton, P. M., W. S. Harris, and L. J. Appel. "Fish consumption, fish oil, omega-3 fatty acids, and cardiovascular disease." *Circulation*, 2002; 106: 2747–2757.

Pischon, T., S. E. Hankinson, G. S. Hotamisligil, N. Rifai, W. C. Willett, and E. B. Rimm. "Habitual dietary intake of n-3 and n-6 fatty acids in relation to inflammatory markers among U.S. men and women." Department of Nutrition, Harvard School of Public Health, 665 Huntington Ave., Boston, MA 02115, USA. tpischon@hsph.harvard.edu.

Rosenberg, I. "Perspective: fish: food to calm the heart." *New England Journal of Medicine*, 2002; 346(15):1102–1103.

Serhan, C. N., S. Hong, K. Gronert, S. P. Colgan, et al. "Resolvins: a family of bioactive products of omega-3 fatty acid transformation circuits initiated by aspirin treatment that counter proinflammation signals." *The Journal of Experimental Medicine*, 2002; 196(8): 1025–1037.

Whelton, S. P., J. He, P. K. Whelton, and P. Muntner. "Meta-analysis of observational studies on fish intake and coronary heart disease." *American Journal of Cardiology*, 2004; 93:1119–1123.

Zhang, J., S. Sasaki, H. Kesteloot, et al. "Fish consumption and mortality from all causes, ischemic heart disease, and stroke: an ecological study." *Preventive Medicine*, 1999; 28(5):520–529.

http://www.mercola.com/2001/apr/25/mercury_fish.htm.

Garlic

Ackerman, R. T., C. Mulrow, G. Ramirez, et al. "Garlic shows promise for improving some cardiovascular risk factors." *Archives of Internal Medicine*, 2001; 161:813–824.

Stevinson, C., M. H. Pittler, and E. Ernst. "Garlic for treating hypercholesterolemia, a meta-analysis of randomized clinical trials." *Annals of Internal Medicine*, 2000; 133(6): 420–429.

http://aic.ucdavis.edu/profiles/Garlic-2006B.pdf., Agricultural Issues Center, UC Davis, January 2006.

www.stevenfoster.com/education/monograph/garlic.html. © 2000 Steven Foster.

Nuts

Abbey, M., M. Noakes, G. B. Belling, and P. J. Nestel. "Partial replacement of saturated fatty acids with almonds or walnuts lowers total plasma cholesterol and low-density-lipoprotein cholesterol." *American Journal of Clinical Nutrition*, May 1994; 59(5):995–999.

Arts, I. C., P. C. Hollman, E. J. Feskens, H. B. Bueno de Mesquita, and D. Kromhout. "Catechin intake might explain the inverse relation between tea consumption and ischemic heart disease: the Zutphen Elderly Study." *American Journal of Clinical Nutrition*, 2001; 74(2):227–232.

Jenkins, J. A., C. W. C. Kendall, A. Marchie, et al. "Dose response of almonds on coronary heart disease risk factors: blood lipids, oxidized low-density lipoproteins, lipoprotein (a), homocysteine and pulmonary nitric oxide." *Circulation*, 2002; 106:1327.

BOOSTER FOODS

The Right Oils

Mozaffarian, D., M. Katan, A. Ascherio, et al. "Trans-fatty acids and cardiovascular disease." *New England Journal of Medicine*, 2006; 354:1601–1613.

Ruano, J., J. Lopez-Miranda, F. Fuentes, et al. "Phenolic content of virgin olive oil improves ischemic reactive hyperemia in hypercholesterolemic patients." *Journal of the American College of Cardiology*, 2005; 46:1864–1868.

Zatonski, W. A., and W. Willett. "Changes in dietary fat and declining coronary heart disease in Poland: population based study." *British Medical Journal*, 2005; 331:187–188.

Tea

Davies, M. J., J. T. Judd, D. J. Baer, B. A. Clevidence, D. R. Paul, A. J. Edwards, S. A. Wiseman, R. A. Muesing, and S. C. Chen. "Black tea consumption reduces total and LDL cholesterol in mildly hypercholesterolemic adults." *Journal of Nutrition*, October 2003; 133(10):3298S–3302S.

Duffy, S. J., et al. (2001) "Short and long-term black tea consumption reverses endothelial dysfunction in patients with coronary artery disease." *Circulation*; 104:151–156.

Harold, N., and P. D. Graham (1992). "Green tea composition, consumption and polyphenol chemistry." *Preventive Medicine*, 1992; 21:334–350.

"Heart Attack Patients May Benefit from Drinking Tea." Harvard Medical School, News Release, May 6, 2002.

Hodgson, J. M., et al. "Regular ingestion of black tea improves brachial artery vasodilator function." *Clinical Science*, 2002; 102:195–201.

McKay, D. L., and J. B. Blumberg. "The Role of Tea in Human Health: An Update Table of Major Flavonoids found in tea." *Journal of the American College of Nutrition*, 2002; 21:1–13.

The Tea Association of the USA: TeaUsa.org, http://www.teausa.com/

UK Tea Council: The Home of Tea, http://www.tea.co.uk/

Flaxseed

Franco, O. H., H. Burger, C. E. I. Lebrun, P. H. M. Peeters, et al. "Higher dietary intake of lignans is associated with better cognitive performance in postmenopausal women." *Journal of Nutrition*, 2005; 135: 1190–1195.

Mayo Clinic, http://www.mayoclinic.com/

The World's Healthiest Foods: Eating Healthy, http://www.whfoods.com/ (Chart on flaxseeds from the World's Healthiest Foods website.)

Legumes/Beans

Balk, E., M. Chung, P. Chew, et al. *Effects of Soy on Health Outcomes*. Summary, Evidence Report/Technology Assessment: Number 126. AHRQ Publication Number 05-E024-1, August 2005. Agency for Healthcare Research and Quality, Rockville, MD. http://www.ahrq.gov/clinic/epcsums/soysum.htm

Bazzano, L. A., et al. "Legume consumption and risk of coronary heart disease in U.S. men and women." *Archives of Internal Medicine*, 2001; 161:2573–2578.

"FDA Approves New Health Claim for Soy Protein and Coronary Heart Disease." US FDA Press Release, October 20, 1999.

Kushi, L. H., et al. "Cereals, legumes, and chronic disease risk reduction: evidence from epidemiologic studies." *American Journal of Clinical Nutrition*, 1999; 70(suppl): 451S–458S.

Marlett, J. A., et al. "Position of the American Dietetic Association: health implications of dietary fiber." *Journal of the American Dietetic Association*, 2002; 102(7): 993–1000.

Messina, M. J. "Legumes and soybeans: overview of their nutritional profiles and health effects." *American Journal of Clinical Nutrition*, 1999; 70(suppl):439S–450S.

Protein in Diet Medline Plus—A Service of the U.S. National Library and the National Institute of Health, www.nlm.nih.gov/medlineplus

USDA Nutrient Data Laboratory, available at: www.ars.usda.gov/nutrientdata

United Soybean Board, Talk Soy, http://www.talksoy.com/

Whole Grains

Jensen, M. K., P. Koh-Banerjee, M. Franz, L. Sampson, M. Gronbaek, E. B. Rimm. "Whole grains, bran, and germ in relation to homocysteine and markers of glycemic control, lipids, and inflammation." *American Journal of Clinical Nutrition,* February 2006; 83(2):275–283.

Jensen, M. K., P. Koh-Banerjee, F. B. Hu, M. Franz, L. Sampson, M. Gronbaek, and E. B. Rimm. "Intakes of whole grains, bran, and germ and the risk of coronary heart disease in men." *American Journal of Clinical Nutrition,* December 2004; 80(6):1492–1499.

Liu, S., H. D. Sesso, J. E. Manson, W. C. Willett, and J. E. Buring. "Is intake of breakfast cereals related to total and cause-specific mortality in men?" *American Journal of Clinical Nutrition,* March 2003: 77(3):594–599.

Sahyoun, N. R., P. F. Jacques, X. L. Zhang, W. Juan, N. M. McKeown. "Whole-grain intake is inversely associated with the metabolic syndrome and mortality in older adults." *American Journal of Clinical Nutrition,* January 2006; 83(1):124–131.

Steffen, L. M., D. R. Jacobs, Jr., J. Stevens, E. Shahar, T. Carithers, and A. R. Folsom. "Associations of whole-grain, refined-grain, and fruit and vegetable consumption with risks of all-cause mortality and incident coronary artery disease and ischemic stroke: the Atherosclerosis Risk in Communities (ARIC) Study." *American Journal of Clinical Nutrition,* September 2003; 78(3):383–390.

EXERCISE

Franco, O., C. de Laet, A. Peeters, et al. "Effects of physical activity on life expectancy with cardiovascular disease." *Archives of Internal Medicine,* 2005; 165:2355–2360.

APPENDIX
THE POLYMEAL:
A MORE NATURAL, SAFER, AND PROBABLY TASTIER (THAN THE POLYPILL) STRATEGY TO REDUCE CARDIOVASCULAR DISEASE BY MORE THAN 75%*

Oscar H Franco, Luc Bonneux, Chris de Laet, Anna Peeters, Ewout W Steyerberg, Johan P Mackenbach

ABSTRACT

Objective
Although the Polypill concept (proposed in 2003) is promising in terms of benefits for cardiovascular risk management, the potential costs and adverse effects are its main pitfalls. The objective of this study was to identify a tastier and safer alternative to the Polypill: the Polymeal.

Methods
Data on the ingredients of the Polymeal were taken from the literature. The evidence based recipe included wine, fish, dark chocolate, fruits, vegetables, garlic, and almonds. Data from the Framingham heart study and the Framingham offspring study were used to build life tables to model the benefits of the Polymeal in the general population from age 50, assuming multiplicative correlations.

Results
Combining the ingredients of the Polymeal would reduce cardiovascular disease events by 76%. For men, taking the Polymeal daily represented an increase in to-

*Reprinted from *British Medical Journal*, vol. 329 (December 2005). © BMI Publishing Group, Ltd. Reprinted with permission.

tal life expectancy of 6.6 years, an increase in life expectancy free from cardiovascular disease of 9.0 years, and a decrease in life expectancy with cardiovascular disease of 2.4 years. The corresponding differences for women were 4.8, 8.1, and 3.3 years.

Conclusion

The Polymeal promises to be an effective, non-pharmacological, safe, cheap, and tasty alternative to reduce cardiovascular morbidity and increase life expectancy in the general population.

INTRODUCTION

Cardiovascular disease continues to be the leading cause of mortality and morbidity in Western populations.[1] Although several risk factors for cardiovascular disease have been identified, its prevention is still suboptimal owing to high costs, low compliance, and side effects of treatment. In 2003 Wald and Law introduced the concept of the Polypill.[2] The advocates of the Polypill selected six pharmacological components that by modifying different risk factors of cardiovascular disease multiplicatively might reduce the levels of cardiovascular disease in the population by more than 80%.[3] In general, the medical community has welcomed the concept but questioned the potential adverse effects and costs of such an intervention.

Our objective was to define a safer, nonpharmacological, and tastier alternative to the Polypill in the general population: the Polymeal. We also wanted to calculate the potential effects of the Polymeal in terms of total life expectancy and life expectancy with and without cardiovascular disease.

METHODS

The recipe

To optimise the Polymeal ingredients we used an evidence based diet conceptual framework, which follows similar principles to evidence based medicine.[4] The constituting elements of a meal or recipe are selected on the basis of the best available evidence; the evidence available for each ingredient is graded according to the level of evidence. We searched PubMed, informed by expert advice, for non-pharmacological ingredients with evidence levels 1 or 2: randomised controlled trials, meta-analyses of randomised controlled trials, and meta-analyses of observational studies.[5] To be included in the Polymeal, the ingredient had to have individually reported effects (not as an element of a diet) on reduction in cardiovascular disease events or modification of risk factors for cardiovascular disease. We checked papers retrieved for further possible ingredients. The following dietary elements met the inclusion criteria to be ingredients of the Polymeal: wine, fish, dark chocolate, fruits and vegetables, almonds, and garlic (Allium sativum).

Efficacy of the Polymeal

We obtained information from the literature on the benefits of the interventions (table 1). Daily consumption of 150 ml of wine reduces cardiovascular disease by 32% (95% confidence interval 33% to 41%).[6] Fish (114 g) consumed four times a week reduces cardiovascular disease by 14% (8% to 19%).[7] For chocolate, fruits and vegetables, almonds, and garlic, we found data on modification of risk factors for cardiovascular disease. One hundred grams of dark chocolate consumed daily reduces systolic blood pressure by 5.1 mm Hg and diastolic blood pressure by 1.8 mm Hg;[8] similar reductions in blood pressure correspond to a reduction in cardiovascular disease events of 21% (14% to 27%).[9] A total of 400 g of fruit and vegetables consumed daily produced a reduction in blood pressure similar to that observed with chocolate (4.0 mm Hg systolic blood pressure and 1.5 mm Hg diastolic blood pressure), so we decided to assume the same reduction in cardiovascular disease effect as assigned for chocolate (21%).[10]

Daily consumption of garlic reduced total cholesterol concentrations by 0.44 mmol/l (17.1 mg/dl),[11, 12] corresponding to 66% of the reduction (0.66 mmol/l) that was found to be associated with a 38% reduction in cardiovascular disease at age 50.[13] Therefore, we considered 66% of the effect previously reported and assumed a reduction of 25% (21.7% to 27.7%) in cardiovascular disease events for garlic. Most of the randomised controlled trials included in the meta-analysis used 600-900 mg/day of dried garlic powder preparations, equivalent to 1.8-2.7 g/day of fresh garlic.[14] We selected 2.7 g/day of fresh garlic for the Polymeal. Consuming 68 g/day of almonds produced half the reduction in total cholesterol (10 mg/dl) observed with garlic,[15, 16] so we assumed a reduction in cardiovascular disease half the one assigned to garlic.

TABLE 1
EFFECT OF INGREDIENTS OF POLYMEAL IN REDUCING RISK OF CARDIOVASCULAR DISEASE

Ingredients	Percentage reduction (95% CI) in risk of CVD	Source
Wine (150 ml/day)	32 (23 to 41)	Di Castelnuovo et al (MA)[6]
Fish (114 g four times/week)	14 (8 to 19)	Whelton et al (MA)[7]
Dark chocolate (100 g/day)	21 (14 to 27)	Taubert et al (RCT)[8]
Fruit and vegetables (400 g/day)	21 (14 to 27)	John et al (RCT)[10]
Garlic (2.7 g/day)	25 (21 to 27)	Ackermann et al (MA)[11]
Almonds (68 g/day)	12.5 (10.5 to 13.5)	Jenkins et al (RCT),[15] Sabate et al (RCT)[16]
Combined effect	76 (63 to 84)	

CVD=cardiovascular disease; MA=meta-analysis; RCT=randomized controlled trial.

We calculated the combined effect of the ingredients of the evidence based diet Poly-meal by multiplying their correspondent relative risk estimates. This is the same method that was used for the Polypill.[2]

Study population

We applied the effects of the Polymeal to a life table built using the Framingham study population. The original Framingham heart study cohort consisted of 5209 respondents (2336 men) residing in Framingham, Massachusetts, between 1948 and 1951. Participants have been examined biannually, and the cohort has been followed for 46 years.[17]

We used follow up data from participants attending study examinations 4 (1956-8), 11 if present or otherwise 12 (1969-73), and 19 if present or otherwise 20 (1985-9). Follow up started at the date of the chosen baseline examination. Each participant could therefore be included more than once but for different follow up periods of no more than 12 years in order to avoid overlapping periods. A total of 9181 participant-observation periods of follow up were available for the analysis.

We used three endpoints in this study: the composite endpoint of incident non-fatal cardiovascular disease (angina, coronary insufficiency, myocardial infarction, con-gestive heart failure, stroke, transient ischaemic attack, and intermittent claudica-tion), fatal cardiovascular disease, and other causes of death. In the Framingham heart study, a panel of three physicians evaluated all events (fatal and non-fatal); agreement of all three was needed.[18] We selected total cardiovascular disease as the outcome (and not coronary heart disease and stroke separated) on the basis of current recommendations in the European guidelines on cardiovascular disease prevention.[19]

Effects of the Polymeal on life expectancy and time
with cardiovascular disease

To translate the effects of the Polymeal on reduction of cardiovascular disease events (table 1) in terms of differences in life expectancy and life expectancy with and without cardiovascular disease, we created multi-state life tables starting at age 50 years and closing at 100 years of age. We stratified the multi-state life tables by sex and created them separately for the general population with and without the Poly-meal. The multi-state life tables included three different states: "free from cardio-vascular disease," "history of cardiovascular disease," and "death." The possible transitions were from "free from cardiovascular disease" to "history of cardiovas-cular disease" or "death" and from "history of cardiovascular disease" to "death."[20] In the life tables representing the population with the Polymeal, we derived the ef-fects by decreasing the rates for the transitions "free from cardiovascular disease" to "history of cardiovascular disease" and "history of cardiovascular disease" to "death" by the estimated risk reduction associated with the Polymeal. We used Excel spreadsheets for all analyses.

RESULTS

Effects of the Polymeal

Combining all the ingredients of the Polymeal resulted in cardiovascular disease being reduced by 76% (95% confidence interval 63% to 84%) (table 1). Whether increasing the amount of each ingredient would increase the effect of the Polymeal is uncertain. On the other hand, decreasing the quantities could be expected to reduce the effects of the Polymeal. Omitting wine from the Polymeal had the strongest effect on the risk reduction of cardiovascular disease (from 76% to 65%). Excluding any of the other ingredients had a lesser effect: 73% reduction without fish, 70% without chocolate or fruits and vegetables, 68% without garlic, and 73% without almonds.

Lifetime effects of the Polymeal

The effect of the Polymeal represented a large increase in total life expectancy and life expectancy free from cardiovascular disease and a decrease in life expectancy with cardiovascular disease for both men and women (table 2). For men, taking the Polymeal would result in increases of 6.6 years in total life expectancy and 9.0 years in life expectancy free from cardiovascular disease. The decrease in life expectancy with cardiovascular disease attributable to the Polymeal was 2.4 years. The reductions were similar for women, although the magnitudes were lower (table 2).

Adverse effects

No proved serious adverse effects were reported in any of the papers selected. For garlic, in addition to body odour, some unproved adverse effects were mentioned: flatulence, oesophageal and abdominal pain, allergic reactions, and bleeding.[11] Fish consumed in larger amounts than recommended as part of the Polymeal has been related to raised blood mercury concentrations, especially with large fish such as shark and swordfish.[7] No association between wine consumption at the level included in the Polymeal and increased risk of breast cancer was reported by the authors of the papers included in our analyses.[6]

TABLE 2 LIFETIME EFFECT (YEARS) OF POLYMEAL AT AGE 50, STRATIFIED BY SEX						
	Total life expectancy		Life expectancy free from CVD		Life expectancy with CVD	
Intervention	Effect	Difference	Effect	Difference	Effect	Difference
Men:						
None (overall)	28.7	Ref	21.0	Ref	7.7	Ref
Polymeal	35.2	6.6	30.0	9.0	5.3	-2.4
Women:						
None (overall)	34.2	Ref	26.9	Ref	7.3	Ref
Polymeal	39.0	4.8	35.0	8.1	4.0	-3.3

CVD=cardiovascular disease; Ref=reference value.

DISCUSSION

The Polymeal is an effective, natural, probably safer, and tastier alternative to the Polypill to reduce cardiovascular disease and increase life expectancy in the general population. The effect was consistent in both men and women at age 50. Adverse effects reported for garlic include malodorous breath and body odour.[13] As garlic is destined for mass treatment, few people will still notice this after a while. No additional adverse effects should be expected from the other ingredients of the Polymeal (in the quantities recommended here) except in people who are allergic to the components. Another advantage of the Polymeal is that its ingredients can be taken combined as a meal or individually at different times of the day. Taking the Polymeal on a daily basis (fish two to four times a week) should be feasible, considering that the ingredients are generally well tolerated and appreciated among the general population. The development and distribution of specific recipes combining the Polymeal ingredients could enhance the compliance of the population.

Costs and precautions

Although the exact price of the Polymeal is unknown and will be country specific, it could be expected to be similar to or perhaps higher than that of the Polypill. By checking a local supermarket in Rotterdam, the Netherlands, we estimated a total price for the Polymeal of €21.60 (£15.20; $28.10) a week (€3.50 for the wine, €6.23 for fruit and vegetables, €2.80 for almonds, €4.34 for dark chocolate, €0.14 for garlic, and £4.60 for fish). Although we do not recommend particular brands, spending more—for example, on your favourite bottle of wine or brand of chocolate— might also be rewarded by an improved quality of life.

The Polymeal should not be combined with additional consumption of alcohol, in order to avoid intoxication and conflicts with friends, relatives, and authorities;

furthermore, additional alcohol consumption could attenuate the effects of the Polymeal and negatively influence other health measures. Driving motor vehicles or performing activities that require high levels of attention shortly after the consumption of the Polymeal should be avoided. Moreover, considering the disturbing adverse effects of garlic, we do not recommend taking the Polymeal before a romantic rendezvous, unless the partner also complies with the Polymeal.

We believe our search was comprehensive and although we looked for additional ingredients to include in the Polymeal, we found no other potential components with a sufficient level of evidence or with clearly reported effects on cardiovascular disease events or on modification of risk factors of cardiovascular disease. Some other ingredients could be added to the Polymeal (olive oil, echium oil, soya oil, soya beans, tomatoes, oat bran, cereals, nuts, tea, chickpeas, and so on), but this will only improve its effect on cardiovascular disease risk reduction.

Concerns might be raised about the validity of the source evidence and the multiplicative model used to calculate effects of the ingredients of the Polymeal. However, these are shared by the Polypill analyses, as we used a similar approach. None the less, a greater possibility of interaction exists between dietary factors as less information is available about underlying mechanisms of action. This might result in an overestimation of the effect of the Polymeal.

Another potential limitation of our study is that no back flows are allowed in the multi-state life tables, and only the first entry into a state is considered. This is not always seen in real patterns of morbidity and mortality.

No contraindications to combining the Polymeal with additional interventions seem to exist. After the daily consumption of the Polymeal, for example, half an hour of walking could prevent further cardiovascular disease events.[21] For those people earnestly seeking to prevent cardiovascular disease, the Polypill can be combined with the Polymeal. The fortification of flour with Polypill ingredients (a statin, two antihypertensive drugs instead of three, folic acid, and aspirin) certainly merits further study. Redundant cardiologists could be retrained as Polymeal chefs and wine advisers.

Conclusions

The preventive strategy outlined here is radical. But the "healthy person" is an outdated concept from the era before scientific prevention. We should recognise that in Western society we all have cardiovascular risk factors, so everyone is at risk, and the diseases they cause are common and often fatal. It may be argued that the Polypill is even more effective, but the Polymeal promises to be an effective, non-pharmacological, safe, and tasty alternative for reducing cardiovascular morbidity and increasing life expectancy in the general population.

We thank the Framingham Heart Study Coordinators for access to the original dataset. The Framingham study is conducted and supported by the National

Heart, Lung, and Blood Institute (NHLBI) in collaboration with the Framingham Heart Study Investigators. This manuscript has been reviewed by the NHLBI for scientific content and consistency of data interpretation with previous Framingham publications. We also thank M E Kruijshaar and L J Veerman for their valuable comments and A A Mamum and F Willekens for their collaboration in the understanding of the life table approach.

Contributors: All authors participated actively in conception and design of the study or analysis and interpretation of data, in drafting the article or revising it critically for important intellectual content, and in final approval of the version to be published. OHF is the guarantor.

Funding: This study was supported by grants from the Netherlands Heart Foundation (grant no 98.138) and the Netherlands Organization for Scientific Research (grant no 904-66-093). OHF, LB, CdL, AP, EWS, and JPM were partly funded by the Netherlands Heart Foundation (grant no 98.138) and the Netherlands Organization for Scientific Research (grant no 904-66-093). AP was also partly funded by VicHealth (fellowship grant no 2002-0191). All authors have acted independently from the funders of this project.

Competing interests: None declared.

Ethical approval: Not needed as this was a secondary data analysis.

1. TJ Gluckman, Baranowski B, Ashen MD, Henrikson CA, McAllister M, Braunstein JB, et al. A practical and evidence-based approach to cardiovascular disease risk reduction. Arch Intern Med 2004;164:1490-500.

2. Wald NJ, Law MR. A strategy to reduce cardiovascular disease by more than 80%. BMJ 2003;326:1419-23.

3. Correspondence. "Polypill" to fight cardiovascular disease. BMJ 2003;327: 807-10.

4. Sacket DL, Straus SE, Richardson WS, Rosenberg W, Haynes RB. Evidence-based medicine: how to practice and teach EBM. New York: Churchill Livingstone, 2000.

5. Oxford Centre for Evidence Based Medicine. Levels of evidence and grades of recommendation. www.cebm.net/levels_of_evidence.asp (accessed 5 Aug 2004).

6. Di Castelnuovo A, Rotondo S, Iacoviello L, Donati MB, De Gaetano G. Meta-analysis of wine and beer consumption in relation to vascular risk. Circulation 2002;105:2836-44.

7. Whelton SP, He J, Whelton PK, Muntner P. Meta-analysis of observational studies on fish intake and coronary heart disease. Am J Cardiol 2004;93:1119-23.

8. Taubert D, Berkels R, Roesen R, Klaus W. Chocolate and blood pressure in elderly individuals with isolated systolic hypertension. JAMA 2003;290: 1029-30.

9. Neal B, MacMahon S, Chapman N. Effects of ACE inhibitors, calcium antagonists, and other blood-pressure-lowering drugs: results of prospectively designed overviews of randomised trials. Lancet 2000;356:1955-64.

10. John JH, Ziebland S, Yudkin P, Roe LS, Neil HA. Effects of fruit and vegetable consumption on plasma antioxidant concentrations and blood pressure: a randomised controlled trial. Lancet 2002;359:1969-74.

11. Ackermann RT, Mulrow CD, Ramirez G, Gardner CD, Morbidoni L, Lawrence VA. Garlic shows promise for improving some cardiovascular risk factors. Arch Intern Med 2001;161:813-24.

12. Silagy C, Neil A. Garlic as a lipid lowering agent—a meta-analysis. J R Coll Physicians Lond 1994;28:39-45.

13. Law MR, Wald NJ, Thompson SG. By how much and how quickly does reduction in serum cholesterol concentration lower risk of ischaemic heart disease? BMJ 1994;308:367-72.

14. Berthold HK, Sudhop T, von Bergmann K. Effect of a garlic oil preparation on serum lipoproteins and cholesterol metabolism: a randomized controlled trial. JAMA 1998;279:1900-2.

15. Jenkins DJ, Kendall CW, Marchie A, Parker TL, Connelly PW, Qian W, et al. Dose response of almonds on coronary heart disease risk factors: blood lipids, oxidized low-density lipoproteins, lipoprotein(a), homocysteine, and pulmonary nitric oxide: a randomized, controlled, crossover trial. Circulation 2002;106: 1327-32.

16. Sabate J, Haddad E, Tanzman JS, Jambazian P, Rajaram S. Serum lipid response to the graduated enrichment of a step I diet with almonds: a randomized feeding trial. Am J Clin Nutr 2003;77:1379-84.

17. Dawber TR, Meadors GF, Moore FE Jr. Epidemiological approaches to heart disease: the Framingham study. Am J Public Health 1951;41:279-81.

18. Stokes J 3rd, Kannel WB,Wolf PA, Cupples LA, D'Agostino RB. The relative importance of selected risk factors for various manifestations of cardiovascular disease among men and women from 35 to 64 years old: 30 years of follow-up in the Framingham study. Circulation 1987;75:V65-73.

19. De Backer G, Ambrosioni E, Borch-Johnsen K, Brotons C, Cifkova R, Dallongeville J, et al. European guidelines on cardiovascular disease prevention in clinical practice. Eur Heart J 2003;24:1601-10.

20. Peeters A, Mamun AA, Willekens F, Bonneux L. A cardiovascular life history: a life course analysis of the original Framingham heart study cohort. Eur Heart J 2002;23:458-66.

21. US Department of Health and Human Services. Physical activity and health: a report of the surgeon general. Atlanta: Centers for Disease Control and Prevention, National Center for Chronic Disease Prevention and Health Promotion, 1996. 361.